Also by Ira Trivedi

There's No Love on Wall Street (2011)
The Great Indian Love Story (2009)
What Would You Do to Save the World? (2006)

INDIA IN LOVE

INDIA IN LOVE

MARRIAGE AND SEXUALITY IN THE 21ST CENTURY

Ira Trivedi

ALEPH

ALEPH BOOK COMPANY
An independent publishing firm
promoted by *Rupa Publications India*

First published in India in 2014 by
Aleph Book Company
7/16 Ansari Road, Daryaganj
New Delhi 110002

Copyright © Ira Trivedi 2014

All rights reserved.

Some names have been changed to protect the identity and privacy of the people whose stories have been included.

No part of this publication may be reproduced, transmitted, or stored in a retrieval system, in any form or by any means, without permission in writing from Aleph Book Company.

ISBN: 978-93-82277-13-2

1 3 5 7 9 10 8 6 4 2

Printed and bound in India by Replika Press Pvt. Ltd.

This book is sold subject to the condition that it shall not, by way of trade or otherwise, be lent, resold, hired out, or otherwise circulated without the publisher's prior consent in any form of binding or cover other than that in which it is published.

*For my beautiful parents,
Mona and Vishwapati Trivedi,
without whom there would be no words.*

CONTENTS

Introduction	1
I: Sex & Sexuality	
The Gathering Revolution	11
The Making of a Porn Star	45
Kinky is Queer	71
Pimps and Hoes	103
The Dark Side	147
II: Love & Marriage	
Love Revolution	173
Matchmaker, Matchmaker	220
The Big Fat Indian Wedding	263
Break-Up	289
Modern Love	324
Epilogue	377
Acknowledgements	385
Notes	387
Bibliography	401
Index	411

INTRODUCTION

For the first time since the Vedic age one of the central pillars of Indian society and culture—marriage—is undergoing drastic change as young adults increasingly choose to marry on their own terms, not settling for marriages that their families have arranged for them. Notions of love are changing as young people date with their parents' sanction and have sex of their own volition. The relations between man and woman in this country have changed more in the past ten years than they have in the previous three thousand. Sex is beginning to escape from underneath the sheets and in to the living room. Traditionally, the mating game began with marriage (arranged by the family based purely on caste and economics) was followed by sex (usually for the first time) and then blossomed into 'love' (if the couple was lucky). That convenient little formula is now being radically altered—from marriage, sex and then love, we are moving to love, sex (or vice-versa) and then, maybe, marriage. Many young Indians from the urban middle class are beginning to believe that love and sex are the only things that matter in relationships, particularly marriage. This unprecedented change in thinking has probably led to more fulfilling relationships than those of the past, but it has also led to multiple crises in our society.

Today, India is at the first stage of a major social revolution. This was catalysed by the explosive economic changes of the past few decades that accelerated the slow cultural change that was already in the making. Now our country is entering uncharted territory.

Most notions related to love and marriage, which were pertinent to our parents and their ancestors, are changing in the modern age. Arranged marriages are shattering, divorce rates soaring and new paradigms of sex and relationships—queer, open, and live-in—are being tested and explored. New values are feverishly in the making, and we live in a state of molten confusion.

The sexual and marriage revolutions are happening simultaneously; it is a circular process rather than the linear progression of the sexual and marriage revolutions that were seen in the West. In India's revolution, the emancipation of women, the break-up of the family as the central economic unit, the redefinition of sexual mores, the shift from arranged marriage to love marriage is all happening at the very same time. This sort of change, happening at cyber-speed, is bound to be turbulent.

◆

Through the course of this book we will hear tales of modern India, an India that is being reinvented on the run by the rise of a newly minted Great Indian Middle Class eager to fit into a globalized world. It will seek to provide a cutting-edge, incisive evaluation of how marriage, sexuality and love work in *contemporary, urban India*.

When I set out to write this book, what I was really interested in were the groups who were driving the changing attitudes to sex and sexuality in modern times, and these were primarily young, urban and middle class. I travelled to all of India's metros and a dozen other cities to collect information and form impressions of the changes that are taking place. I became convinced that I needed to probe deeply into middle-class attitudes towards my subject, because what the middle class thinks and feels today will become the norm tomorrow, especially given the way the world is evolving.[1] In India, today, the middle-class population stands at 420 million of the total population of 1.2 billion.[2] It is estimated that 90 per cent of the Indian population will be middle class by

2039[3] and that by 2027, India will have the biggest middle-class population in the world.[4] In other words, in roughly a quarter of a century, or in the course of another generation, India will have added one billion people to the middle class—almost double its current population.

It is this middle class that will finally break through the age-old caste system of India. The similarities amongst India's middle class across the country are greater and perhaps more binding than the traditional forces of caste and religion that have shaped the country for millennia. While change has been slow to happen until now, there are signs that economic growth and education are helping to bring down age-old social barriers.[5]

Focusing on an urban, youthful, middle-class demographic makes sense, especially in the context of this book, as it will be more representative of the India of the future than any other demographic. I've already mentioned how middle class the country will be in the future. As to how urban it will be—at the present time, India is urbanizing at breakneck speed. In the next fifteen to twenty years, India will see the largest migration in the history of the world from rural to urban; thirty-one villagers will show up in an Indian city every minute over the next four decades—700 million people in all.[6] I strongly believe that urban youth are the early adopters of most trends especially when it pertains to lifestyle trends. Aspirational rural youth, in their turn, crave the lifestyle of their urban counterparts and it is becoming less difficult and more enticing to move to the city. The geographic pattern of India's income and consumption growth is shifting too.

India is also one of the world's youngest countries and its sexual revolution too is of the young. India's current population includes 315 million people who are under twenty-five[7] and by 2020 India is slated to be the youngest nation in the world, with an average age of twenty-nine, compared with thirty-seven in China and the United States, forty-five in parts of Europe and forty-eight in Japan.[8] It is an unprecedented demographic condition in its history, and in absolute numbers it is unprecedented anywhere in the world. This demographic dividend is driving this revolution along with other factors, and will continue to drive it in the future.

◆

As a result of technological, economic, political and legislative changes over the past decade, the choices, freedom and experiences of the present generation have been radically different from everything that has preceded them. Technology in particular has been a major game changer. Cable television, Facebook, Twitter, YouTube, chat rooms, online porn and the like have teased the imagination of a young India, expanding her horizons and aspirations with the click of a button. India already has the third largest internet user base, 100 million people strong, just behind China and the USA. In the next three years the number of internet users is expected to be in excess of 300 million. Economic development has aided the sexual revolution too, with consumerism being an integral part of it. With further industrial development, rural to urban migration, nuclearization of families, and the rising divorce rate, the proportion of single-member households is likely to increase steadily along the lines of the industrial West.[9]

◆

Besides the fact that no books existed for the general reader on the sexual revolution taking place in the country today, there was a more personal reason why I wanted to write such a book. This was because I wanted to try and chronicle the way in which the personal relationships of my friends and I were changing. After riding the free-for-all dating rollercoaster of the United States, I had moved back to New Delhi, five years ago, to live with my parents. One of the main reasons for my move was to organize my chaotic personal life. It seemed to me that everyone that I knew in India was quickly finding suitable men, getting hitched and settling down. I was in for a shock when I moved back. The country I had grown up in, left, and had now returned to, felt intimately familiar but also completely unknown. I found myself living in a bizarre mélange of traditional Indian culture where arranged marriage was expected but also where a Big Apple style dating culture was the norm amongst the *same* people. So someone could be meeting prospective partners for marriage through the arranged marriage process, while dating and mating rampantly on the side. I was intrigued to see how marriage continued to play such a totemic role in the lives of so many of my peers—not just the to-be-wedded, but their families as well. The furore and grandeur that accompanied the whole business of marriage in these times was baffling to me. Equally interesting was how romantic love was being redefined for an entire generation.

Through the stories that I capture in this book, I explore the apparent polarities—tradition and modernity, arranged marriage and internet dating, pornography and a deeply conservative attitude—that seem to be present simultaneously within our society.

◆

This book is divided into two sections and ten chapters. Each chapter comprises three strands—personal narratives, conversations with experts and extensive analysis based on research. Though I study the topics I've chosen in a variety of ways, perhaps the *most* cogent and insightful aspects of the book are to be found in the personal narratives that I recount—carefully chosen from over 500 that I've listened to and documented. These narratives have allowed me to look at the revolution from within, through the eyes of the people who are the protagonists of the grand drama, whose stories and experiences are representative of the change.

The first part of the book will focus on India's sexual revolution.
The profane and the holy coexisted harmoniously in ancient

India, as even the most cursory look at our heritage will tell the interested observer. So how did we get into a situation where for the longest time the moral police subjected everything they could to the most puritanical forms of censorship? Even today, the darkest and most excessive forms of sexual perversion and violence could be said to be the manifestations of a society that has been sexually repressed for decades. I will be examining these and other aspects of the new Indian sexuality in this section.

The dramatic shift in traditional values related to sex and sexuality is visible everywhere you look. Premarital sex in urban areas is skyrocketing—an estimated 75 per cent in the eighteen to twenty-four age bracket.[10] Sex is rampant in urban high schools, and it is no longer unthinkable for thirteen-year-olds to be dating, and for sixteen-year-old high school students to be having sex. Sex is finally out of the closet and on to the streets. On a short drive through urban India one is bombarded with titillating sexual images—of scantily-clad women sucking on popsicles in an ice-cream ad, an actress spread-eagled on a washing machine, or a couple on the verge of sexual congress in a deodorant ad. The same overt sexuality is present in Bollywood movies. Sex scenes are common on the same screen that even a decade ago censored French kisses. Women are gyrating in the most sexual of ways in G-rated movies, and Indian designers now include the stringiest of bikinis in their annual offerings. Pornography is widely available, with a recent Google survey declaring that Indians are ranked number six in the world for online porn views. Homosexuality was decriminalized in 2009 for the first time in a hundred years, although a controversial Supreme Court ruling a few years later reversed that, only to have it roundly condemned in most sections of society, and there is a flagrant gay party scene in the bars and bathhouses of metro cities. For gay men, sexual encounters are a click of a button away. Sex for sale, for both men and women, is easily available, including a new host of sex workers from Indian college girls to middle-aged house-wives, and reputable five-star hotels across Indian cities are being used as modern-age harems.

Unfortunately, some of the things that India is holding on to are incompatible with its newfound pleasure principle. With all the liberties and exploration the sexual revolution has brought and will continue to bring, there will be a flipside; the dark side of the sexual revolution.

In many parts of India, sexual ideals and practices that are reminiscent of a patriarchal and repressive past are upheld. There is a fierce backlash against the sexual excess, and there is a growing tension between the old and the new. There is a dark underbelly to India's sexual revolution as she is caught in a quagmire of her own making. For example, baby girls and female foetuses continue to be killed and the sex ratio continues to plummet. Government documents explicitly say India does not 'need' sex education. Instead, they recommend Yoga and Naturopathy. Organized spaces for young people to discuss sex and gender are few and far between.

◆

The second part of the book will focus on India's love and marriage revolution.

Immense upheavals are afoot in middle-class India. One of the first customs to explode with the generational divide is arranged marriage as young people begin to date and marry partners of their own choice. Today's lovers are eager to obey the will of love, embracing the romantic excesses that earlier generations had warned against. The marital relationship between husband and wife has been romanticized in ways that would have horrified our ancestors who believed that love was one of the by-products of marriage, not the reason for it.

The move of the Great Indian Middle Class towards marriage based on love represents a much larger social revolution—a love revolution that will forever change not only the way that love and sex are handled, but also family life and social structures. Love matches have risen from just 5 per cent of Indian marriages to 30 per cent in the past decade.[11] Some polls suggest an even higher rate in the metros. This is not unnatural. Indeed, the love revolution that India is going through has already occurred in large chunks of the world and has forever changed the way that Europe and North America view marriage.

In a reflection of the times, the break-up of marriages is an inevitable part of the social revolution and divorce rates are soaring. And while up until now the preferred ideal relationship for young men and women has been marriage, this is changing too. Live-in relationships, open marriages, hook-ups, serial-marriages, and other permutations and combinations that may not even be strictly legal are being experimented with, and it is safe to say that a decade or so from today the relationship map of urban India will look very different from the one we see today.

Like a shy, but eager newly-wed bride, the country is slowly shedding her chastity belt. The one certitude I discovered in the course of writing this book was that this upheaval is not temporary. We are never going back to the India of our past. The sexual revolution has begun, it is gaining pace, and nothing can stop it.

I
Sex & Sexuality

THE GATHERING REVOLUTION

> Because the Goddess has come to the great mountain Nilakuta to have sexual enjoyment with me she is called Kamakhya, who resides there in secret. Because she gives love, is a loving woman, is the embodiment of love, is the beloved, she restores the limbs of Kama and destroys the limbs of Kama, she is called Kamakhya. Now hear the great glory of Kamakhya, who, as primordial nature, sets the entire world in motion. —*Kalika Purana* (KP 62.1-3)

The Goddess Parvati was deeply in love with Shiva, and she performed tens of thousands of years of penance, meditating on one foot and doing strict fasts to win his love. Eventually her efforts paid off, and she got married to her beloved.[*]

Parvati was thrilled about her marriage but her father, Daksha, the king of the mighty Himalayas was not. He strongly disapproved of his daughter's strange husband with his ash-smeared body, necklace of skulls and wayward, pot-smoking friends. After his daughter's marriage, King Daksha decided to have a yagna to which he did not invite his frightening son-in-law. Parvati, deeply insulted by her father's action, committed suicide by throwing herself into the sacred fires of the yagna.

On hearing of Parvati's death, Shiva flew into a terrible rage

---

[*]The footprint of this meditation still exists in the Kanya Kumari temple in Tamil Nadu.

and beheaded his father-in-law, replacing his head with that of a goat. He then danced a terrible dance of destruction throughout the universe, with the corpse of his beloved partner on his shoulders. His anger was so intense that it threatened to destroy the entire universe. Lord Vishnu, the preserver, was forced to interfere. To appease Shiva, Vishnu flung his sacred discus at Parvati's corpse; sliced into fifty-one pieces, each body part was consecrated and fell to earth as a Shakti peeth, where the Devi would live on and be worshipped. These Shakti peeths are important places of Hindu worship and are scattered around the country. In Kurukshetra (Haryana) where one arm of the Goddess fell, the temple is constructed in the shape of a giant arm. In Taratarini in Odisha where the Goddess's breasts are said to have fallen, two hills are considered to be sacred breasts, and pilgrims drink milk out of a giant cup as prasad. The most famous and powerful amongst all the fifty-one Shakti peeths is the Kamakhya temple in Assam where the yoni (vagina) of the Devi is said to have fallen.

Perched at the summit of the Nilachal hill beside the sacred Brahmaputra River in Assam, the Kamakhya Devi temple has been revered for 1,200 years as one of India's most frequented Devi temples, and the country's most powerful centre of Tantra. The Kamakhya Devi Temple is the source of the Yogini Kaula, one of the oldest forms of Tantra, a form of Hinduism which dominated the country from the sixth century onwards. The Tantras—a large body of texts, composed between about 650 CE and 1800 CE proposed strikingly transgressive ritual actions which violated all conventions of Hinduism and advocated engaging in activities such as drinking wine and menstrual blood, eating meat, and having sex with 'forbidden' women, such as women married to other men.[12]

The Kamakhya Devi temple is the top tourist attraction in Guwahati, and even on a Tuesday afternoon the approach to the shrine is choked with traffic, people and animals. My fellow pilgrims are an eclectic bunch—raucous families, wandering sadhus, and an inordinately large number of young couples. I strike up a conversation with a young man from Patna who is here with his young wife and I discover that that they, like many others, have come to the temple to pray for a child. The Kamakhya Devi is not just the Goddess of sex, but also of fertility.

The most arresting visual at the temple is that of goats. Hundreds of goats roam around freely in the temple complex. Most of them are baby goats, but there are a fair number of adults too, of varying heights and girth, some with long beards, others with big horns. All of them are black or white and as I later learn—male. The goats wander confidently around the temple complex, blissfully unaware of their imminent death, bumping into pilgrims, head-butting each other, and defecating with abandon.

According to the rules of sacrifice in the ancient scripture *Kalika Purana,* birds, tortoises, alligators, goats, boars, buffaloes, iguanas, deer, crows, yaks, black antelopes, hares and lions, fish, human blood, and, in the absence of these, horses and elephants, are all acceptable offerings to the divine Goddess. Thankfully human sacrifice was outlawed in 1835 (though I heard rumours of it happening furtively) and now only male animals are sacrificed, most commonly goats and pigeons, and on major festival days— buffaloes.

A visit to the Goddess is not for the faint-hearted. I see more than one bleating sacrificial lamb being dragged to its death, and am witness to the assassination of tearful baby goats and unassuming pigeons. Their heads are severed from their bodies by a leviathan butcher whose white clothes are tinged pink with baby goat blood and who, without a flicker of an eye, chops off goat heads and screws off pigeon heads as easily as bottle caps. I discover that all of these goats have been ritually bathed, worshiped and purified with mantras before being executed. Their heads will be mounted at the altar of the Devi, while their bodies will be sent to the temple kitchen where goat meat will be distributed to the pilgrims as prasad.

I wander around the temple premises, noticing some interesting stone carvings on the walls—that of a woman in a squatting position who appears to be giving birth, and another of a fierce pregnant woman with a quiver of arrows at her side. I am taken by surprise when a man with his hair coiled into thick braids and a discoloured loin-cloth covering his body comes up behind me and furtively whispers in my ear that for ₹300 he will organize a special puja for me, one that will guarantee not only a speedy marriage but also the birth of a rajkumar. Fifteen minutes later, I find myself face-to-face with a ten-year-old girl in her school uniform; she is meant to be the incarnation of the Goddess. The loin-clothed man is serving as the priest. The ritual begins with me washing the girl's feet, pouring water on them from a bowl meant to be the yoni, or female genitals of the Goddess. I then make a border around the girl's feet with red dye; this is meant to portray blood. The bowl of water is then placed between the girl's feet and I'm made to repeat mantras said first by the priest and then I pour water, rice, or flower bits over the girl's feet. The concept of this puja is that the Goddess will enter into the body of the virgin girl and bless me. After a quick ten minutes, my man gives the girl ₹50 and she goes scampering away to school.

As for me, I am purified and ready to enter the sanctum sanctorum of the temple, an underground cave housing the main idol. After alternately pushing and waiting in a queue for three hours, I finally descend into the sanctum sanctorum of the Devi. The cave is small, and many fervent pilgrims use force to kowtow before the Goddess and get a sip her purifying waters. If it weren't for the sheer cushion of all the other human bodies holding me up, I could easily be crushed underfoot.

The main idol is a block of stone with a curious vagina-like cleft running through it called the yoni. It sits in a pool of water formed by a natural spring running beside it. Devotees touch the stone with their hands and take the water from the spring, drinking it and sprinkling it over their heads.

Once a year, during the Ambubachi festival, the water in the pool turns red because of an increased supply of iron flowing through it, signifying the holiest of days for the temple, the days of the Goddess's yearly menstruation. The Ambubachi festival is considered the most auspicious time of the year for devotees because it signifies fertility and a woman's power to reproduce. During this time, farmers in the region stop their work, many people fast, and some don't even comb their hair as a form of penance. This practice of earnest worship during the Goddess's menstruation is in sharp contrast to most temples in India where women are forbidden from entering when they are menstruating.

I wriggle my way out of the crowded underground cave, and make my way to a nearby tea-stall, where I befriend the young vendor, Darshan, whose full-time occupation I discover is priest-in-training; he runs the tea-stall on the side. He is friendly and forthcoming, and he agrees to talk to me, speedily putting his younger sister, a smiling teenager, in charge of his stall; we seat ourselves next to a lazy, large-eyed billy goat and get talking.

Eight generations of Darshan's family have been priests at the temple, and he has been reading Tantric texts since he was very young. The thoughtful young man tells me that the temple gets many visitors from the West who come to learn about Tantra, though unfortunately Tantra in the West is associated almost exclusively with 'Tantric sex'.

He explained to me that Tantric rituals were a lot more than just sex. In fact, sex was just a means to an end, a means of awakening latent energies in the body and of attaining spiritual liberation; female power or shakti was at the centre of all their worship and rites. For example, powerful female yoginis would drink a cocktail of semen and menstrual blood and use sexual rites to awaken the kundalini shakti.

After speaking to Darshan, as I wandered around, I began noticing how much sexual symbolism there was at the temple—from the figures carved in the wall, to the worship of blood, particularly the Goddess's menstrual blood, to the sexually explicit lore and myth attached to the temple. I found it ironic that in a country where today prudish parents, governments, and various institutions have almost suffocated sex out of existence, here sex was not just accepted, but worshipped by millions.

♦

The temple of Kamakhya Devi is just one example of India's rich sexual past. From the time of the *Rig Veda* (1500-1000 BCE) to the age of the *Kamasutra* (ca. 300 CE) and to the courts of the Rajput and Mughal kings many centuries later, from the elite down to the peasant, in ancient Indian culture, sex was not taboo. It was discussed openly in books, religious and fictional, and depicted in paintings, hymns and folktales, which celebrated 'women with breasts like mangoes'[13] and their numerous lovers. Many Hindu gods and goddesses were depicted as romantic couples, and ancient Indian temples, such as Khajuraho in Madhya Pradesh, and Ajanta and Ellora in Maharashtra are full of images, often erotic and sexually explicit, of sacred gods, goddesses and apsaras (heavenly nymphs).

From the earliest times, Hinduism has been characterized by two simultaneous forces: erotic and ascetic. The early religious texts, the *Upanishads* were the first texts to introduce this dichotomy—the path of the householder where the goal is the worldly pursuit of family, work and so on, and the other path, that of the renunciate, where the focus is on spirituality and attaining liberation from the cycle of life, death and reincarnation. This tension, between sex and celibacy, between the sensual and the spiritual, appears throughout the vast realm of Hinduism, and manifests itself in a multitude of forms.

The Shiva lingam, perhaps the mostly widely worshipped and venerated Hindu symbol illustrates this tension. The lingam or the sexual organ of Shiva first appears in the *Mahabharata* (300 BCE to 300 CE). The same phallus is seen as both as a potentially procreative phallus and a pillar-like renouncer of sexuality.[14] In Hinduism, Shiva is seen as the perfect husband to his wife Parvati, the adulterer who chases the divine Mohini, as well as the ultimate renunciate. He is worshipped, celebrated and accepted in all these forms.

The two Hindu gods who have crossed over from religion and myth and have arguably had the greatest impact on Indian society are Rama and Krishna, both of whom have appeared in seminal texts over the centuries. Rama and Krishna live on in the daily lives of hundreds of millions of people everywhere in the country, participating in their hopes and joys, sorrows and grief, and in their song and dance. They have been assimilated into the Indian psyche as no other deities have been and have had a tremendous effect on shaping the Indian perspective of love and relationships, their appeal transcending religious affiliations and regional boundaries.

As with generations before me, I too grew up listening to stories of Rama and Krishna and they formed my first impressions of love and marriage. Both Rama and Krishna are avatars of Vishnu; they are born on earth in the form of men to rid the world of evil. Though they are essentially the same, they have strikingly differing outlooks towards love, marriage and sex, mirroring the schizophrenia of the Indian mind. Krishna is as playful as Rama is serious. He is known for mischief and romantic dalliances with Radha and the gopis. Krishna is a prankster and eternal schemester whereas Rama is dogmatically righteous and moral. Rama has only one wife, whereas Krishna has 16,108. Rama is fair-skinned whereas Krishna is dark. Krishna is leela purushottam, the Supreme Being, whereas Rama is maryada purushottam, the epitome of propriety. Both Rama and Krishna illustrate a holistic worldview about what constitutes the ideal life, but it is Krishna who is said to be the purna or complete avatar of Vishnu, combining in himself all the sixteen rasas whereas Rama lacks shringar—the erotic element.

Let's first take a look at Rama—the seventh avatar of Vishnu, the eldest son of Dasharatha, the King of Ayodhya who had four sons by three wives. Rama marries Sita, who was miraculously born from the earth to King Janak. The love story begins when Ram goes to Janakpurdham, the kingdom of Janak, to compete for the hand of Sita. There he defeats many powerful and eligible princes by lifting the Shiv Dhanush, Shiva's sacred bow, and wins Sita as his bride. The blessed life of Rama takes an unexpected turn when he is banished to the forest because of a ploy hatched by his stepmother Kaikeyi, so that her own son Bharata can become king. Sita follows her husband into a dangerous exile of her own volition, setting the standard, so to speak, of wifely loyalty, patience, unconditional support and sacrifice.

During the last year of their fourteen-year exile, Ravana, the demon king of Lanka, kidnaps Sita, beguiling her through his wizardry. Rama embarks on a mission along with his loyal brother Lakshmana and the monkey god Hanuman to rescue Sita from the island of Lanka. Rama kills Ravana, fulfilling the principal reason for his birth—to rid the universe of the tyranny of Ravana. The story does not end here. A tragic twist to the tale occurs when the people of Ayodhya question their queen's chastity. After all, she was kidnapped by a demon king and spent some time in Ravana's kingdom. Though it breaks Rama's heart to do so, he sends Sita away because Rama believes that his foremost duty as a king is towards his subjects and it is his dharma to maintain a moral standard in his kingdom.

King Rama separates from his queen even after she passes an agni pareeksha, or the test of fire—a metaphorical test of virtue. In the end Sita walks into a fire, performing self-sacrifice. Rama continues to rule Ayodhya with a broken heart for the next 11,000 years.

Rama focuses obsessively on duty. He loves Sita dearly yet is obliged to send her away. Sita remains devoted to her husband, come what may. She is the epitome of female purity, virtue and sacrifice complementing the qualities of her husband—the 'perfect man'. These character traits are important to understand because they are at the heart of the epic and its somewhat dogmatic function to inculcate morality in society. After all, the *Ramayana* is not just an epic of adventure and love, though it is that too, but a revered religious text that many people consider a guide to life.

Rama and Sita's romantic equation sets high standards for lovers in this nation. First, because the romantic relationship has to be validated by the sacred act of marriage, and a happily married couple stands for the most successful of love stories. Second, it asks of each partner a steep price for conjugal conduct—husbands must be willing to wage wars for the sake of their wives, and women must follow their men into exile. Third, the couple must be ready to make sacrifices for the sake of society, even at the cost of the marriage itself.

The Radha–Krishna love story is far more radical given that it is one of passionate love and a consequent disregard for conventions. As the diametrical opposite of the disciplined, sensible Rama we have Krishna, the eighth avatar of Vishnu. Krishna spends his childhood incognito in the idyllic village of Vrindavan where he discards all semblance of princely propriety. He is an incorrigible, lovable playboy who consorts with his love Radha and the other village girls in the meadows of Vrindavan. The notes of his flute are carried along the ripples of the sacred river Yamuna while he sings and dances his ways into the hearts of all those around.

The Radha-Krishna relationship is a brazen one and the couple breaks many social conventions at once. They engage openly in numerous sexual encounters including the one most celebrated, the ras lila, the antithesis of domestic bliss. Throughout the course of their village romance, Krishna and Radha are not married; they never speak about marriage, or get married. In his teenage years, Krishna leaves his birthplace to kill the demon Kamsa— the purpose for which he is born on earth, and to take up his princely duties—never again to return. Eventually Krishna becomes the King of Dwarka, and marries 16,108 women.

Krishna is the ultimate lover and the greatest part of erotic literature in ancient India deals with his stories. His ras lila with the gopis—the cowherdesses of Vrindavan—described to be sexual congress, is mentioned in the *Harivamsha*, which was composed before the fourth century CE. The Sanskrit classic, *Gitagovinda*, written by Jayadeva in the twelfth century CE was the most important landmark in the development of Krishna's role as lover. In this text, Krishna's sensitivity to the needs and feelings of women is portrayed beautifully. In the last canto of the text, which is said to be written by Krishna himself, Radha, in languorous post-coital bliss, commands Krishna to paint her feet, comb her tresses, and do whatever she commands him to do. (The story goes that Jayadeva had gone to the river for his bath when Krishna assuming his form completed the last couplet of his work and ate the food prepared by his wife. When Jayadeva discovered the stanza completed and his food eaten, he interpreted it as divine sanction). The impact of the *Gitagovinda* was extraordinary and within just a century or two of its having been written, it acquired enormous popularity and influence. From the fourteenth to the sixteenth centuries, several writers continued Jayadeva's romantic legacy. As Pavan Varma writes in *The Book of Krishna*, 'the cumulative result was that the love lore of Krishna and Radha moved out from the sanctum sanctorum of the temple to the dust and din of daily life. Their erotic love play made a transition from the refined if passionate milieu of Sanskrit poetics to the earthy and seductive medium of the lingua franca of the masses.'[15]

I always wondered why Krishna never married Radha and when I explored this I discovered that several sources give different reasons.[16] Some say that Radha was already married, others say that Radha and Krishna had a spiritual love that had nothing to do with marriage, while others say that by not getting married they were making a statement. Perhaps my favourite reason was told to me by a roving swami in Vrindavan: a Vaishnavite council, comprising high-level saints, met in the seventeenth century to reach a final verdict on Radha's relationship with Krishna. They concluded that Radha must be Krishna's lover because it was not possible to have the degree of passion that they shared in a husband-wife relationship. The Krishna-Radha love story never culminated in marriage, yet it remains the most celebrated story in the life of Krishna. Paintings, miniatures and statues aside, there are numerous temples across India that have the couple installed as deities—the only example of a romantic relationship not involving formal marriage being worshipped in a gloriously public way. The Radha–Krishna relationship has also influenced many movements in art and literature, the best-known being the Bhakti movement of which Meerabai, a Hindu princess from Rajasthan, was one of the most significant figures, known best for her devotional poems and songs. Besides the *Gitagovinda* by Jayadeva, several religious and artistic movements looked to the Krishna-Radha romance for inspiration—Vaishnava poetry by Govind Das, Gyan Das and Mukund Das are some other popular ones, though many, many more exist. In the sixteenth century CE, a number of love cults with Radha and Krishna as their presiding deities emerged. One major figure in the movement was Chaitanya Mahaprabhu whose followers worshipped him as an incarnation of God. It is said that he longed for Krishna just as a lovelorn Radha did.

It was time to see for myself what strange love stories were taking place in the country today. At the campus of an engineering college in Delhi, I am judging the Mr and Ms Rendezvous competition, where students from all over India participate to win the coveted titles and be declared the most eligible bachelor and bachelorette on campus. Here I meet Prayag, who captures the title and steals the show with his energetic, albeit heavily accented rendition of Michael Bolton's 'When a Man Loves a Woman', which would have made Bolton proud.

Prayag, twenty, is in the final year of his engineering course.

He is good-looking in a dorky sort of way, with a thin, lithe body (from his years playing state-level badminton) and glasses framed in thick, red plastic. He sings, plays the guitar, and is also an expert chess player. His family lives in Nagpur and is strictly middle class: his father has a government job, and his mother is a housewife. His parents are keen that he take the IAS exam but young Prayag aspires to more. He wants to be an entrepreneur; it is his dream to become the country's next tech tycoon. For my parent's generation, and the one before that, a government job was considered the epitome of success. Not anymore. Most of the hundreds of young people whom I interviewed consider government jobs to be dull and boring. Job security, health insurance, benefits, prestige—these things don't matter so much. What seems to matter above all is money, which allows them to indulge in the country's burgeoning consumer culture.

On a sunny winter day in Delhi, I sit with Prayag and his new girlfriend Pia at the canteen.

Pia, a third year student, is studying computing and mathematics. She is plain-faced, her most dominant feature being her long, thick, frizzy hair with bangs that touch the frame of her glasses. After a courtship that included dates at McDonald's and Pizza Hut (where they always split the bill), Prayag captured her heart and 'proposed' to her, she became his girlfriend. Prayag is Pia's first boyfriend.

As we sit and talk, a pretty girl strolls by. She has bright blonde highlights in her hair, and is dressed rather provocatively—in an abbreviated skirt and a tight top that shows off her generous breasts. Prayag bristles like a hound in heat, and turns reflexively to stare at her. Pia doesn't notice this; she is busy prattling away to a classmate of hers. Prayag furtively whispers to me that the name of the girl who has walked past us is Charu. She is a humanities student and is hot stuff on campus. I casually ask him if she has a boyfriend, and he nods vigorously.

'She does,' he says, his eyes continuing to follow Charu's progress.

'You like her?' I tease him. Prayag tears his eyes away from Charu and looks guiltily at the floor.

'No, ma'am,' he says finally.

'Why not? She's pretty,' I whisper, making sure Pia, plain as a chapatti, cannot hear us.

'She is not a good girl,' he whispers back, cool and granular, his tone different from the flushed teenager of a few seconds ago.

'What do you mean?' I ask him wondering what misdeeds Hot Stuff Charu could possibly be up to.

'She's just, how do I say this, a bad girl, if you know what I mean,' says Prayag.

He explains in his normal voice, as Pia has just wandered off with her girlfriend: 'There are girls who are good, and then there are girls who are bad. Pia is a good girl. Charu is a bad girl. I mean, I guess, there *are* girls who are in-between. Sakshi was like that, but she was really special. I guess other girls can be too.'

Sakshi is someone Prayag speaks of often, his first girlfriend, a girl whom he fell deeply in love with, but who after three months, left him for a friend of his from Delhi University.

Prayag says he loves Pia too, though they have been dating only for a month. But he says that he could never feel for anyone the way he did for Sakshi.

Prayag, like many of his contemporaries, has grown up dividing women into two categories: 'good girls' are not sexually forthcoming or active and 'bad girls' are and while he lusts after the latter, he could not imagine being romantically involved with them. During his campus courtship of Sakshi, though, he had been forced to redefine his ideas about the sexuality of modern women. Sakshi seemed to Prayag like his mother—idealistic, strong and trustworthy, but at the same time uncommonly sexy, with her 'traditional' good looks, slender, graceful figure and large breasts. To Prayag, Sakshi was the perfect Indian woman, just the right blend of conservative and modern. She wore salwaar-kameez to class but managed to look sexy in the well-fitted, low-cut outfits, with their diaphanous dupattas. Her hair was lustrous and long, and she kept it in a loose, long braid with escaping wisps that created a halo around her head, giving her a beatific aura. After his three-month relationship with Sakshi he knew though she was seemingly modest and conservative she was capable of posing in the nude in dorm rooms, performing fellatio in empty classrooms, and conducting a secret affair with another boy while being committed to him. A lovelorn Prayag was torn—how could he love a 'bad' girl so intently.

Many of these views by my fellow Indians on 'good' and 'bad' stem from a deep sense of sexual repression. For example, masturbation, which most sexologists consider to be healthy, is considered by most to be terrible—something which you must never talk about, or no one should see you do. Even something sexually titillating, like a woman wearing a short skirt, or talking to someone of the opposite sex is looked down upon. On the other hand, the celibate—the holy man, the virgin bride—are considered good and pure. It is this innate repression, this mistrust of the sexual which is then thrust on to women, or men, and relationships.

Prayag's confused views on sex are typical of the average urban Indian, broadly speaking. There appear to be two paradigms of good and bad, 'fast' and 'slow', pure Sita and frolicking Radha.[17]

As scholar Heidi Pauwels observes in her comparison of the two: 'If Sita is Rama's wife, Radha is Krishna's love. If Sita is chastity incarnate, Radha is sensuality incarnate. She is Krishna's paramour, and in most interpretations, their relationship is a clandestine one.' Whereas Sita is legitimately married, Radha is said to be married to another while she conducts her romance with Krishna though this is a hotly debated issue. 'If the mutual love of Rama and Sita is an example of happy monogamy, Radha's relationship with Krishna is famously fraught with the issue of his unfaithfulness and her jealousy of his other loves and wives. If Sita is a queen, aware of her social responsibilities, Radha is exclusively focused on her romantic relationship with her lover. Thus we have two opposite role models. Hindu women then have to navigate between ideals from both ends of the moral universe: the loyal, chaste wife and the adulterous lover.'[18]

What of the modern Indian woman then? She constantly struggles with the pulls and pushes of both extremes. On the one hand owning up to the desire to have sex would make a girl bad. Refraining from sex before marriage is a way to show virtue and commitment; you are expected to wear your virginity like a badge of honour. On the other hand, in some circles that are considered 'cool', the notion of purity and virginity is an atavistic notion of the past. Today's urban Indian girls, like Prayag's first love Sakshi and his girlfriend Pia are stuck somewhere in between. They are no longer like Sita enclosed in a Lakshman Rekha when her mate leaves to hunt, but are more like a modern day Radha, hanging out with her lover in malls and running out of her dorm room for a midnight rendezvous. And, like Radha, sex is typically not casual or adventitious. It is something that is done when you are deeply in love, in a committed relationship that one hopes will lead to marriage. Statistics published in a 2007 report on Youth in India, published by the Ministry of Health and Family Welfare, prove this: 61 per cent of men in urban India want to marry their premarital partner (42.3 per cent men do end up doing it), while 78.2 per cent of women intend to marry their partner (86.3 per cent end up doing it). This extensive study showed that the majority of youth who engage in a premarital romantic partnership had expectations of a longer-term commitment. The hook-up and one-night stand culture still seems to be rare in India and though there is burgeoning curiosity about sex among the country's youth, they appear to want to experience it within a serious relationship.

Traditionally, Sita has been looked upon as the female role model. She is gracious, inspiring, pure and, most importantly—sacrificing. But today the Indian woman is beginning to protest against this long-standing role model which both men and women have idealized for centuries.

◆

Besides these religious underpinnings to the country's sexual heritage, the most famous treatise on love, that had its origins in ancient India was of course the *Kamasutra*—the famous exposition on lovemaking and repository of wisdom—erotic and more. As scholar Wendy Doniger writes in her book *On Hinduism*, 'It [Kamasutra] is a book about the art of living—about finding a partner, maintaining power in a marriage, committing adultery, living as or with a courtesan, using drugs—and also about the positions in sexual intercourse.'

Vatsyayana, the author of the *Kamasutra* (kama means sensuality and sutra means rules of), lived during the third century CE in the city of Pataliputra, which later became the home of the highly cultivated and eroticized Gupta court. It is unclear whether Vatsyayana himself was as highly sexual as the *Kamasutra's* protagonist, the nagaraka, who can be thought of as an urbane playboy. Some maintain that Vatsyayana was actually a virgin yogi. Regardless, he wrote his book out of a concern that sexual learning in his time was slowly disappearing.

Through depicting the life of the nagaraka, the *Kamasutra* offers suggestions on many subjects, from how to freshen the breath by chewing betel leaves to how to treat a prostitute. But it is, of course, an enormously detailed manual on every aspect of lovemaking. Vatsyayana describes twenty-six different styles of kissing and details on how to arouse each part of the body. He discusses the types of sounds one makes during sexual intercourse, how to begin and end lovemaking, and how to use the nails and teeth as a source of pain to further stimulate the body. He discusses the sexual compatibility of individuals depending on their body and genital size and the intensity of desire. Vatsyayana mentions homosexuality, and writes about the importance of women's pleasure in a way that implies that women could benefit from reading the *Kamasutra*. He discusses the G-spot and the woman's climax. To pleasure the woman, he advises a man to use his index and middle fingers inside the vagina while rubbing the clitoris with his thumb.

We have to keep in mind that the *Kamasutra* was passed along as an oral tradition, so it was subject to a lot of interpretation along the way. Yet the fact that it has survived for so long (for over 2,000 years) and has been a resource for other erotic commentaries is proof enough of its immense value.

However, in Hinduism kama is only one of three goals (trivarga) of human existence of which the other two, dharma (duty) and artha (purpose), are often given more importance because of their emphasis on duty towards society.

It is clear that dharma was more important and complex than artha or kama,[19] and the liberal and sensuous strand running through ancient Indian society had to contend against law-givers, scholars and teachers who wanted to mould society in quite different ways. One of the most well-known dharmashastras is *The Laws of Manu* (in Sanskrit the *Manusmriti*) composed around 100 CE. It is said to be written by Manu, but that is almost certainly a pseudonym[20] since Manu is the son of the Self-born One, the Creator, the Indian version of Adam, a mythical construct but not a god; the one who defines the beginning of the human species.[21]

Manu's monkish attitude was at the opposite end of the spectrum from Vatsyayana's *Kamasutra*. Manu saw sex as a strictly procreative, monogamous activity, as opposed to the pleasure-giving experience Vatsyayana encouraged. Vatsyayana writes that a woman who is not pleasured may hate her man and leave him for another while Manu states: 'a virtuous wife should constantly serve her husband like a god, even if he behaves badly, freely indulges his lust, and is devoid of any good qualities'. Whereas the *Kamasutra* has an entire chapter on 'Other Men's Wives', *The Laws of Manu* warns 'if men persist in seeking intimate contact with other men's wives, the king should brand them with punishments that inspire terror and banish them'. Vatsyayana saw adultery as merely a means of providing pleasure, while Manu worried about the possible uprooting of the caste system should pregnancy occur with an unknown father of the wrong caste.

Manu's was not the only text opposing the erotic views of the *Kamasutra*. Many Hindu texts of the time like the *Bhagvad Gita*, composed a little before the *Kamasutra* (all dates in ancient Indian history are vague, so we don't know for sure) denounces indulging in the senses as being evil. Ironically the *Bhagvad Gita* is a discourse given by the grown-up Krishna, who once frolicked with cow-girls in Vrindavan.

Buddhism and Jainism, religions which were flourishing in the third century, rejected the physical world. Ashvaghosa's *Life of the Buddha* which may be a hundred years or so older than the *Kamasutra* warns that 'the one who they call Kama-deva here-on-earth, he who has variegated weapons, flower-tipped arrows, likewise they call him Mara, the ruler of the way of desire, the enemy of liberation.' For Buddhists, Mara was the ultimate tempter and was even known as the lord of death.[22]

Semen was widely regarded as an enormously precious substance, and meant to be preserved. The most famous example of the power of semen is Shiva, who is often represented as an erect phallus, a symbol of power and fertility. Shiva holds back his seed so his 'lingam' remains erect as a potential destructive force. Semen retention by celibacy was further impressed upon in Ayurveda, an ancient Indian system of medicine which advised limiting sexual intercourse to two or three times a week during youth and once or twice a month later on.[23] Fortunately, the heavy-handedness of texts like *The Laws of Manu* were offset from time to time by the works of famous playwrights like Kalidasa whose fourth century *Raghuvamsa* is a masterpiece of erotic verse.

◆

The definitive history of Indian sexual culture is yet to be written. And to do that, anyone who attempts to research the history of the country's sexuality in the ancient or medieval period is doomed to grow increasingly frustrated as I did. Certain periods are well documented, but vast portions are maddeningly vague. Finally, I turn to James McConnachie, British author who has written a well-regarded book on the *Kamasutra* entitled *The Book of Love: The Story of the Kamasutra*, to get a better understanding of the country's sexual beginnings, so to speak.

'There is a massive gap in history,' he begins. 'We just don't know much about India's sexual history. Piecing together India's sexual history is really a struggle, especially because it is so vast, and while we have some pieces of the puzzle, there are so many that we do not have.'

I am glad I am not the only one who felt that way. Sources from the same time period were often fundamentally at odds with each other—some were highly erotic, others religious, and then there was the material that was both religious and erotic.

McConnachie tells me about sexual culture in India's medieval period (eight to eighteenth century CE). He explains the 'twin-tracks' mindset which dominated much of this period. Essentially he described the erotic-ascetic tension that I had found throughout my research. One line of the twin tracks says that sex is religious, sacred and profound, whereas the other line says that sex is just sex.

'My assumption is that in the medieval period, sex was largely used by religious thinkers as a metaphor. Sex was spiritualized, and made into something sacred. We have sex explicit on temple walls, in Tantric texts, and in theatre. But at the same time, you get the odd poet who goes down and dirty, and then you get the handbook on sexual postures,' says McConnachie.

While the Tantric shastras from the Kamakhya Devi temple saw sex as sacred, we also had texts like Amaru's eighth-century

Amarusataka, a famous erotic love poem. Other well-known erotic works from the medieval period include the *Ananga Ranga* (*Stage of Love*) written by Kalyana Malla in the fifteenth century. The *Koka Shastra* (fifteenth or sixteenth century CE) was a well-known sex manual that referenced the *Kamasutra* and predicted how a woman would be as a wife and sexual partner.

The Mughal period (1526-1857) saw the creation of a new, less conflicted sexual culture. From the twin-tracks mindset, there was now a middle-track mindset. Even though Islam has a mild anti-sexual element, and had its ups and downs so far as society's attitude towards sex and sexuality was concerned, during most periods of Mughal rule, sex wasn't frowned upon. In fact, the Mughal period had a more balanced view on sex and sexuality than the era that had preceded it. The sexually explicit artwork of the time shows that sexual love in most Islamic societies was marked by a cheerful sensuality.

McConnachie explains further, 'What really strikes me about the erotic miniatures and writings of the Mughal era is that despite being separated from the *Kamasutra* by more than 1,000 years, and by religion and culture, they show us a strangely similar world to the one we see in the *Kamasutra*—they show us sex that is unabashedly luxurious, resolutely non-spiritual, filled with sensual pleasure—and slightly acrobatic!'

There was however a slight disruption in the 'middle-track' sexual culture with the more erotic productions of the Rajput ateliers of northwestern India which created an entire sensual genre in the fifteenth century with an erotic hero, the nayaka, and heroine, the nayika sometimes referred to as Krishna and Radha.

The real change in sexual mores seems to have come about with the advent of the British in the eighteenth century; they brought new energy to the twin-track conflict culture.

'It was a marriage of two cultures—Indian and Victorian, which were oddly similar, and had the same deep-set tension. For all their prudery, the Victorians were surprising salacious, and were responsible for printing and publishing enormous numbers of sexual texts. The two cultures met each other through British imperialism and colonial adventures and brought the same problems together. They didn't destroy anything, they just gave a new energy to something that had always been there,' explains McConnachie.

Unfortunately the ascetic side of Indian and Victorian culture was what prevailed, especially when the British discovered the high-priest of prudish values—Manu.

The Laws of Manu was one of the first Sanskrit texts studied by the British; they borrowed freely from it to frame legal and administrative systems for India. In truth, *The Laws of Manu* were just one of the texts referred to in ancient India, but through the British, Manu became the ultimate voice of authority, deeply infiltrating contemporary Hindu culture, building into it many negative assumptions about lower castes and women that sharply restricted their freedom, regulated their behaviour and blocked their access to social and political power.

Those regulations were taken by the British to be universal, applying to all 'Hindoos'. Part of this impulse stemmed from the push to establish uniform laws—which was also going on in Britain at the time.[24]

To find out more about British Victorian influences on India's sexual culture, I speak with Wendy Doniger, perhaps the world's greatest living authority on Hinduism.

'In the late eighteenth and early nineteenth centuries, the downhill sexual journey began. It was the Protestants with the British that [did] the harm, though the Christian missionaries had some influence too. The Protestants were a different crowd, they were Victorians... And worst of all, they were Puritans,' says Doniger.

'How did the British force their beliefs on to the Indians?' I wonder aloud.

Doniger explains it wasn't just the British who were responsible for disseminating the prudish Victorian attitude to sex but the anglicized Indian elite too, who in their eagerness to please their masters, preached these new values to the Indian middle class, who in turn broadcast them widely throughout the nation.

'Europeans liked Indian philosophy, like the *Bhagvad Gita*, but they made fun of the sexier temple carvings and gods. The Hindus wanted to be respected by the Europeans and to seem more like them. It wasn't everybody; it was largely the people who spoke English,' says Doniger.

McConnachie agrees with this view. 'Wendy is spot on about motivations for Hindu reformers—wanting respect. The British came with all these preconceptions about lascivious Orientals, who were seen as over-erotic, or actually feminine in a way that made them supposedly unfit to govern. So showing yourself to be asexual or anti-sexual or puritanical also showed you were fit to run your own country. Masculinity was seen to be about self-control—just as it had been for Shiva.'

Professor Geeta Patel (a college professor who first inculcated my interest in South Asian sexual history) agrees with this view. 'Doniger is right that Indians absorbed something and made it their own. This is called hegemony. And perhaps because we always know that one particular picture is shaky, we hold on to it more tightly. The result is we give up our own histories and, with it, all the possibilities that one can see in them.'

The stifling of sexuality thus received the sanction of many others, including eminent Bengali reformer, Raja Rammohan Roy—best known today for his efforts towards the uplifting of women with his anti-sati and anti-child marriage movements. Roy was the founder of the Brahmo Samaj that propagated a new kind of Hinduism influenced by Hindu Vedanta, Islamic Sufism and Christian Unitarianism. However, Roy was a great admirer of British Victorian values, and his views on sexuality were, as a consequence, influenced by them.

Roy's most influential successor was Swami Vivekananda, who carried on the ideals of the Bengal reforms with a movement called Sanatana Dharma (Universal Dharma) which many Hindus still embrace today. He preached the importance of chastity and of Hindutva, or the 'Hindu identity' to his followers, which continues to have a perceptible influence on art, film and literature.

Another great son of modern India who had a dampening effect on sex and sexuality was Mahatma Gandhi, who passionately preached celibacy. The Mahatma took a vow of celibacy at the age of thirty-six and his conflicted views on sex are apparent in his memoirs where he writes with anguish about his battle with his own sexuality. He declares he was tormented by sexual passions, which he described as uncontrollable. Gandhi also said women were the embodiment of sacrifice and non-violence, as also the keepers of purity.[25] Rather surprisingly, the Mahatma felt that, in some ways, women had to be careful not to invite sexual abuse. During his time in South Africa, Gandhi saw a young man harassing his female followers. Instead of punishing the male, Gandhi personally cut off the girl's hair.[26]

Influenced by the likes of Victorians, and the British Raj in general, as well as some of the country's most iconic leaders like Mahatma Gandhi, Raja Rammohan Roy, and Swami Vivekananda, Indian society of the early twentieth century became decidedly illiberal, a far cry from the country that had given rise to the *Kamasutra*.

◆

I realize that India's sexual past is not so different from the present. The sexual tension, the dichotomy, hypocrisy, irony—call it what you want—has been there from the beginning and continues to flourish. There are these extreme views on sex at either end of the spectrum, and those are the ones that have survived.

McConnachie explains with an analogy: 'Indian history has always been varied. It's like being in a big garden with one spectacular flower. We look at that flower because it is most interesting. But at the end of the day, it is just a single flower.

The *Kamasutra*, for example, is that magnificent flower in a vast garden. How people read the past was based on their politics. Some people turned to Manu, while others to the *Kamasutra*. A country which has a deep literary past gives you a variety of options and you can weed history anyway you want. The truth is that we simply cannot come to big conclusions about a big culture.'

◆

Today, however, the pendulum appears to be swinging back towards a more relaxed attitude towards sexuality, especially in urban India. And it has done so in double quick time, for even when I was becoming sexually aware, not so long ago, things were very different. Like most Indian kids who came of age in the '90s, I thought sex was bad, something so awful that it must never be talked about. No one said so explicitly—it was just understood, maybe because it was never talked about.

Even in my high school, in the middle India town of Indore, sex was never discussed, not even amongst the closest of my friends. When I went to the US for college, I was far behind the curve in terms of experience, since most girls had already had their firsts and many more. I pretended my way through conversations on sex, shy to admit to my new American friends that I was a virgin, afraid to reveal that I'd only had my first boyfriend the summer after I'd graduated (thank god I had quickly kissed him).

Today the scene has changed out of all recognition. Indeed, it is women who are at the heart of this cultural change as they come to terms with their desire and challenge stereotypes of the 'good' Indian girl. Recently, I spent the day at an all-women's college campus in New Delhi speaking with young Indian women about their sexual habits. I listened as they expounded confidently and expertly on their sexual experiences. From the hundred plus accounts that I listened to that day, it appeared to me that sex on campus was the norm rather than the exception, and many girls admitted to having lost their virginity before they started college. On urban college campuses across India especially in metros, premarital sex seems to be rampant. Free from the clutches of family and the mores of middle-class India, girls are keenly interested in sexual exploration. This sense of experimentation is mirrored in the bustling nightlife and social scene—in nightclubs, bars, hookah lounges and cafes where young people mingle freely. As one eloquent interviewee at St. Xavier's, Mumbai, once a strict Catholic college, put it to me, 'If you aren't doing it here, you just ain't cool.'

CHENNAI

I visit Prayag a year after he graduated from his college. Much has changed in his life—he has found a tech job in an multinational company in Chennai. He is clean-shaven, the fuzzy hair that sprouted on his chin shorn away. He goes to the gym now and takes protein supplements and has gained some weight. Wonder of all wonders, he is even using deodorant, something which he never did earlier, and this makes spending time with him more tolerable.

Prayag comes to pick me up from the airport on his new cherry-red motorbike, a Hero Honda Achiever, which he has bought with his signing bonus. He is definitely feeling and looking more confident than the pale, sleep-deprived ghost I had last seen in Delhi.

The first thing that Prayag tells me with a toothy grin is that he is no longer a virgin; he has finally had sex with his girlfriend of three months, Samyukta. Though Prayag has had girlfriends in college, he never had sex with any of them. His most sexually aggressive moment had been when he had demurely kissed Pia on the lips, a moment he would never forget. Sex, he says, has been simply amazing and he feels transformed, physically and mentally.

For their first time, Prayag and Samyukta rented a hotel room in a three-star hotel. They began the night by watching a Hindi film, then had a meal at the hotel restaurant, and finally made their way to their room. Despite Prayag's meticulous preparation that involved watching thousands of hours of porn, the first time was difficult. It was hard to get the condom on, and when he finally did, it was so tight that everything felt painful. To add to this, he couldn't manage to slide in his organ as smoothly and painlessly as he had observed in the movies. Somehow they had managed to do the act, but it was a frustrating experience. Thankfully, Samyukta was as willing to practice and improve as he was, and soon they had managed to achieve pleasurable union.

In Chennai, Prayag lives as a Paying Guest (PG) with a local family. His parents insist that he live in this strict environment (he has to be home by 9 p.m. on weekdays) mostly because of the vegetarian food that the host family offers him. Retaining vegetarianism is of crucial importance to Prayag's parents because it implies that he abides by the values with which he was raised, of which vegetarianism is the touchstone. Prayag could care less about these values; it turns out he has recently taken to eating meat and loves his butter chicken whenever he goes out for a meal.

Prayag takes me to his congested apartment, where he has a small, bare room that shares a thin wall with the owners of the apartment—a stodgy, Tamil couple.

Is this where he has sex, I wonder, thinking how uncomfortable it must be.

Thankfully, Prayag tells me that he is not allowed to have friends visit, so he usually goes to friends' places or Samyukta's apartment (which she shares with four roommates) to do the deed. He tells me that he plans to move out of the 'shit hole PG' as soon as he can convince his parents about his 'dedication' to being a vegetarian.

Though it only 8 p.m. and not quite dark yet, Prayag insists on taking me to Climax, the most happening 'disc' in town, which is in one of Chennai's many new malls. On our evening out, I finally meet the girlfriend, Samyukta, a sweet-faced, dark-skinned girl with taut, tidy features. She is from a small city close to Chennai and works as a receptionist at Prayag's company. She is dressed in a pair of tight jeans, high heels and a tight t-shirt. She is very much in awe of Prayag, of his engineering degree, of his senior position (relative to her) at the company and, most of all, of his newly purchased motorbike on which he drops her home every day.

Prayag knows the doorman at Climax, so the cover charge is waived for all of us. I notice the charges: entry is free for women, ₹200 for a couple, and ₹400 for a 'stag' or a single man. Men pay a premium for being single.

The nightclub is packed, mostly with stags, but there are also co-ed groups. The box-shaped club features a bar made entirely of red and black plastic, a dance floor with swirling strobe-lights, next to which a tired looking DJ plays his tunes in a rickety red-coloured booth, and a few black, sticky pleather couches.

Despite the early hour and the tawdry settings, Climax is rocking. There is a palpable energy in the air, and if not for the skewed sex ratio, a good party might have been on the cards.

Undeterred by the gender imbalance, Prayag and Samyukta head straight to the dance floor where they immediately start dancing frenziedly and expertly to the popular Bollywood and Tollywood tunes that are blaring from the speakers. I too am encouraged to dance, and Prayag, Samyukta and I form a small circle. Samyukta is quite a talented dancer, and she jumps up and down, twirls expertly, whooping along with the music. Prayag is awkward on the dance floor and has one move only, a march-along that he performs with confidence, looking proudly at Samyukta, who has upstaged us all with her prowess.

At 10 p.m. the music is abruptly switched off, and the lights are turned on. We all gaze around in alarm, squinting in the sudden harshness of the white lights. I am told that nightclubs in Chennai shut at 10 p.m., which explains our early arrival. We shuffle our way out of the club, and make our way to the next party, which Prayag promises will be as happening as Climax. I notice that Prayag is drenched in sweat from his vigorous marching.

Not long after I find myself in a small, dark, shabby apartment. Music plays from a laptop, and a squat bottle of Old Monk rum sits on a table with some plastic cups and mixers. The sex ratio is much better, and groups of boys and girls huddle together on mattresses thrown on the floor. A few people crowd around a small glass hookah taking turns with the pipe, inhaling expertly and blowing out perfect rings of smoke.

The scene is typical of a college house party and Prayag tells me that most of the people here are recent graduates like himself, working in various corporations dotted around the city.

Prayag pours us all drinks. I notice that he pours more rum into Samyukta's than into our cups—the standard ploy to get the girlfriend drunk. Samyukta sips on her strong drink, half a plastic cup of rum diluted with a splash of water. After taking a gulp she tells me, curling up her button nose, that she doesn't like the taste of alcohol, but likes the high that it gives her.

Some marijuana is brought out, and a young man expertly rolls a joint and passes it expeditiously around the small group. Everyone takes a drag. Soon Prayag is drunk. I recall that Prayag never drank in college.

He tells me with a certain drug- and rum-infused swagger: 'I never thought I would be a chick-magnet, but I am now. I was always the dorky boy in school, but working hard has got me places. Ira, life is just ammmazzzing.' (He'd stopped calling me ma'am once he graduated.)

At 3 a.m., the party is still whirling on. I have just woken up from a short nap induced by second-hand pot smoke. I take in my surroundings. What had seemed like a fairly innocuous party now seems a rubbish pit. Prayag, my ride home, is passed out on the floor. Samyukta is sitting in a corner smoking a cigarette and giggling with a nondescript young man. I doubt I will find taxis at this time in the morning so I decide to go back to sleep until daybreak when I can make my way home.

As daylight streams into the apartment, I wake up. In the morning, the apartment looks even more squalid, and all the remnants of the debauchery are evident. Snoring men are passed out on the booze- and food-stained floor. The long empty bottle of alcohol lies abandoned in a graveyard of cigarette butts. Samyukta must have found a ride home because I'm the only girl left. I chastise myself; old habits die hard, and despite being much too old for these sorts of situations, at a college-like party like this, be it Boston or Chennai, I am still the last woman to leave.

I shake Prayag awake. His breath smells rancid, and he rubs his bloodshot eyes. He wears contact lenses now, and one has fallen out, so his vision is blurred. We try looking for the missing lens on the floor, but given the mess in the apartment and our less than ideal physical condition, it is an impossible task. Prayag comes out to help me find an auto to get me home and we fall into a rather bizarre conversation about his relationship with Samyukta.

'I won't marry Samyukta because she had sex with me. If she had sex with me, then that means that she can have sex with anyone.'

'Prayag! That's ridiculous. She had sex because you wanted to!' I say indignantly.

'But if she had sex with me, then she will have sex with other guys also. Her mentality is like that only,' he says sheepishly.

'What is her mentality like?' I ask.

'She has a cheap mentality. She roams around with fast girls, so she may be fast too.'

'Are you saying that Samyukta is a "bad girl"?' I ask.

He looks at me blankly.

'Remember our bad girl, good girl classification?'

'Huh?' he says, confused.

It seems that the 'good girl, bad girl' formula that Prayag had used for many years has been forgotten. With the change in his personality, he has also changed his vocabulary. However, while speaking with him, I discover that in essence things have remained the same. Now girls either have a 'cheap mentality' or a 'healthy mentality'. Girls who have a cheap mentality tended to be 'fast' which basically meant 'fast' to have sex and therefore not worth marrying.

I say to Prayag, 'Samyukta is a fast girl so you don't consider her worth marrying? But you also claim to love her, how does that work?'

A hung-over Prayag is strained by this conversation. 'It's all confusing for me. I don't know about all this stuff. Better to focus on career than to think of love-shove and all,' he says wearily.

◆

> No people in the world are more confused in their attitude toward sex than we Indians. Our cherished ideals bear little resemblance with our patterns of sexual behaviour; our fantasies, heavily influenced by our mythology, impinge on our subconscious and add to our confusion because they contradict each other. A land of phallus-yoni worshippers laud the virtues of virginal chastity, renunciation of sex and brahmacharya. —*Khushwant Singh*

Prayag is not alone when it comes to muddle-headed views on sex and love. Since time immemorial, across cultures and continents, a woman's virginity has been prized, treasured and conserved. Indian tradition too has always propagated a patriarchal culture through its extreme, almost obsessive, paranoia about the virtues of female chastity.

As I interacted with Prayag, what the scholar Wendy Doniger had explained to me became self-evident. 'In most of the history of Hindu culture, a girl must be a virgin [at the time of her marriage], or all hell breaks loose, and you get your money back,' she had said. And, as we have seen, Hindu culture has played a very large part in shaping Indian culture and Doniger's contention is borne out by Hindu scriptures from the very earliest times. The *Rig-Veda* talks about the blood of deflowering of the first night and how dangerous this blood can be. If clothes get stained with blood, they must be given to the priest to be taken care of, else they will destroy anybody that they touch. In *The Laws of Manu*, serious fines are imposed on people who destroy the virginity of a girl. The *Arthashastra* contains guidelines on what to do if virginity is lost and declares that a marriage is invalid if the girl is not a virgin and if blood is not shown on the sheets of the wedding night. An entire book in the seven-volume *Kamasutra* is devoted to the kanya, or the virgin, making sure a man is circumspect with a girl on her wedding night. The *Kamasutra* essentially says that a girl is a virgin on her wedding night, so you must make her a happy person, or else you'll destroy the marriage for the rest of her life.[27]

Through this age-old emphasis on chastity, a man exerts control over a woman. A woman is not allowed to experience sexual pleasure until she marries her husband, and when she does, she is only allowed to have sex with one man—her husband—and bear his children. So despite India's shifting sexual landscape, guilt, contradictions, conservative attitudes and shame towards sex remain. Many of the young women that I spoke to on college campuses spoke of the constant struggle between their views on sex and those of society. I was fascinated by their views on the young men they dated and whom they hoped to marry one day. Because of the environment they were rooted in, to many of these young women, virginity continued to matter, though they were no longer virgins and they were afraid that their prospects of marriage would be diminished by their sexual activity.

As a result, labiaplasty or tightening of the labia, is a highly sought-after surgical procedure in the country. Dr Krishna, a practitioner in New Delhi, says that in his clinic alone, the number of procedures has gone up from one a month in 2010 to over six every month in 2012.

Mumbai-based cosmetic and plastic surgeon Dr Manoj Manjwani says he is seeing a growing number of patients for hymen repair surgery every each month.

Less drastic 're-virginization' techniques for women include vaginal tightening creams, such as the popular 18 Again, and numerous Ayurvedic and herbal remedies that are now flooding the market.

Given the confusion and tension surrounding sex and chastity, Prayag's mindset is not difficult to understand.

◆

A few weeks later, back in Delhi, I get frantic Facebook messages from Prayag. He has found out that Samyukta was not a virgin when they had had sex. Samyukta's Facebook chat records with an ex-boyfriend revealed this crucial information. He was, at first, violently angry with her, threatening to kill her, and then threatening to kill himself. When she stopped answering his calls, he camped outside her apartment. An increasingly beleaguered Samyukta lodged a police complaint against him and then a restraining order.

After his initial rage at Samyukta's infidelity, Prayag is now depressed. Over the phone he tells me that he has stopped going to work, so he has been fired. He has been kicked out of the vegetarian household and is crashing at a friend's apartment. He says he loves Samyukta, but he can't forgive her. I tell him to forget about her and to move on, but he says he cannot, that he loves her too much. Maybe Samyukta feared this extreme reaction from Prayag and that is why she kept her secret. Prayag sobs on the phone as he speaks to me, then he begins crying uncontrollably, and finally he becomes hysterical and hangs up.

A few months later, I am glad to find out that Prayag has managed to get his act together. He seems to be holding up, still traumatized by the series of events, but not as deeply depressed.

He and Samyukta have un-friended each other on Facebook, and are disconnected on all other social media but he has found out through a common friend that she is engaged to her distant cousin, a love-cum-arranged marriage. He has found a job in Hyderabad, where his parents have insisted on a vegetarian PG, which has an even stricter curfew than the last.

Prayag's reaction may seem unwarranted, but it is not uncommon. I am relieved that he has not resorted to more extreme measures. According to a police report, the state of Tamil Nadu has the highest number of what the police term 'love failure suicides', with over 5,000 cases reported each year. According to police officials, many youngsters get involved so deeply in relationships or become so possessive about their partners that a rejection takes on life-threatening significance.[28]

Most Indian girls that I know, including myself, have dealt with obsessive Indian male behaviour. I have noticed that the smaller and more conservative the town, the more drastic the behaviour. In my high school in Indore, every single girl I knew, irrespective of physical appearance, had at some point in her school life been the object of obsessive male attention.

In the recent blockbuster movie *Raanjhanaa*, the main character, a young Hindu boy, is obsessed with a teenaged Muslim girl, who is sent out of town when it is discovered that she is flirting with a Muslim man. When she returns to her home town all grown-up, her girlhood paramour is still waiting for her, while she has totally forgotten about him. He continues to serve and love her despite the fact that his love is unrequited. At the end he dies for her, but it is not in vain, because at least he had loved.

In a culture inexperienced with love and romance, sadly, it is Bollywood and other regional cinema that influence the romantic ideals of most young people. In a typical Bollywood love story, the hero aggressively pursues his love-interest, teasing her, chasing her, harassing her, displaying his love for her in front of her friends; the hero, who is usually an obsessive romantic will not accept no for an answer, and eventually wins her over. In a society in a state of flux, young people like Prayag, Pia, Samyukta and others often act in strange and confused ways, taking their cues from movies or magazines or the internet or their equally muddle-headed peers, while at the same time attempting to reconcile the new ways with traditional modes of behaviour.

Hopefully, over time, the benefits of the gathering sexual revolution will become apparent and society will become a little more open and equal. But it is early days yet.

THE MAKING OF A PORN STAR

Overlooking the magnificent expanse of the Bay of Bengal, perched on the shores of the Chandrabagha beach in the eastern state of Odisha stands the Sun Temple of Konark. It was built by King Narasimhadeva I of the Eastern Ganga Dynasty around 1250 CE in praise of the Sun God, using 1,200 craftsmen over a period of twelve years. The grand temple is designed in the form of the gigantic chariot of the Sun God pulled by seven horses to represent the seven days of the week. It has twenty-four wheels, representing each hour of the day. The Sun Temple is the best-known example of the Kalinga School of Indian temple art and is famous for its imposing dimensions, design and for the thousands of erotic sculptures adorning its walls.

It is a popular tourist attraction and my tour guide and I share the spacious temple premises with hundreds of visitors—turbaned farmers, camera-wielding Japanese tourists, red-faced men and women with British accents, and honeymooners. My tour guide, a tired-looking, unshaven, rather scruffy-looking man who smells strongly of alcohol, begins narrating by rote the history of the temple in broken English. He points out the numerous images on the temple walls—celestial nymphs, mythological creatures, and triumphant elephants that march around the entire base of the temple; he intermittently points out maithunas—amorously intertwined figures of couples copulating.

'Homo,' he says, pointing to two apsaras, their faces peaceful and serene as they engage in intercourse.

'Doing secretly in night,' he adds, showing me some rats, which are part of the scene.

Since I am interested in the maithunas, I tell my tour guide to focus on 'love scenes only'. In Tantra, the maithuna is a sexual ritual and the most important part of the grand tantric ritual known as the panchatattva.

Animated now, the guide points out the diminutive but intricate sculptures of women performing fellatio on men, men performing cunnilingus on women, men having sex with men, of women having sex with women, men with many women, one woman with many men, and even men and women with animals. The tiny erect organs of the male figures, carved in sandstone, are visible even after hundreds of years. The serene expressions on the faces of these statues in sexual congress suggest a sacred, meditative experience as opposed to something hedonistic and sybaritic.

As I pass a large carving of a trio in an erotic position, I catch two young Indian men pointing towards it and giggling. When they see me photographing the sculpture, they shut up and look shamefaced. I also notice a bewildered villager staring at an erotic image that depicts a well-endowed apsara in a coital position with a man. I watch him poke the large stone breast with his finger, and then amble away, the expression on his wrinkled, weathered skin unchanged. Thousands of tourists, both old and young, from every level of society walk past the temple walls. I wonder what they really make of all the explicit erotic imagery, beyond their visible embarrassment or their studious ignoring of what stares them in the face. The most famous representation of Konark—the giant wheel—which has been endlessly represented on stamps, currency, posters, and advertising usually has the erotic imagery carefully blurred away. I remember a blog I came across where a housewife turned amateur sculptor had displayed her objet d'art: a homemade Konark Wheel. I noticed that she too had replaced erotic artwork with images of deities. Though our erotic past stares us in the face, mixing freely with sacred temples, we simply choose to ignore it. 'Here the language of stone surpasses the language of man', Rabindranath Tagore once said about the Sun Temple. And indeed it did.

Ancient India was a highly sexualized society, and the erotica depicted in art was an integrated part of our past. Sex continued to be a major part of the philosophical and religious life of the country well into the Middle Ages, from around the tenth century to the sixteenth—a period of renaissance in erotic art and literature. During this time, the Sun Temple of Konark, the temples of Khajuraho in Madhya Pradesh and many other structures celebrating sex as a joyful union with the divine, were built across the country. And then everything that had to do with sex and sexuality went into steep and precipitous decline. We have examined some of the reasons earlier in this chapter. The consequences of the closing down of the exuberant sensuality that once reigned continue to play out today. One of the worst outcomes has been the repression and moral policing of Indian society to an outrageous degree, which has resulted in all sorts of imbalance.

One of these is an excessive consumption of pornography, a hallmark, I discovered, of a once repressive society in a terrible hurry to shed its inhibitions. The world of online pornography is overwhelmingly affordable, accessible and acceptable, a fact corroborated by seven Indian cities ranking amongst the top ten in the world for online porn traffic. Google trends reported that the search volume index for the word 'porn' has doubled in India between 2010 and 2012, which makes sense, given that one in five mobile users in India wants adult content on their 3G-enabled phones.[29]

Statistics say that three in five Indian men approve of pornography and the proportion of those actually watching porn is higher, with nearly three in four declaring that they watch porn.[30] Indian women too are watching porn, and over 55 per cent of all women say their sex partners approve of pornography.[31] Porn pervades all parts of urban India, with Ahmedabad in Gujarat having the highest percentage—78 per cent—of both men and women watching and approving of porn.[32] A surprising statistic is that 25 per cent of all pornography-watching women in Jaipur and 16 per cent in Patna watch porn *without* the knowledge of their partners, showing that women are becoming more sexually curious, and that porn is not just a male domain anymore.[33]

Though the publishing, possession, making, selling or distribution of pornography (including transmitting of 'obscene material in electronic form') has been banned in India since 1969, with a penalty of imprisonment up to three years (or five years for the offence of child pornography), today's technology allows anyone with an internet connection access to porn.

To find out more about pornography in India, I began by watching locally made porn. Most of the 'blue films' that I watched featured a glum, washed-out Indian woman having sex, often with a foreign man, in a dingy flat. The plot, storyline and acting were non-existent. For example, a sex scene would begin in a bathroom where the woman soaps herself and bathes using water from a plastic bucket. She would then go into a dimly-lit bedroom to have intercourse with the man. There was no aesthetic element to these videos, no music and not much vocalization, except for whimpering moans from the woman and the occasional grunt from the man. The women in the videos usually wear granny panties or nightgowns and the men a pair of trackpants, while the shoot locations are often shabby and dirty. Far from being arousing, the porn that I watched was violent and disturbing.

Since watching blue films had been such an unpleasant experience, I decided to learn more by speaking to Ashim Ahluwalia, the producer-director of the 2012 film *Miss Lovely*, based on his extensive research into the Indian porn industry in the early 1990s. Ahluwalia confirms that my views on Indian porn were correct, and that many people referred to them as 'nicotine-patch porn' since they seemed designed to turn you off porn. He adds that Indian porn has no genres, unlike most western porn. Most 'desi sex' is straightforward, quick sex with no deviations such as anal sex or any other fetishes being explored. Most Indian blue films have abysmally small budgets and are shot in empty flats with the cameraman usually being one of the participants. The actresses are typically from small towns and poor families. Many start off in films with minor roles and get into porn when their careers in mainstream cinema fail to take off. Typically, these girls are looking for 'fame' in modelling or acting.

Though the Indian porn industry is in poor shape today, it has not always been this way, laments Ahluwalia. The pioneers of porn were southern filmmakers from Tamil Nadu and Kerala in the late 1970s and early 1980s. The liberal censors in these states and the availability of infrastructure to support cheap film production led to the birth of the Indian porn industry. To pass censor boards, the first pornographic films did not show hard-core porn. But to titillate audiences, theatre owners and distributors added 'bits', that is, random pornographic sequences from foreign films. Indigenously made 'bits' featuring Indian actors soon began appearing in these films, as cheap recording technology made shooting scenes easy. This practice was so common in Tamil Nadu and Kerala that 'bit cinema' became its own classification, and these films became so popular that audiences would refuse to watch films without 'bits'.

As documented in *Miss Lovely*, the 1980s were the 'golden age' of Indian sleaze. Indian popular cinema began to feature more explicit material across a wide range of genres, with a definite aesthetic element. A whole string of Tarzan and cavemen films were made, as well as many outlandish horror films involving sadism, rape and necrophilia. According to Dr Meena Pillai, a cultural critic at the University of Kerala, the films of the 1980s that were labelled as pornography were less about nudity and graphic sex than they were about female sexuality. These films typically featured a voluptuous, sexually aggressive woman as the main character. In such a soft-core film, the woman was the lead, she was in command and chose her own sexual partners.[34]

The advent of hand-held video cameras changed the porn industry of the 1980s. Porn films were shot using hand-helds, thus making them cheaper to shoot, dirtier, and bereft of creativity. Locally shot hard-core porn began to be previewed in video parlours across India where audiences crowded into a room by the side of the road and paid a few rupees to watch these films on a small TV. Soft-core films with 'bits' continued to be shown in theatres, though with much less frequency. By the late 1990s the entire scene changed as the arrival of the internet brought with it an entire universe of pornography. Soft-core films diminished in popularity, and video parlours showing blue films continued, as they do today, catering mostly to the poorer sections. The internet had killed the Indian porn star.

◆

One evening a group of young Indian men, engineers and tech-nerds, relaxed over drinks and, as is not uncommon to such an evening, their conversation eventually moved to porn. Indian women are known the world over for their beauty and sensuality and though several Indian girls had become international beauty queens, there was no singular Indian porn star. Upset by this, the young men decided to create their own dream girl, the kind of Indian woman who would titillate their senses, provoke their passions, and who they could spend long, peaceful masturbatory hours with. Thus was born a lollapalooza of a woman—Savita Patel aka Savita Bhabhi, a Gujarati bhabhi, a Wonder Woman-lookalike with breasts that would put Pamela Anderson to shame. She donned a navel-baring sari with a cleavage-sporting blouse along with the trademark features of a good Indian wife—sindoor, bindi and mangalsutra. What started as banter amongst a group of drunken young men became an instant online hit. Based on the life of a hot, sex-hungry Indian housewife, the online comic-strip struck a chord, and within the span of just a few episodes became a country-wide sensation with half a million daily visitors.

Savita Bhabhi is the good Indian housewife who lives in a small town and cheerfully takes care of her home, husband, in-laws and numerous visiting family members. But she also has a raging sex drive, loves the taste of semen and is bored silly with her workaholic husband. In her free time, she seduces door-to-door salesmen, servant boys, young relatives and even her husband's colleagues, luring them into having hedonistic sex with her. As cartoon porn, Savita Bhabhi is mediocre at best—the script is laughably simplistic, the artwork amateurish (to the extent that Savita Bhabhi looks different in each cartoon) and the plotline crude, yet it is hugely popular. The success of Savita Bhabhi, it seems, lies in the distinctly local flavour of the comic strip that readers relate to.

In one episode Savita Bhabhi is shown having sex with a variety of service-providers, men whom Indian women typically visit every day. Bhabhi has sex with the local kirana-wallah in the storeroom and also with the kulfi-wallah whom she asks to insert the kulfi into her vagina. In another episode, Savita Bhabhi contests the Mrs India pageant where a judge, an uncanny Amitabh Bachchan lookalike, asks for sexual favours that she is more than happy to dispense. In another episode, 'The Perfect Indian Bride', Bhabhi convinces her nephew to have a quick arranged marriage to a girl by proving to him that Indian women are hardly sexually demure.

A journalist aptly describes Bhabhi: 'Her long dark hair parted dutifully in the middle, bright red sindoor and a mangalsutra dangling between oddly heavy bosoms, Savita Bhabhi was pornographic, but not quite. The cartoon comic strip may have inspired fantasy for a few, but for most, it poked fun at the coy Indian attitude towards sexuality, at our discomfort with any bold assertion of the sexual. The more virgin and demure she appeared, the more kinky and lurid we wanted her to be. When the Traveling Bra Salesman rang her doorbell, or when cousins visited from a world afar, no surprise that Bhabhi quickly discarded all pretence of "*sharam*".[35]

Savita Bhabhi forms a part of her reader's daily existence as she exists in the realm of their possibility. She plays off common Indian fantasies: of the young man lusting after the neighbourhood bhabhi, or the new sister-in-law who is strictly off limits. 'This layered response to a bhabhi or sister-in-law just does not exist in the west. So Savita Bhabhi really is an Indian product.'[36] Sociologist Patricia Uberoi 'cites the '90's Bollywood smash hit *Hum Aapke Hain Kaun*, a family film that sanitized a range of erotic relationships in popular culture. The film carried a whole erotic register just below its surface: the *bhayya-bhabhi* relationship was usefully immortalized in songs and purple sarees.'[37]

For Bhabhi there is no romance in sexual encounters. There is no hugging, no kissing, and no 'I love you' except with her husband, with whom she is never depicted having sex. Unlike Western pornography, there is always bristly pubic hair in sight, on both the men as well as on Bhabhi. Though Savita Bhabhi initiates the sex, it is the man who takes over, and traditional male-female sexual roles are followed. Savita Bhabhi pleases men by performing fellatio, and then begs them not to ejaculate inside her, but on her breasts or in her mouth since she enjoys the taste of semen. In her own words, she says, 'Nooo don't cum inside me... I want you to shoot it on my face.'

'"A woman once thanked me for showing Savita reaching an orgasm in every episode," says Deshmukh, the pseudonym of Puneet Agarwal, the creator of Savita Bhabhi. "I can wager that many husbands have asked their wives about female orgasms and how they can help them reach it after reading the comic." It may be self-serving, but according to Deshmukh, his pneumatic housewife has helped us 'take a small step in bridging the gap between male and female sexuality.'[38]

Deshmukh says that he wanted to show that sex is not only a male thing, and that it is 'a two-way street', especially since close to 30 per cent of the viewers are female. He is trying to focus on female pleasure in the coming stories, which I notice are getting more sexually equal, with men performing a lot more cunnilingus on Savita Bhabhi.

Unfortunately, in June 2009, the Indian government sent a letter to all internet service providers asking them to block savitabhabhi.com. The ban was the result of complaints from women's groups who charged Savita Bhabhi with representing the 'demon of impurity'.[39] There was a large public outcry, mostly virtual (since this is where Bhabhi's fans existed) against banning Savita Bhabhi, as millions of readers were left in the lurch.

Fortunately for her fans, a few months after the ban, Savita Bhabhi was back in action, re-emerging on a different website under a paid subscription model. Today, Savita Bhabhi episodes are released every few weeks, and the creators have even started a new series titled Savita@18, based on Bhabhi's teenage exploits. Bollywood, too, has taken note and a movie starring Rozlyn Khan is in the works.

Porn shifts the way people think about sexual relationships, about intimacy and about women. Savita Bhabhi is a satire on Indian society and showcases the contradictions of a repressed, yet overly stimulated society in a laughably simplistic way. Even though Savita Bhabhi is just a toon porn star, she represents the Indian woman who is proud of her sexuality and is willing to flaunt it. Savita Bhabhi also undermines the patriarchal view that every traditional Indian woman has to be 'pure' which is the literal meaning of the name 'Savita'.

According to creator Deshmukh, 'India is a sexually repressed country and for it to break the shackles, it is the women of India who are going to have to come out first. We are already seeing this, and hopefully SB will do her bit to help in this revolution.'[40]

Today, besides home-grown pornographic icons like Savita

Bhabhi, western imports are beginning to make their appearance as well. India has its first Playboy bunny, Sherlyn Chopra, who rose to national fame after her appearance on the cover of *Playboy* magazine, and Sunny Leone, a porn-star of Indian origin, has become enormously popular and is now appearing in mainstream Bollywood films. Realizing the untapped potential of a virgin market, *Playboy* is opening its first club in Goa, where the first Indian Playboy bunnies have specially designed bunny costumes—a two-piece outfit and sheer skirt along with the traditional bunny accessories of cuff, collar, bow tie and bunny-tail. According to a company statement, 'this new costume is a celebration of India's rich culture and the Americana of the classic Playboy Bunny Costume'.

◆

With the advent and penetration of broadband internet and affordable cell phones, sex is now just a click away. Social media websites like Facebook and Orkut, others specifically tailored for dating, and yet others for sexual encounters like PlanetRomeo have made sex easily accessible. Neuroscientists Dr Sai Gaddam and Dr Ogi Ogas studied the online sexual behaviour of 100 million people across the world by analysing internet data in their book *A Billion Wicked Thoughts: What the Internet Tells Us About Sexual Relationships*. Gaddam's and Ogas's studies indicate that Indian searches for sexual content demonstrate a lack of sexual experience; 'how to kiss' is one of the more popular searches in India compared to searches from Western countries, which are less instructional and more exploratory—like 'anal' or 'bondage'.

Gaddam and Ogas also found that the sexual material that people in India searched for was titillating rather than being explicitly pornographic because of the sexual naiveté of the searchers. Common plotlines of popular porn films revolve around fantasies of first sexual experiences, uncommon themes in countries where attitudes towards sexual relations are relaxed and liberal.

Indians are aroused by culturally specific content. For example, the fetishization of the belly button was much more common in the Indian subcontinent than anywhere else in the world, and internet searches like 'wet sari hot navel songs' and 'wet sari in rain' were popular searches on YouTube.

But the internet alone apparently isn't enough satisfy the Indian appetite for sexual fulfilment. Sex toys are the latest craze in India, and Chinese products have flooded the black market. The adult product market in India is estimated to be US$221 million (₹1,377 crore) against a global market of US$21.8 billion (₹1,35,830 crore) and this is expected to double to US$453 million (₹2,821 crore) in the next three years, exploding to around US$1.6 billion (₹9,967 crore) by 2020.[41] Experts attribute this boom to the growing number of people who want to experiment in their sex lives. Statistics too show that currently just 9 per cent of Indians use vibrators compared to 21 per cent globally although 57 per cent Indians say they'd be interested in trying sex toys if they had access to them.[42] Though Chinese sex toys appear to be new entrants to India, the truth is the concept of sex toys is ancient. In the *Kamasutra*, Vatsyayana advises his readers to use wooden penises to please women, and for men who don't have access to women, he advises using stone sculptures of women. These ancient erotic paraphernalia sound curiously similar to dildos and inflatable latex dolls, two fast-selling varieties of sex toys.

The sale of sex toys is illegal as defined by Section 292 of the Indian Penal Code which defines 'obscene' as 'a book, pamphlet, paper, writing, drawing, painting, representation, figure or any other object if it is lascivious or appeals to the prurient interest', so sex toys are only sold on the black market. Prices for sex toys are unregulated so profit margins on these products can be huge. Where there is a demand, the enterprising Indian is never far behind, so as sex toys catch on in the country, many entrepreneurs are jumping on to the sex toy bandwagon—some more successfully than others. In Mumbai, a fifty-year-old NRI from the US was arrested at the airport for smuggling sex toys including sex games and high-end lingerie worth ₹3.5 lakhs.[43] Even in smaller Indian towns, sex toys are fast becoming popular, and recently a stash of contraband sex toys was recovered from a hardware store in Rajkot, Gujarat.[44] Realizing the potential of the sex toy industry, Samir Saraiya, an ex-employee of Microsoft quit his job to start an online sex shop. He has an exclusive agreement to sell global lingerie and sex toy brands through his website thatspersonal.com. The lawyer representing the online store hopes to circumvent the law, as their products do not carry graphic or pictorial descriptions, which can be classified as 'obscene' by Indian law.

SEXCAPADE

One of the biggest centres of the sex toy trade in the country is Palika Bazaar in Delhi. On the day I visit, with my boyfriend Vinayak in tow, I notice there isn't a woman in sight. The dim cavernous shopping corridors are lined with small shops that sell a range of goods from black market electronic items to fake Jockey underwear, astrology services, porn videos and sex toys. The place is packed with groups of loitering young men who throw me lascivious stares. I am glad that I have had the foresight to bring a male companion with me for this expedition.

Our first stop is a small video stall that looks illegal enough to source what we are looking for. The placard outside the shop reads 'Rainbow Videos' which I quickly discover has nothing to do with homosexuality. Vinayak asks the salesman if he has porn. He quickly pulls out a pile of DVDs in plastic covers and beckons for Vinayak to sit next to him on a small stool behind the counter so he can show him his wares. Vinayak points to me, and I go take a seat with some hesitation.

He points to the fuzzy pictures on the pirated movies.

'This is top-class desi porn. Only Indian girls and twelve hours non-stop.'

'Is this, uh, XXX?' I ask

'Yes, ma'am, don't worry, this is five times X. You won't miss out on anything!' he replies jauntily.

After we choose a couple of DVDs, for which we pay an exorbitantly high price (and later discover that we have been ripped off), Vinayak asks him with hesitation if he has any of 'those kinds of toys'. He gives Vinayak a slimy smile.

'Yes, sir, just wait one minute.'

The salesman makes a couple of phone calls and five minutes later a man carrying a black garbage bag approaches us.

Again he asks me to sit on the stool next to him. He begins to pull out a variety of sex toys from the bag. 'For female only,' he says. The range of the penis-shaped vibrators and dildos is astonishing. They come in blocks, in squares, shaped as sausage-like human organs; they are made from plastic, from silicone, from rubber, and other unidentifiable materials; they come in a spectrum of colours—in fluorescent pink, in black, in skin tones and rainbow colours. As I look at these pieces the man continues to comment on his wares.

'Ma'am, this is best quality. Just see how bendy. 100 per cent silicon,' he says, twisting the dildo 180 degrees to demonstrate its flexibility.

The prices that the man quotes to us are outrageous, starting from ₹5,000 for a plastic vibrator, and going up to ₹10,000 for top-quality silicone. We've been fleeced once, but not again. I do not purchase these expensive toys, but I do find out more about who buys them. Our salesman tells me that the most common purchaser of sex toys is the single Indian male, though, at times, they come with their female partners. Single women customers, or groups of girls are rare, though he has had a couple of foreign women customers. As I glance around the seedy market with its squadrons of greasy, hovering men, I can see why women might not want to come here.

Vinayak and I stroll around the market, still on the hunt for sex toys, and are surprised at how big it is. The deeper we go into the dizzying, concentric maze, the sleazier the stores seem to become. Vinayak asks a young loafer—a Justin Bieber lookalike, no older than seventeen, with tight jeans and the band of his underwear showing—where we can find sex toys. He asks us to follow him, and we are led to a small storefront decorated with a variety of statuettes of Indian gods. The sickly sweet smell of incense pervades the air. In a similar fashion to the previous salesman, he too asks me to sit next to him on a small stool. He makes a few phone calls and soon a man with a black garbage bag appears.

The faux Justin Bieber is an aggressive salesman, and as he shows me a variety of dildo-cum-vibrators he comments lovingly on his products.

'Ma'am, what quality!' 'Ma'am, this one is 100 per cent Japanese technology.' 'Arre, ma'am, this one is to love only,' he says fondling a large black dildo, which he proceeds to demonstrate, strapping it on and thrusting back and forth.

He too quotes outrageously high prices, and when I tell him that I am in the market for something cheap, he brings out a variety of small, dinky toys—a keychain vibrator, a vibrating cock-ring, and even a delay spray to be used by men.

After a lengthy negotiation, I am sold a dildo-cum-vibrator for ₹1,000, down from the initial price of ₹15,000. As we are leaving, the faux Justin Bieber yells after us.

'Ma'am, what about sir? Let me show you an amazing piece for him.' Out of sheer curiosity we go back to the stall, where he pulls out a giant block of silicone with a slit down the centre. There is some black, curly pubic hair near the mouth of the slit, indicative of a vagina. I examine what I think is fake pubic hair and when it comes off easily, I suddenly realize that this hair isn't necessarily synthetic or part of the toy. I quickly hand the toy back to the whippersnapper salesman and rush out of the store as fast as I can to find the nearest bathroom.

•

Sex toys and porn aside, there are other indicators of how rapidly the sexual revolution is being monetized. Take the condom industry. Time was when there were only a couple of brands of condoms available in the country, the most popular ones being manufactured by the government, called Nirodh, and the other by a private manufacturer, aptly named Kamasutra. Today, the scenario has changed considerably. Condoms are readily and invitingly available in all shapes, sizes and flavours, including a paan-flavoured condom.

The current market size for condoms in India is US$120 million (₹747 crore) and is growing steadily every year.[45] Sales in the contraceptive category grew around 30 per cent last year compared to the 15 per cent growth in food products, hot beverages, hair and personal care products. The market is forecast to double to US$234 million (₹1,458 crore) in 2015 and grow to nearly US$715 million (₹4,454 crore) in 2020.[46] A manager at the popular chain of Twenty Four Seven convenience stores in Delhi disclosed that at his centrally located store, condom sales were highest on a Saturday night and that several of his customers were young women. An estimated 77 per cent of single women use the morning-after pill while 26 per cent married women do the same.[47]

Other products associated with sexually active behaviour are also becoming popular. For example, vaginal beautification is becoming increasingly important to Indian women. Brazilian wax, a process in which all the hair in and around a woman's vaginal area is removed, is now common in the beauty parlours that pockmark India's urban landscape, when less than five years ago, the procedure was relatively unknown to Indian women. I remember a visiting American friend asking for one at a New Delhi parlour, and getting a look of disgust in return. Today, across cities in India, Brazilian waxing is becoming common. During a recent trip to Haridwar, a city on the Ganga most famous for holy water-cleansing dips, a beautician at a parlour asked me if

I had a boyfriend and if I would like a Brazilian wax all in the same breath. Indians have even taken hair removal one step further. Laser hair removal parlours have become almost as ubiquitous as beauty parlours. A manager at a nation-wide chain told me that permanent hair removal in the bikini or vaginal area is the single most popular item on their menu.

Other types of vaginal beautification include 'vajazzling' a process of decorating the vagina with diamonds, crystals and other sparkly stones stuck on by glue. The procedure lasts until the hair on the vagina starts growing back. 'Clitter', or glitter for the clitoris is the cheaper form of vajazzling.[48]

Some experts blame easy availability of Western pornography online for making women want to beautify their vaginas. Surveys reveal that 34 per cent of Indian women in metro areas watch porn[49] where they see clean-shaven vaginas. Thinking that this is what it 'should' look like, women are opting for these processes.

Women are also becoming more interested in what they wear to bed and the resulting growth in the lingerie market has taken India by storm—the organized lingerie market has almost doubled from ₹780 crore in 2003 to ₹1,645 crore today.[50]

In 2012, by the time the iconic push-up brand Wonderbra was launched in India, all its pre-launch stock on display was sold out. Nearly 100,000 women from across the country had pre-booked their orders online. Several other brands have made their debut since, and online lingerie stores like Pretty Secrets and Zivame are gaining popularity.[51]

Less than ten years ago one could only find granny panties in large clothing stores, and for 'fancy' underwear one had to visit small shops selling goods like make-up and nightgowns. When you asked them for 'fancy' underwear they whisked you to the back of the store and surreptitiously pulled out plastic boxes of lacy Chinese underwear in risqué styles and patterns. Today, malls across the country have several lingerie stores, and India has more than thirty foreign and domestic brands of women's lingerie. Men's briefs too have taken on a new dimension with more than one company selling 'sexy' underwear for men.

Rajiv Grover, COO, Genesis Colours Pvt Ltd, which markets the brand Bwitch, says that its primary target audience of fifteen-twenty-five-year-olds is open to new styles. 'The younger generation wants to flaunt innerwear,' he observes. 'There was a time when bra straps were hidden as much as possible. Now women love to show them off. Lingerie has become a fashion accessory and is not a need-based product anymore.'[52]

Through the course of her two-decade career, lingerie designer Suman Nathwani has seen some shifts in India's lingerie market. When she first started: 'White was equated with virginity back then. A girl who wore white was nice and sweet, while wearing lace or bright colours was considered loose,' she says. 'Red was reserved only for the first night, and black if you wanted to seduce your husband.'

The scene today is a little different. Says Nathwani, 'So many women in their forties walk up to me and ask for sexy lingerie tips to dress up their figures. They don't want to be shy anymore.' She finds that animal prints and neons go well with Indian skin tones and are usually in demand. 'You can mix and match them. Leopard and zebra prints are also such a draw.'[53]

SEX CLINICS

While we have examined some of the newer signposts that point to the country's incipient sexual awakening, one of the more ubiquitous and longest-lasting fixtures of its urban landscape that relate to sex and sexuality is the sex clinic. Any drive through the outskirts of urban India will feature posters and hoardings advertising doctors and clinics treating 'gupt rog' or secret (read sexual) illnesses. In a country where proper treatment and counselling are not readily available for sex-related ailments, all sexual problems are usually taken care of by the ubiquitous 'sex clinic'. These sex clinics offer a variety of services to clients, mostly Ayurvedic and herbal, the most popular of which are cures for sexually transmitted diseases, impotence, premature ejaculation, ways of enhancing sexual performance and methods of acquiring male progeny.

In New Delhi there are quite a few sex clinics concentrated in the crowded old locality of Daryaganj; I discover that there is no direct or easy way to get there. I first take the metro, then a motorized rickshaw, then a man-powered rickshaw, and then walk to find my way to a crowded street which is the sex clinic row of Delhi. The best known sex clinic in the city is Sablok Clinic which sports a large glossy signboard with colourful flashing lights. The first image that comes to my mind when I see it is of Las Vegas with its long, twinkling, casino-lined streets. A blown-up wedding photo of a happy couple smiles down at visitors from the Sablok signage, though the glass covering is damaged and a crack runs through the middle of the once happy couple—not the picture of matrimonial bliss that it is meant to portray.

My photographer friend Vijay and I walk up a flight of stairs to enter a large and well-appointed office with plush carpets and pinewood panelling. We have timed our visit for 6.30 p.m. on a Saturday evening, hoping to observe and speak with patients, but much to our disappointment, even at our carefully chosen hour, the clinic is deserted. I ask to see the doctor, but the receptionist tells me that I must first pay the ₹500 consulting fee. I explain that I am a writer working on a book and I want to interview the doctor. The receptionist looks excited, goes inside the doctor's office and quickly beckons us inside.

The doctor is a corpulent, ferocious-looking man with loose-hanging jowls and emerald-green eyes. The walls of his office are dominated by two large portraits of his male ancestors around which are strung plastic-flower garlands. He seems pleased to give us an interview. He begins by telling us that Sablok is the oldest and best sex clinic in India, founded in 1928 by his grandfather. The 'secret' knowledge that he disperses has been passed down from his ancestors to him, and he uses his powers to help Indian society.

The Sablok website has a paragraph on masturbation:

> Masturbation or Hand Practice is the ejaculation of Semen with the help of hand starts mostly due to bad company... Gradually they get so much accustomed to this bad habit, that it becomes too much difficult for them to get the rid of this. When they grow up they feel that they are too weak to enjoy their happy married life. Due to excess of masturbation their genitals (penis) do not develop fully. Masturbation has many negative effects—physical weakness, lack of self-confidence, irritating & frustrating temperament, frequent night discharges & weakening semen passing before or after urination. Masturbation is not a good habit and it must be avoided to make the life happier & healthier.

Among other ludicrous suggestions the website also declares that 'night discharge' can be cured by walking barefoot in the morning on green grass. I inquire if the views on the website are his own.

'Yes,' he declares. 'Masturbation is the worst habit of Indian men. It spoils their married life, it also causes many diseases. It must be avoided fully and I have a very good Ayurvedic cure for it.'

The doctor tells us that Sablok's 'specialty' is in curing fertility problems and homosexuality through Ayurvedic potions. Vijay is proudly gay, so when the doctor declares that homosexuality is unnatural, he gets provoked. Much to my chagrin, Vijay and the doctor get into a testy argument.

'Doctorji, homosexuality is *very* natural. In fact it has been around for ages, and even been mentioned in our holy scriptures,' declares Vijay.

'All nonsense. Homosexuality is a matter of the mind, and happens in our society because boys don't get to hang around with girls. But, as I said, it can be cured by lowering the male testosterone through herbs.'

'How would you then explain homosexuality in the West, where boys and girls do "hang around" together, and that too from a very young age!' retorts a fuming Vijay.

The doctor replies with a guffaw. 'Ha! The West! Those countries are polluted and have *too* many problems. I have many customers who come from there to get treated. *I* know.'

Vijay turns around, and not so subtly declares to me, 'This guy is *so full of shit*!'

Vijay is a passionate gay-rights activist and his feelings have been hurt. I am speechless, and before I can think of something to pacify him, the doctor says calmly, 'Are you a gay, young man? Don't be shy. I can cure you, just come behind the curtain and let me do some examinations.' The doctor rolls up his sleeves and gets up from his chair.

Vijay screeches, 'But I don't *want* to be cured!'

Before Vijay can say more, and before we get into trouble—because I can see where this is going—I drag him out of the clinic, and the doctor is left standing by the examination bed.

After Vijay calms down, he refuses to go to any more sex clinics. I beg and plead with him, and he finally agrees to come with me to the neighbouring sex clinic: Chetak Sexologist.

We enter a small, single-room office, which is empty save for a man burning incense sticks in front of a small statue. There are no patients in sight.

'Could we see the doctor?' I ask.

'Who is the patient?' asks the young man.

'It is us,' I say. 'We are, uh, a couple.'

'I am the doctor. Please wait till I finish my puja.'

Vijay and I first pay the ₹200 fee and then tell the doctor that we are a newly married couple for whom sex is painful.

'It's painful for me to have sex,' I tell him.

'Hmm…it must be tight,' he says pointing to my vagina, but looking at Vijay.

'What do I do?' I ask.

He thinks for a second. 'Well... I will give you some medicines to make it less tight, but best for you is to go to a gynae [short for gynaecologist].'

'Any you recommend?' I ask.

'Go to Laxmi Nagar, there are many gynae over there,' he says.

Laxmi Nagar in New Delhi is an area infamous for quacks and shanty abortion clinics.

I must have looked confused, because he continues, 'They can do a simple operation, only takes half an hour. They just cut a few things, and put a band aid, and you are done.'

'Uh, and this will make it less tight?' asks Vijay.

'Yes, they cut it and loosen it. After that, great sex,' he says, giving Vijay a sneaky little smile.

He then prescribes a herbal potion for Vijay that flaunts a bull on the bottle and promises to increase virility. The bill is ₹600. We swiftly take our leave.

♦

Sex clinics were once the go-to places for all sexual problems, but today it appears that they are losing ground. After depressing hours spent surfing the farrago of nonsense, half-baked truths and misconceptions that these clinics peddle on the internet, I hope that greater access to information will help dispel many of the myths that distort sex and sexuality.

SEX DOCTOR

To get an overview on the major sexual trends within urban Indian society, I decide to meet with India's most eminent sexologist, Dr Kothari.

Dr Kothari was India's first sexologist. In many ways this man whose inspiration and hero is Vatsyayana, *is* the modern-day Vatsyayana. Dr Kothari is the only person in the world who has served three successive terms as chief advisor to the World Association for Sexual Health. He is also the man who held the first Annual Conference on Orgasm in India. He established the first department of sexology and sexual medicine in South Asia and has the largest private collection of erotic ancient Indian artefacts in the world. Dr Kothari has done much for sexual medicine in India, especially with his path-breaking studies on the female orgasm and minimum penis size for female satisfaction. Given his credentials, it is impossible to write about sexual behaviour in India without speaking of Dr Kothari who, over the course of his forty-five-year career, has examined over 50,000 cases of sexual problems in the country.

I meet Dr Kothari in his small South Bombay office, which looks and feels even smaller because it is crammed with so many erotic objects. Dr Kothari apologetically confides that he can't keep any of his erotic objects at home because they tend to distract the help, so he stores everything here. He shows me his latest acquisition, a beautiful seventeenth-century sculpture where a man is having simultaneous intercourse with five women—with his penis, two index fingers, and his toes.

Dr Kothari discovered his passion for sexology over fifty years ago after going through sexual anxieties of his own. He saw a man masturbating next to him at a movie theatre, and was shocked by the size of his penis, which was much larger than his own. He thought he had an undersized penis, so he went to quacks and sex clinics across the city, but no one was able to quell his anxiety. Young Kothari was studying to be a medical doctor at the time so, in his desperation, he decided to specialize in sexology to discover the truth for himself. After completing his training in the US (because India offered nothing like it) he went on to become India's first medically qualified sexologist.

I ask Dr Kothari how Indian sexual behaviour has changed over the past decade.

'The sexual landscape in India has changed tremendously, and women are at the heart of the change. They are becoming more sexually assertive and are reclaiming their sexual rights,' says

Kothari, with a look of pride on his wizened face.

'Earlier, many Indian women didn't know what an orgasm was, and they asked me what it felt like. I told them that it's like sneezing—unless you experience it, you'll never understand! Today my female patients ask me why they *haven't* had their orgasms! They demand pleasure.'

He adds, 'Men too are realizing that women have sexual needs. In the past, typically, Indian men didn't like performing cunnilingus on women. It was a patriarchal mindset; they thought it was dirty or beneath them. I had to explain to them that foreplay was most important.'

I understand from Kothari that across age groups, sexual experimentation and sexual expectations have increased. Indians, especially Indian women, are more sexually aware and *expect* sexually fulfilling relationships. The change is definitely more pleasurable, but it has also brought with it confusion and sexual anxiety, which sometimes creates rifts in relationships.

Until a decade ago, most of Dr Kothari's patients were male; women rarely saw him, and if they did, it was always with their husbands. Today, over 30 per cent of his patients are women whose relationships are on the verge of breakdown because of lack of sexual compatibility.

Dr Kothari explains, 'Sex in India has typically been only procreational and recreational. Today, there is a new dimension, and sex has become relational. Sex has become an important marker of how good the relationship is.'

In the West, there has always been a lot of emphasis on sexual performance and on being 'good' in bed, whereas in India, sex has so far not *defined* relationships in the way that it has in Western countries. Psychologist Sudhir Kakar explained to me how the traditional Indian view of sex is more holistic than the Western view where sex is all about the physical act, which may or may not have love attached to it. In India, on the other hand, sex, love and marriage have always been a sacred, one-package deal.

According to Kothari, though, it seems that all of the old views of sex are changing and we are beginning to move towards a more Western model where sex, marriage and love don't necessarily have to be associated with each other.

I ask Kothari about the most common sexual problems he comes across in his profession. He explains that Indian culture, like so many ancient cultures, is shrouded by myths accumulated over years, centuries and generations. It is practically impossible to launder an Indian mind of superstition and fantasy and this, Dr Kothari reveals, is the most pressing predicament of Indian sexual behaviour. Perhaps the most contentious were fallacies related to masturbation and penis size. 'No other activity has been so wrongly condemned but as universally practised as masturbation. People in India have a lot of guilt about masturbation. They feel that masturbation causes acne, homosexuality, and even diseases like tuberculosis! I even have people come and tell that the cure for masturbation is to have sex with a virgin!' says Dr Kothari.

He adds, 'I tell people that the penis does in a vagina what it does in the folded palm. There is no such thing as "excessive" masturbation. The tongue doesn't become weak in a talkative person, just like a penis doesn't become weak with masturbation or intercourse. The view that masturbation is something unhealthy needs to be extinguished because it can be a positive, healthy way to channelize desire.'

The other problem, one that he too faced when he was a young man, was 'bigger is better'. 'What is important is how good your performance is and not how long or how big your penis is. The normal sexual length of the vagina is six inches, only the outer third has nerve endings, the inner two-thirds is virtually insensitive. For adequate sexual gratification you need to be two inches plus, when erect of course,' he says passionately.

Most sexual problems arise, he says, because of lack of sexual education, and exposure. Kothari flares up when he speaks to me about quacks and sex clinics which were once the only places to get sexual help.

'These phonies promote all the wrong things; sex clinics are shams and should simply be outlawed! They dole out magic sex potions, spread myths about sex which then *lead* to sexual problems even if people don't have any,' says an inflamed Dr Kothari, who has encountered his fair share of sex clinic quacks over the course of his career.

I am curious to know what the main differences are in sexual problems and behaviour between India and the West.

According to Kothari, the West is more sexually advanced so their problems too are more advanced and complicated. Like Gaddam and Ogas, whose internet searches had revealed sexual naiveté, Dr Kothari too has found that Indians are 'sexually ignorant and unschooled'.

He explains with an example.

'A couple was married for twenty-one years yet could not consummate the marriage. They went to sex clinics, psychiatrists and physicians but nothing seemed to work. Finally they came to me. I explored their desire, erection, intromission and orgasm. The male reported enough desire and adequate quality of erection but was unable to penetrate. I asked them about their position during sex. It turned out that he was performing by keeping his legs outside hers, and was unable to insert his penis properly into her vagina. They weren't able to have sex, simply because of improper positioning,' Dr Kothari says to me with a sigh, shaking his head in frustration.

'Indians are sexually naive, but also superstitious, and carry heavy mental baggage when it comes to sex. If only we could dispel some of the myths and madness, India would be a sexually healthier country.'

Before I leave, Dr Kothari sums up a lifetime's worth of findings in a sentence: 'Indian sexual problems are between the two ears and not between the two legs.'

◆

As we come near the end of this brief journey through some aspects of this country's new stirrings of sex and sexuality, it would be instructive to look at a recent survey by the contraceptive company Durex which brought to light an alarming paradox. While 68 per cent of Indians claimed to be happy with their sex lives, only 46 per cent confessed to regular orgasms. Another survey done in the same year by a leading Indian magazine pointed out that only 8 per cent of females always reach orgasm during sex.[54] As I delved deeper into statistical data on sexual behaviour, I discovered that the numbers just didn't add up, and also seemed to be pointing in many different directions. Some showed that Indians were sexually adventurous and satisfied with their sex lives, others seemed to show that Indians (especially women) were stuck in Victorian times. What was especially noteworthy was that we seem confused and contradictory when it comes to having opinions about sex because there is a war between the conservatism of the recent past that is being contested by the rising sexuality of the present and our ancient traditions.

All in all, it would be a good thing if the corset that binds Indian society were to loosen. Sexually liberal societies do not tolerate rape, violence against women, child molestation and sexual harassment. Surprisingly, even conditions like neurotic sexual behaviour and nymphomania have been detected as being more prevalent in conservative societies than sexually permissive ones. At the same time, the spread of HIV/AIDS, the breakdown of the family unit and other societal problems can be features of societies that are more permissive. Striking the right balance is not always easy, and cannot be mandated by the state or by any other authority; it has to evolve over time. The next decade-and-a-half will therefore be critical for Indian society to develop along the right lines as we shall see in subsequent chapters.

KINKY IS QUEER

IN COLD BLOOD

On the night of 14 August 2004, Pushkin Chandra and his boyfriend Kuldeep picked up two men from Connaught Place. The first stop for the motley group was a farewell party for Danish expat Uffe Gartner on his penultimate night in Delhi. Of the quartet, only Pushkin knew Uffe, a colleague of his at the United Nations. The other three young men were 'vernac' or vernacular (in popular gay terminology—men who come from lower-class backgrounds and do not speak English); Kuldeep, unemployed at the moment, was the son of a peon, and the other two were street cruisers with no identifiable source of income who only met Pushkin and Kuldeep when they wanted to have sex. These three men were completely out of place in the posh, expat crowd that Uffe had invited to his party. Pushkin, an empathetic young man of thirty-eight, named after his father's favourite Russian poet, Alexander Pushkin, observing their discomfort, suggested that they leave and go back to his place.

The next morning Pushkin and Kuldeep were found murdered. They were naked, their hands and feet tied with rope, their throats slit. There was blood everywhere. Several of Pushkin's belongings, including his DVD player, mobile phone, handy-cam, camera and cash had been stolen. The motive of the cold-blooded murder, it seemed, was only petty theft.

That night Sid too was at Uffe Gartner's farewell party. He

had been a regular attendee of the Saturday night parties and orgies that Uffe frequently held at his house, and was sad that this friend of his would be leaving India forever. For twenty-four-year-old Sid, who had only recently moved to Delhi from Punjab, Uffe's parties had been a gateway to the good gay life in Delhi. Through Uffe's parties, he had met many of his new friends—the fashionable, chic, gay men of the city whom he idolized.

Pushkin's murder had irrevocable consequences on Sid's life. On the morning of 16 August, as Sid nursed a terrible hangover from two back-to-back nights of partying, his father, the retired principal of a secondary school, entered his room. He held the morning's paper open in front of him.

'Tell me, son, that party that you went to on Saturday night, you said that it was thrown by a Danish friend of yours.'

'Haan, Papa,' grumbled Sid.

'You mentioned his name was something like Uf?'

'Haanji, Papa,' Sid muttered under his breath, wondering about his father's sudden interest in his social life.

'Do you know a man called Pushkin?' his father asked curiously. Now Sid took notice. How could his father know his friend Pushkin?

His father looked expectantly at him.

'Um, yes... Why?'

'Pushkin Chandra was murdered yesterday after he left one Mr Uffe Gartner's gay orgy party,' his father read aloud from the newspaper that he held in front of him like a shield.

Sid's head spun, he could feel all the blood draining from his face. It was a double whammy. Pushkin, his friend, was dead, murdered, and now his authoritarian father knew he was gay.

'The newspaper says that this Uffe Gartner had gay parties every Saturday. You too go out for late nights on Saturday. Why in the world are *you* going to these gay parties?' asked his father with a look of genuine confusion on his face, his chalk-white moustache twitching from side to side, the way it did when he was especially perturbed.

Sid didn't know what to say. He had been meaning to discuss his homosexuality with his parents for over six years, ever since he had discovered he was queer, but he had been unable to muster the courage to do so. Today of all days, what with a terrible hangover, and news of the ghastly murder, no, he could not have this conversation today. The only thing that came to Sid's mind was to run away, as far away as he physically could, from his parents and his house.

As Sid sat on the lawns of Nehru Park, a park that he frequented to pick up men, he wept for his friend Pushkin, bemoaning the death of the exuberant, handsome young man. He remembered the looks that he had exchanged across Uffe's living room with the tall, fair, young man, and the one dance they had shared on a hot Saturday night. As Sid grieved, he heard the joyful moans of men having intercourse in the bushes. He promised himself that from this day on he would always, come what may, remain true to himself.

◆

'I smell homophobia,' whispers Sid in my ear as we sit in a classroom in New Delhi. Sid, who is now a lawyer and human rights activist with the Naz Foundation, an NGO active in fighting for the rights of the gay community, conducts sessions on sexuality for groups across the country. Keeping the promise he had made to himself in the aftermath of Pushkin's death, Sid quit his job at a homophobic corporate law firm in 2008 to join the Naz Foundation in a fight for his rights. Today, he is talking about LGBT rights to a group of sixty district court judges. It is a varied group, some judges appear to be young, some are old, there are a substantial number of women, both old and young.

I have accompanied Sid here as his AV person, and I flip his slides as he speaks passionately about LGBT rights in India. As Sid goes through the slides, I see the stone-faced judges becoming increasingly uncomfortable. Most people refuse to look at the fairly innocuous images on the slides—of two men holding hands, of two men hugging—things that even straight Indian males do plenty of. Sid has moved on to the subject of HIV/AIDS and begins talking about anal sex. At this point, a choleric-looking judge with a fuzzy, dark beard jumps up from his seat.

'You! Shut up! You cannot use terms like that in front of us. We are judges!'

'Sir, are you talking to me?' Sid asks calmly.

'Yes! Of course! How can you talk about this? Don't you know who we are!' says another judge.

'Uh… That is *why* I am talking to you about sexual rights,' Sid says. 'It's important for you to understand. Surely you talk about sex in cases that come to you. Rape, for example. It is part of the dialogue.'

'But rape is something natural! The things you are saying are unnatural and disgusting.'

Now Sid is pissed off. ' Oh, honey…' he mutters, and he continues now in a louder tone, matching the volume of the judge. 'For your information, homosexuality has been decriminalized as per the ruling of the Delhi High Court, and rape is not natural. You, of all people, should know this.'

'You don't know anything, you good-for-nothing-gay,' screams the judge.

I notice several of the women judges hiding their faces behind their dupattas.

'You, sir, can leave this lecture immediately. If any of you feel like this gentleman here, then you are welcome to leave too!' Sid screams back.

At this point, the choleric judge, who was the first to take offence at Sid's presentation, storms out of the room, and a group of his friends quickly shuffle after him.

Sid is clearly shaken by all this. His face has turned grey, and tiny beads of perspiration erupt all over his forehead despite it being cool inside the room. Several of the other participants look unembarrassed by the outburst, they just continue to look at us blankly, as if nothing at all has happened.

◆

Prince Iravan refused to die a virgin. His father, the warrior prince Arjuna, one of the five mighty Pandavas, had been told that if he wished to win the biggest war in the history of humanity, the war of Kurukshetra, he would have to sacrifice his beloved son to the goddess Kali. Iravan would die for honour, as it was his duty and his dharma as a royal prince, but to die a virgin, to have never felt the touch of a woman on his skin—he wasn't prepared to do that. The unhappy prince asked to be married to a virgin bride, but no woman was willing to marry a man doomed to die after just one night. What were the Pandavas to do? As always, when in a quandary, they sought the counsel of the wily cowherd Krishna, their most astute advisor and well-wisher. Krishna used his divine powers to transform himself into a beautiful young woman named Mohini and pleasured Prince Iravan on his last night on earth. Matters took their course, Prince Iravan was beheaded and Krishna, who had taken his virginity, mourned him like a devastated widow.[55]

Hindu mythology is peppered with numerous such stories. Shiva, one of Hinduism's three main deities, is represented as half male and half female in one of his popular avatars—Ardhanarishvara. In the epic *Mahabharata*, the Princess Shikhandi marries another woman. Later, Shikhandi is changed into a man but her marriage to a woman as a woman remains valid, illustrating that a marriage conducted by customary Hindu rites remains valid regardless of gender. In the aristocratic courts of ancient India, eunuchs, or the third race, held an unusual sway over kings and were important and effective advisors in government. The *Kamasutra* too speaks freely and openly about homosexuality.

In Hinduism, non-vaginal sex is not looked upon as evil or

criminal, but merely as a minor taboo, which, like other taboos, may be broken by those with divine powers or by ordinary people under special circumstances. Unlike the homophobia that prevailed in Europe and North America through much of their past, where sodomites were punished by persecution, torture and execution, Indian history offers us no such experiences. Author Devdutt Pattanaik studies homosexuality in ancient India through three different sources: temple walls, sacred narratives, and ancient law books.[56] In the course of his research, Pattanaik finds several erotic images, ranging from dignified same-sex couples exchanging romantic glances to wild orgies involving warriors, sages and courtesans on the walls of Hindu temples. Indian epics and chronicles are replete with references to same-sex intercourse. Most common are stories of gender conversion, of women turning into men and men turning into women. The beautiful temptress Mohini, an incarnation of Vishnu, is so attractive that she has Shiva shedding semen, eventually leading to the creation of mighty gods like Hanuman and Ayyappa.

Hindu law books like *The Laws of Manu* (once again) oppose freewheeling homosexual sex but in a mild way (unlike Christianity which punishes sodomy by death) with penalties like cold-water baths. In the bible, the Book of Leviticus states: 'If a man lies with a male as with a woman, both of them shall be put to death for their abominable deed; they have forfeited their lives'. It establishes the death penalty as the proper punishment for sodomy.[57]

In her two-decade-long research, scholar Ruth Vanita has found that same sex love 'including invisibilized partnerships, visible romances, and rituals such as the exchanging of vows, has flourished in India without any history of punishment'.[58] All ancient sources suggest that there was a distinct place for homosexuality in ancient India. Mughal courts had an accepted queer culture which merged with Hindu culture. Transgenders (hijras) held important positions in the Mughal court, and dominated both the bureaucracy and court hierarchy in Mughal regimes.

Homophobia entered India unofficially through the ecclesiastical route from England and officially through the IPC (Indian Penal Code). Under colonial rule, the minor strain of homophobia in Indian tradition became the dominant ideology. The law prohibiting homosexual sex was set in stone in Section 377 of the IPC in 1860 by Lord Macaulay, notorious for his prudish views on sex. According to Section 377 'whoever voluntarily has carnal intercourse against the order of nature with any man, woman, or animal shall be punished with imprisonment for life, or with imprisonment of either description for term which may extend to ten years, and shall also be liable to a fine'.

Several nineteenth-century Indian social reformers and nationalists left out erotic aspects (particularly of homosexuality) in their translations and publications of literature to pander to British ideals of the time. Homophobia became deeply intertwined with modern nationalism, and many prominent nationalists were against it, forgetting the many references to homosexuality in both Hindu and Muslim traditions. So as the wheels of history turned, despite the liberalism offered to us by our ancient scriptures, homophobic culture become deeply embedded in the Indian mind, becoming most evident in the middle classes who shaped public opinion. Even though the United Kingdom, the principal architect of our modern homophobia, legalized homosexuality between consenting adults in 1967, we continue to cling to homophobic Victorian mores.

Today, as part of the sexual revolution, homosexuality is finally coming into its own in this country. Rainbow-coloured festivals and parades are being organized and thousands of young people in their twenties and early thirties are coming out of the closet. Lesbian groups are budding across the country in second-tier cities like Baroda, Puducherry and Vishakhapatnam. The gay social scene is spreading across the country with professional party-organizers, a flagrant nightclub culture, house parties and social clubs with names like Desi Dykes and Boyzone springing up everywhere.

As author Manil Suri wrote in a poignant piece:

> Ever since the Delhi High Court's 2009 ruling struck down a law instituted under British rule to criminalize homosexual activity, media coverage has been sweeping away decades of invisibility. Not only do participants openly announce their sexuality on the streets, many are comfortable enough to be documented on videos for the web. A recent YouTube posting shows a queer flash mob regale a crowd of onlookers outside Dadar, one of central Mumbai's busiest train stations. *Time Out Mumbai* published an entire issue on the queer community in the city this past January—a month that also saw a book launch for *Out!*, a fiction anthology from 'The New Queer India.[59]

India's Queer Revolution can be attributed to changes in the political, technology, financial and media landscapes.[60] Public discourse on homosexual issues has led to the emergence of gay rights groups across the country that work openly on issues of sexuality, sexual rights and sexual health. The growing movement for awareness and prevention of HIV/AIDS has played an important role in the homosexual discourse and vice versa and organized political activism has led the fight to decriminalize homosexuality.

Technology has given Queer India a place to connect: the internet has been a game-changer, as has the cell phone. Decreased internet and cell phone costs as well as increased coverage mean that more gay people have access to worldwide queer resources as well as numerous websites to locate casual partners. The anonymity offered by the internet and cell phones allows people to create unique identities and lead dual lives. The Indian male can now be a queen on the internet and a king in his homophobic household.

INDIA'S REIGNING QUEEN

'It's a crazy world out there, and you can get anything. Name it, and you have it. There are su-su ranis [golden shower queens or those who like to urinate on you or vice versa], chutney ranis [ass lickers], dhakka starts [guys who like receptive anal sex] and muscle marys [gym boys for hire]. The nautanki-ranis command big prices [they dress up as brides and you are supposed to rape them]. There are policeman for hire [ghodis] and special married men [pao-bhatas and double-deckers] who want you in bed with their wives by their side!' explains Ashok Row Kavi, the first man to talk openly about homosexuality and gay rights in the country, and founder of Humsafar, a male sexual health NGO and editor of India's first gay magazine, *Bombay Dost*.

He continues, 'The smaller the town, the bigger the circuit they seem to have. I remember going to Jaipur where the reigning queen got a salute from every cop at each traffic signal we whizzed past. It's wilder in the cow belt. Once I was in Vrindavan, the abode of Lord Krishna, and I spent the entire time fucking men, and it was all done in the spirit of free love. In Moradabad, a whole dharamshala was used for an orgy and some holy soul tipped off the police who came and joined in, and then arrested the poor guys!'

Ashok believes that that the cheap and wide access to internet and cell phones is really the impetus behind the queer revolution in India. He offers further details: 'The Internet has changed everything...yes, everything. So has the mobile. You go on PlanetRomeo, and there are around 90,000 men cruising at any one time in India on the net. Of these, 9,000 are from Bombay alone—*every single day.* Everybody has a bogus name, and suddenly I've discovered that older men are at a premium,' says the sixty-five-year-old with a naughty grin.

'I've seen young college guys in Cafe Coffee Day cruising on the net, hooking up, rushing out to meet their "contacts", getting into the car and returning within forty-five minutes,' says Ashok.

It is impossible to separate the issues of HIV/AIDS and homosexuality. HIV/AIDS has provided a platform on which to fight for sexual rights, and a way for activists to garner the support of governments and international organizations. Ashok has been a pioneer of the movement for the prevention and control of HIV/AIDS and was part of a technical group reviewing numbers and budgets for the Indian government's AIDS control arm. I ask him about the current situation.

According to recently published government figures there are an estimated 2.5 million gay men in India, of whom 7 per cent are infected with HIV. Speaking about these numbers, Ashok is visibly angry; he insists these numbers were cherry-picked by the government. He spits out his words, 'All we have done is reduce the number so that the government could work with the budgets. We first gave a number using the Asian figure of 5 per cent of the sexually active male population being homosexual but when I presented these numbers, the Director-General of NACO (National AIDS Control Organization), shouted at me: "Go back to the drawing board." Apparently, it was felt that the number being mentioned was too low.'

'Off I slunk back to my office room and looked at the number of gay men on public sex sites seeking sex. Even that figure was too high, so we came up with new numbers. That was the 2.5 million, which is now in every NACO record.'

According to Ashok, the HIV/AIDS situation in India is pretty dire today, though the government projects things to be under control. 'Most gay men refuse to use condoms. Over 50 per cent of the men on sex sites are married to women and more than 35 per cent don't even have a sense of identity as gay men [they just fuck men because they love it]. They have sex with women because they want to 'prove' their masculinity. Just imagine the bridge population infecting women.'

Ashok believes that the crux of the Indian sexual problem lies in the male psyche. And, if we were to study this all-powerful psyche, then a lot of our problems could be solved. He says, 'There is a huge dysfunction in the male psyche in India—the sexual repression is shocking. I've seen men masturbating in cinema halls openly during the item numbers that come on screen. Like giant prisons, there is practically an "enforced homosexual behaviour" syndrome at work here, as there are not enough females to go around.

'The problem is that nobody understands the male psyche, and no one has tried. The truth is that men will do *anything* for the pleasure principle. I remember one gorgeous guy who expected me to urinate on him while he masturbated, so I asked: "What's in it for me?" And the bugger went blank. So I left him there in the bar like a dead dodo!'

◆

On a perfect spring day in March of 1994, volunteers from the ABVA (AIDS Bhedbhav Virodhi Andolan, or the AIDS anti-discrimination movement) showed up at the gates of Tihar Jail to distribute condoms to male prisoners. There had been an inordinate number of HIV-positive cases reported amongst the male inmates, and ABVA thought it necessary to take action. The Delhi police did not allow the ABVA activists entry into the prison, stating that the jails were gender segregated, and that by allowing condom distribution, they were abetting an act made criminal by Section 377 of the Indian Penal Code. The enraged ABVA filed a petition in the High Court of New Delhi challenging the antiquated 377, pointing out that it blatantly violated constitutional rights of life, liberty and non-discrimination.

As is usual with courts in the country, the case filed by the organization was delayed for many years. It finally came up for hearing seven years after it was filed in 2001, when it was dismissed because representatives of ABVA (a poorly financed organization run by volunteers) were unaware of the court date and did not show up for the hearing. At the same time, cases of police harassment against homosexual people had been increasing in cities across the country. Two incidents in July 2001, commonly known as the 'Lucknow Incidents'—a set of raids on a public park frequented by gay men, and on the offices of two NGOs working on safe sex issues—made it necessary to take action. This was when the Naz Foundation (India) Trust led by Anjali Gopalan got involved and along with the Lawyers Collective filed a public litigation case in the Delhi High Court in late 2001.

Several prominent personalities who supported homosexuality, like author Vikram Seth, academic Saleem Kidwai, actors Rahul Bose and Pooja Bhatt, and ex-Miss India Celina Jaitly, supported the petition by signing a document titled 'Voices against 377'. The petition became a movement and for the first time in the history of modern India, the LGBT community and their supporters came together to fight for the revoking of Section 377. The public litigation argued that Section 377 had a deleterious effect on HIV/AIDS, a disease that was spiralling out of control across the country, with some Indian experts estimating that between twenty and fifty million Indians were infected with the disease.[61]

After seven long years of trials and tribulation, and much deliberation, the case finally came up for hearing in 2009. In a historic judgment delivered on 2 July 2009, the Delhi High Court overturned the 150-year-old Section 377, and consensual homosexual activities amongst adults were declared legal. In a brave judgment, a bench of Chief Justice Ajit Prakash Shah and Justice S. Muralidhar declared that if not amended, Section 377 would violate Article 14 of the Constitution, which states that every citizen has equal opportunity of life and is equal before law.

Although the prime minister extended his support to the judgment, an astounding nineteen petitions were filed by religious, political and conservative groups in the Supreme Court of India, stating that homosexuality was a Western import and sullied Indian culture. Unfortunately the Bombay High Court ruling was overturned by a two-judge bench of the Supreme Court towards the end of 2013. The Supreme Court judgement was greeted with outrage across the country, with the government filing a review petition against the Supreme Court's decision. The fight carries on, and the encouraging thing about the whole sorry affair is the scale of support the gay community has received from many sections of Indian society.

'WE ARE LIKE THAT ONLY'

I am sitting in a terrace garden as lush and verdant as a rain forest, nestled between three multi-coloured stray dogs and a pint-sized tabby, all of whom live amicably in this small home along with their owner. As the director of the Naz Foundation, Anjali Gopalan has dedicated a decade of her life to fighting for homosexual rights, and is the country's most prominent voice for gay rights and for the repeal of Section 377. Anjali is a stout, unassuming woman with a hard, angry face, and a brush of short, grey curly hair, who doesn't like to talk about herself. I have had to chase her for months simply to have a conversation, but after her initial wariness, she has proved to be quite accommodating (she is especially happy to talk about her garden and her dogs).

Anjali and I walk over to the Naz Foundation care home for HIV-positive children which she runs. The home is a small, tidy building with thirty beds. The kids love Anjali and crowd around her when she arrives, tugging at the bottom of her kurta, clinging to her legs, others raising their arms, asking to be held. Anjali is radiant, glowing with delight.

'Children have a way of changing your life. People used to tell me, "You are single. What will happen when you are older?" I am one of those women who went from being a single woman to having an incredible extended family. How many can say that?' she says with a smile.

In 2000, when Naz was still operating out of Anjali's home, a four-year-old male child was left at her doorstep. He was HIV-positive, both his parents had died of AIDS, and he had a brother who was HIV-negative who had been adopted by an uncle. No orphanage would have this child, so Anjali had no choice but to take him in. 'I thought it was common sense to take care of someone. As time went on, we got more children. I was getting into trouble. People told me to stick to advocacy, not to run institutions. I would ask them, "Why not? We were changing the system, but what were we doing for those who needed the system the most?" People told me, "What's the point? How long will they live?"'

She introduces me to a well-dressed young man who seems to be in charge. He comes up to her, touches her feet, and then hugs her. 'This is our oldest, the four-year-old who was left on our doorstep. I feel bad for those people who abandoned him. Those people who never called even once to see how he was doing. If only they saw him today, what regrets they would have,' she says proudly.

As we walk around the care home, from bed to bed, Anjali introduces me to each child, from toddlers all the way to teenagers. She talks to me about the sexual health training that she does across the country, and the gamut of problems that she sees mostly because of lack of education and narrow-minded thinking that people disguise as 'culture'.

'People say that India has a culture, and that we must protect it. But having a rich culture comes with a shitload of problems. We are in transition, a state of flux, and a state of molten confusion. Despite all the years that I have been doing work in sexuality and HIV/AIDS, people still take my breath away with their crappy, narrow-minded thinking. *"We are like that only,"* they say to me, refusing to change and accept, and that explains everything, at least to me.'

'I AM WHO I AM'

Sree realized that she was lesbian the day she got married. Though she tried to consummate her marriage, lying naked next to her husband night after night, she could not have sex with him.

Sree tried stripping down to the clean cotton underwear that her mother had bought for her to wear after her marriage. He stroked her breasts and fingered her, which she somewhat enjoyed, but the minute he brought his penis (an organ which she thought was the ugliest part of the human body) close to her, she felt disgusted and moved away. She had told Prakash that she enjoyed oral sex, that she wanted him to perform cunnilingus, but he had looked at her in disgust and told her that he would never do that to a woman. He had asked her politely at first, and aggressively later, as if it were his right, that she perform fellatio on him. But the thought of bringing that demonic organ anywhere close to her mouth made Sree want to throw up. The thought of having sex with a man was repulsive to her. On the other hand, her husband Prakash had only sex on his mind. At twenty-five, he had never had sex before and badly wanted to—this was one of the main reasons that he had agreed to a speedy marriage with Sree, though he didn't find her particularly attractive.

After a few months of trying, they both gave up. Prakash went back to masturbating daily and Sree resorted to conjuring memories of the best moments of her life—when she had shared her dormitory bed with her first love, and how they had together achieved the greatest pleasure that she had ever felt in her life. Attractive and energetic, Sree has short, cropped hair styled into spikes and a large OM tattoo on her athletic arms. Kalashree (Sree) Suwarnkar was born in 1984, the same year as me, in interior Maharashtra in Latur, and brought up as most girls in traditional, middle-class families in small-town India are—with idealistic notions that marriage and fidelity are the most important parts of a woman's life.

Growing up, Sree found herself attracted to women. Much to the wrath of her mother, she was a tomboy, refusing to grow her hair long, preferring to wear shorts, pants and jeans as opposed to long-skirts or salwaar-kameez. Even as a young girl

Sree masturbated regularly to images of women—actresses, female cousins, girlfriends—visualizing them dancing to the Bollywood tunes that she loved.

Sree was a happy-go-lucky girl who hated studying and remained a mediocre student throughout school and college. She much preferred the extracurricular and sports activities that were on offer, which she was better at than the boys. She began her first sexual relationship in college in Pune with her best friend. At that time, she didn't know that she was lesbian, or even what being lesbian meant. All she understood at that age was that it was natural and enjoyable to pleasure her best friend.

Her parents began looking for a suitable match for Sree the day she turned twenty-one. The thought of marriage to a man seemed unattractive and unnatural, yet it felt even more unnatural not to follow her parents' instructions, so she agreed to marry Prakash, a twenty-five-year-old man from her Maratha community with an M Tech degree and a job at an engineering firm in Bangalore.

It was only after a year of marriage, when Prakash and she had already separated, that she began to explore her sexuality again. Encouraged by the new sexual confidence that the internet lent her, Sree became increasingly bold. She was thrilled to find that there were other women like her, and she joined the online community to chat with single women looking for relationships. She watched lesbian porn, found a lesbian group in Bangalore she attended meetings with, and even had a few online sexual encounters with women.

Two years after they got married, Prakash and Sree filed for divorce. Sree then moved to Nasik, where she lives a single, independent life working at a battery factory as a technical manager. Sree speaks to me candidly about her failed marriage.

'I tried to convince my parents about my divorce, but they did not listen to me at all. They told me to fulfil my marital duties, to force myself to have sex with Prakash. My parents were worried, especially because both my brothers weren't married, and they thought that if I got divorced it would ruin my brothers' chances.' Rather than being deterred by the negative reaction of her parents, Sree was convinced that she must remain loyal to herself and to her sexuality, so she applied for a divorce without the consent of her parents.

'Those were the most difficult days of my life; my parents were just not willing to listen to me. A lot of situations arose in which suicidal thoughts were in my mind,' says Sree grimly.

'My parents want me to have long hair and to wear salwaar-kameez. I don't like to do things like this. Main jo hoon, main hoon (I am who I am),' says Sree with a look of conviction in her eyes.

Sree talks to me about her current relationship with Sapna. Sree met Sapna online, they chatted online for a few weeks, and then started talking on the phone. After two months, Sree went to Pune to meet her.

'We met at a McDonald's in the mall and we got along so well that we went for dinner. The hotel where we went for dinner had a disco, and we danced all night. How we danced that night, it was amazing,' she says remembering the night wistfully.

She tells me shyly, twirling a golden band with a tiny diamond that she wears on her finger, that she has recently gotten engaged to Sapna. She hopes to move to Bombay to live with her as soon as she finds a new job.

Sapna comes from a middle-class family and works in interior design. She is out to her parents and family. I ask Sree how Sapna's experience of being open has been.

She shrugs. 'She is the oldest daughter, and supports her family. She even pays for her sister's education. Also, they love me a lot, so maybe that is why the experience has been good,' she adds with a laugh.

She recalls the time when Sapna's sister was in the hospital and Sree went and spent days by her side, like any good family member would do. At the end of it, Sapna's parents told her 'Sree is our jamai' and that to Sree was the kindest thing she had ever heard.

Sree shows me pictures of her engagement party in Pune where she exchanged rings with Sapna. Sree wears a tank top, and has large tattoos on both arms. She is sitting on a motorbike, and Sapna, a fair, dewy-faced girl with long dark hair, sits behind her wearing a pair of jeans and a petal-pink kurta. Friends crowd around them—cheerful, happy, accepting young men and women.

'Main jo hoon, main hoon' is Sree's mantra. Perhaps the biggest blow to a patriarchal society is when a woman makes sexual choices for herself, not just choosing her own partner, but also the *gender* of that partner.

Sree is a cultural rebel, an agent for sexual autonomy and social change, who, in the face of overwhelming opposition and intractable circumstances, has begun to fight to realize her dreams. It is heartening to see the change, and though the battle is a long way from being finished, at least it has finally begun.

SANGINI, MY LIFE PARTNER

The small apartment that Sangini is run out of is crowded with people and animals. The primary residents are two lesbian women, Maya and Bitoo, and their pets—two mongrel dogs and a small turtle that sits placidly in a corner taking stabs at a wrinkled piece of bhindi, occasionally nudged at by the dogs. There is also a small army of all-male support staff who look after the house and do admin work for Sangini. Lastly, there is the recent stowaway: a shy, pretty young girl, who looks not a day over twenty-one. This apartment is used for a variety of different purposes: as a home for Maya and Bitoo, as a kitchen for the small catering business that Maya has started, and most importantly, as the headquarters for Sangini, India's most prominent lesbian group, run as a part of Anjali Gopalan's Naz Foundation. More inconspicuously, it is a shelter for lesbian women who have run away from repressive conditions at home.

'The biggest change that I have seen over the past few years, especially since the [Delhi High Court] judgement on 377, is that women are coming out so much younger. A decade ago, if women came out at all, it would be in their forties, after marriage and kids. Not anymore. Now most women who come to us are in their twenties,' says Maya, as we talk in her cheerful, crowded living room. She is a counsellor, listening to the hundreds of women who need someone to speak to and occasionally she helps women who have mustered up the courage to run away to find a new place in the world.

I immediately think back to the other Maya I'd spoken to a little earlier. Maya Sharma is a prominent lesbian activist in India who runs Vikalp—an LGBT organization based out of Gujarat. Maya told me how she had married and borne a son because she thought it would give her maturity and respect. Maya came from an educated middle-class family and it was impossible for her to imagine breaking away from her family, for where else could she go? How could she survive? It was only later, at forty, when she starting working, first as a paid volunteer in a women's organization, and later in labour unions that she found the courage to leave her husband, and come out about her homosexuality. 'Why are Indian women coming out at a younger age today?' I ask Maya.

'Women are becoming financially independent and more confident about leading their lives on their own terms. The internet has given them access to information about groups like us who are out there to support them.' She adds with a chuckle, 'Also, finally, Indian women are just not ready to take shit anymore.'

I spot Sangini's latest stowaway in the hallway. She is fashionably dressed in a pair of tight jeans and a figure-hugging polo t-shirt with a pair of matching, long, dangly earrings. She is organizing all her things into a gigantic pink suitcase. Another equally large suitcase lies unopened next to it. From the number of things this young lady has with her, it looks she is planning to be away for a long time.

'Women decide to run when their families begin to put unprecedented pressure on them to get married,' Maya says. This is when they contact Sangini. The first thing that Sangini does when someone wants to run away is try to resolve differences with their families. If discussions break down, then they plan the escape. The fugitive-to-be begins to send her belongings in small instalments to the Sangini headquarters (this apartment), so that she can travel light on the big day. Calls are avoided because they can be traced, and only email is used. Bank accounts are slowly emptied out so that the fugitive's location cannot be traced through bank transactions. Sangini also helps the runaway with her job search because financial independence from parents is critical to the success of the escape. The lesbian network in India, though nascent, is getting more organized and better able to help those who seek it out. The number of lesbian organizations is growing as the number of women joining these organizations is increasing. There are LGBT groups present in Mumbai, Kolkata, Bangalore and Baroda (amongst many others) and these groups often coordinate with each other to form a cohesive network of assistance. Most importantly, more Indian women are working and financially independent, and this makes it possible for them to think of a life outside a traditional heterosexual marriage.

As I leave, I see the fugitive sitting at the dining table, her arms folded tightly, and her head down. She is crying softly. Even though I don't know who she is, where she is from, or what her problems are, I feel for her. It takes a lot of courage for an Indian woman to run away from home. I remember my only attempt of running away when I was visiting my parents after my first year of college. After the short stint of independence at Wellesley, I had felt oppressed in my parents' home in small-town India, and after a particularly trying fight, I had decided to leave. Though I had planned my midnight escape meticulously, I only got 100 kilometres away in a shared taxi before two carloads of family members found me and brought me back home. I still remember how scared, terrified and alone I had felt during those six hours of flight. When they found me crouching in a car, a part of me had never been more relieved. When I got home to the screaming and scolding, there had been hugs, kisses and waterworks of joy.

I wished there was something I could do to help this runaway, but I knew that Maya wanted to conceal her identity until her situation was resolved. I want to tell her that after the long, difficult battle is fought, there will be beautiful moments of freedom, happiness and love, and that she too will be found.

THE QUEER REVOLUTION

In his hometown of Phaltan (100 kilometres from Pune; population of about 53,000), Kapil Ranaware is a local celebrity. He is the first boy in the history of the town to clear the IIT-JEE, perhaps the most difficult college entrance exam in the world, which 500,000 students take every year. Every mother in Phaltan wants her son to be like Kapil. They all send their sons to the same schools, the same tutors, and even the same temples where Kapil is rumoured to have prayed. But Kapil has a dirty little secret that he is desperate to tell, but may never be able to share with his family. He is gay.

Kapil did not know that he was gay, or even what homosexuality was till he was fifteen years old. It was only after the tenth standard, when he moved to Pune to begin the strict two-year training for the IIT-JEE exam, and stumbled upon gay porn on the internet, that Kapil realized that he liked men. He always knew that he was different from the other boys. He was teased for being effeminate, for laughing differently, for walking differently, and he had never understood what the big deal about girls was. Now he was beginning to realize why.

Ultimately, Bollywood showed Kapil the way. *Dostana,* a 2008 blockbuster film featuring actors Abhishek Bachchan and John Abraham, brought the topic of homosexuality into the mainstream.

Millions of families across the country watched this film together, many understanding for the first time what being gay was. In the film, the two actors pretend to be gay so they can share a flat with a girl. While watching the film, Kapil noticed that he was wildly attracted to the hunky John Abraham. He also found nothing amusing about two men loving each other. His friends, on the other hand, made fun of the gay men and ogled the actress Priyanka Chopra. Kapil seriously began questioning his sexuality, and scoured the internet for any information that he could find.

Kapil studied hard, landing a 2,000 rank amongst the 500,000 students who took the IIT-JEE exam, securing a seat in the biotechnology department at IIT Delhi. Kapil loved IIT Delhi: it was like an all-boys' school (the sex ratio at a typical IIT is ten boys to a girl) and he saw many cute boys that he immediately liked and wondered why his fellow students complained about the lack of women. Here at college, Kapil had the freedom to explore his sexuality. He had free internet, his own mobile phone, and he was far away from the clutches of his parents' morality.

Social media presented a turning point for Kapil. The internet gave him access, and Facebook gave him a new identity: he could be anyone, anywhere, at any time. He cruised freely online—miles, even countries away, for information and for men—which gave him access to unlimited sexual partners, from Delhi to Pune and much to his surprise, Phaltan.

The first time was painful for Kapil. It was during his second month at IIT, he was seventeen, and his lover, twenty-three. He found him on Facebook, and the only criteria for Kapil was that his lover have a place to have sex, and that he wasn't far away. Though Kapil didn't enjoy the sex, he was interminably relieved that there were others out there like him, that he was not 'defective' or have a 'disease' as some blogs had indicated.

Kapil kept the gay part of his life secret, operating through fake Facebook accounts. He discovered that there were all sorts of gay people—old, young, and many who were married to women.

A fellow cruiser introduced him to PlanetRomeo; this website transformed the way he cruised online, opening up a new host of opportunities. On PlanetRomeo he could search for men by location, he could see their pictures, their likes, dislikes, and even their preferred sexual positions.

Over the two years that Kapil has been at IIT, he has begun to enjoy his furtive, often vigorous sexual encounters. He seeks out men in his own age group, preferably students who live close to the IIT campus. Not much conversation is had during the encounters, and often condoms are not used. Kapil has never had a desire to meet any of the men again, or to pursue a romantic relationship, except once, when Cupid struck.

Kapil met the man whom he called Robby on PlanetRomeo. Instead of having sex, Robby and Kapil spoke all night, falling asleep naked, holding each other. They kept in touch online until Kapil declared to Robby that he loved him, and wanted to be in a relationship. But Robby didn't want a boyfriend. He was going to get married soon to a woman that his parents had arranged his marriage to, though he would continue to have sexual encounters with other men.

Kapil's first love hit him hard, like first love often does, and he started thinking carefully about his future. He knew that he wasn't a liar like Robby; he would never get married to a woman when he loved a man. He had to be true to himself, and to do this he would have to tell the world that he was gay.

Kapil's most striking features are his eyes—round as saucers, with a permanent, almost ghoulish, blank look. He has craggy yellow teeth, with two canines that jut out like fangs from the sides of his mouth. His hair is cut short, and he has grown the fingernails of his pinkie fingers an inch-and-a-half long. Most of the time that we talk he looks blank, but occasionally he breaks into a squeaky sigh, or a laugh, transforming his face from a ghoul's into a happy elf's.

I met Kapil through a focus group that I conducted on the

IIT campus to discuss love, sex and relationships with students. My first question to the group had been, 'Who here wants to be in a relationship?' Every hand had shot up. I asked why and the answers were varied—someone to talk to, emotional support, someone to have fun with. A boy sitting in the front row who had been listening intently raised his arm, and told me in broken, heavily accented English, 'I want to be in a relationship, but not with a girl, but with a boy, because I'm a gay.' I was taken aback, this wasn't something that I had expected. At the end of my session, I asked the students, casually and cautiously, expecting at least a few positive answers—how many of them had had sex? Out of all the students in the room, only one had raised his hand confidently. It was Kapil, the boy in the front row.

I began visiting Kapil frequently at the IIT campus at night, when he had finished with his classes. We would sit at a small tea-stall that stayed open all night, eating Maggi noodles and drinking sweet tea from the machine. Of the 5,000 students at IIT Delhi, Kapil was the only openly gay person, though he told me that he know of more than 200 gay men on campus, courtesy social media, and he suspected that there were several hundred more. He had a few friends in the gay community at IIT, but most of the time they ignored him because they didn't want anyone to suspect their 'wayward' sexual orientation.

Kapil came out five months before I met him by posting a message on Facebook, which read:

> 'Thought a lot about it, nearly 20 days and nights full of introspection and it was hard to accept myself the way I was especially because of the homophobia around. But finally I accept and tell the world that I am a GAY! People like Ashok Row Kavi are inspiration for me and why should I feel ashamed of myself when homosexuality has been there since ages plz note this is NOT hacked status.'

Despite his cautionary footnote, Kapil's friends flooded his hostel room, telling him that his Facebook account had been hacked, and that the hacker had proclaimed him 'a gay'.

'I told them that I was the one who posted it, and that I was really a gay,' Kapil said one evening as we sat chatting at the tea-stall.

'And how did they react?' I asked.

'Initially they were shocked, but when they realized that I was serious, they became curious. The first question that people asked me was "Do you find me attractive?" They asked me how sex was, how we had sex, how I felt after sex, and what positions I liked.' Sex was clearly on their mind—with man or woman.

Much to Kapil's pleasant surprise, his coming out process had been smooth. His friends at IIT, in Pune, and even in Phaltan have accepted him, telling him that his being gay was no big deal. 'I realized that everyone was cool about it. No one mocked me, no one laughed at me. I was totally shocked, I thought it would be *much* worse,' Kapil said with an elfin smile.

Kapil's acceptance amongst his peers is no exception to the norm. Of the 5,369 men and women surveyed by a magazine in 2010, 17 per cent approved of homosexuality[62]—a figure that increased from the magazine's previous survey in 2000. This may seem low, but in a country that has previously been fiercely homophobic, it is a positive step. Perhaps what is more telling, however, are my conversations with young people across India. There has been a distinct generational shift—partly due to more gay people coming out as a result of decriminalization of homosexuality in 2009—and as straight people see gays leading positive lives, people appear to have become more tolerant. Fifteen years ago, anything even alluding to homosexuality was highly taboo, and was kept hushed. It is only recently, with the growth of a robust, liberal media and the advent of technology that the gay movement has found a voice and an entire generation is growing up with more liberal views than before.

Understandably, the biggest opponents to Kapil's homosexuality are his parents. He wants to tell them, but he is not sure if they will understand, and if so, how they will react. His mother doesn't even know what the word gay means. The only person that he has told in his family is his sister. Kapil doubts that she takes him seriously. He tells me that his sister understands because she has had an inter-caste love marriage, but she also does not know much about homosexuality, and she hopes that Kapil's sexual orientation will change. I notice that this is a common reaction of the older generation that Sree and Kapil's parents belong to.

'I thought that I would come out to my parents. I wrote a letter, I rehearsed everything. I decided that I would call them so many times, but then at the last minute I chicken out. I just don't have the guts,' says Kapil.

'Maybe they'll understand, like your friends did,' I tell him optimistically. 'At best, they may just feign ignorance.'

'No, Ira ma'am, I don't think so. There is so much societal pressure, especially from relatives. We live in Phaltan, and I am a Maratha. We are proud people. Maybe I'll tell them when they put pressure on me to get married or when I find someone that I love.'

As Kapil speaks, a perspicacious passage from my friend Anita Jain's memoir, *Marrying Anita: A Quest for Love in the New India*, comes to mind: 'In the West, people are obsessed with sex, so they focus on what sexual acts are committed in homosexual relationships. In India, the focus is marriage, and society is more concerned with maintaining the family structure and less with what is being done in the bedroom. I've heard some gay men tell me that their parents don't care what they do or with whom as long as they end up getting married.'

Homosexuality in India is accepted as long as it does not interfere with reproduction and the family process. Sex and marriage seem to be disconnected—so as long as the son marries and has children, he can do whatever he wants in the bedroom. As long as homosexuality is 'masti' or fun, it is okay, but the minute it becomes an identity—like it is slowly becoming for Kapil—then it becomes a problem.

It was late now, almost 2 a.m., and Kapil and I were the only ones left at the tea-shop. There were still some students hanging around outside their hostels, mostly groups of boys. We walked past a male trio who snickered when they saw us. Kapil increased his pace and I almost had to run to keep up with him. He was staring down at the road and was suddenly quiet. I asked him if something was the matter.

'One of those guys is a gay. I think he is cute, and he likes me too, but he doesn't want to hang around with me because I am open. He makes fun of me so that people don't think that *he* is a gay,' he said to me in a whisper, peering over his shoulder to make sure the boys were distance away.

He added wistfully, 'Ira ma'am, sometimes, I feel really alone. I am bored of all this sex stuff, and I wish that I could have a boyfriend like you.'

PEGS AND PINTS

On a Tuesday night in Delhi, the party is at Pegs and Pints. On the dance floor the men dance fervently, violently, khuley aam, to the music. Outside, it is a Delhi winter night, cold and foggy, but inside the temperature is soaring. There are a lot of bodies and a lot of heat. Men grind pelvis-to-pelvis, dry hump, and make out on the dance floor, fumbling with each other's privates.

The bar is small and packed with men—most are dancing, while others stand on the margins of the dance floor carefully scoping out the crowd for men they can take home. There are a few flamboyantly dressed transvestites and only a handful of women. Any place in New Delhi that is packed with men at midnight, especially where alcohol is flowing, a woman has numerous reasons to flee immediately, but here I feel strangely safe. I gleefully notice that not a single man is staring, looking, or even paying attention to me.

Kapil and I have come to gay night at Pegs and Pints with a mission to land a boyfriend for Kapil. At least that *was* the plan. On the dance floor, Kapil is a beast. He is a fluid and nimble dancer, and he hops, skips and gyrates confidently to the music, though in curious juxtaposition, his face and saucer eyes remain as expressionless as always. I am amazed at what a good dancer he is and how confidently and unselfconsciously he is dancing—all by himself. He doesn't seem interested in meeting anyone. The music here is great, a mix of English pop and Bollywood tunes, though the latter are clearly the rage. When the DJ plays Bollywood music, the dance floor goes crazy, and it is almost a little dangerous to be on it with all the flailing arms and legs. Kapil knows all the words to the songs, both English and Hindi, and he mouths them as he dances. I join Kapil on the dance floor. At first I dance cautiously, I am the only woman on a floor full of men, but then I too let my hair down and dance exuberantly to the music. I can't remember the last time I danced like this.

'I would be careful if I were you,' says a slinky man with a lizard-like face pointing his cigarette towards me. 'Many of these men are bisexual, and someone may jump on you. They can get violent here, that time of night is approaching.'

The man who is being so solicitous is Manish, the queen of the club. He organizes weekly gay nights at clubs around Delhi. Though Delhi's gay scene is getting hot now, Manish tells me that the *real* party had been in Bombay, the nucleus of India's gay scene. Manish remembers that time fondly. The first gay nightclub to hit the scene in the mid-1990s was Voodoo, a discotheque in South Bombay where Manish lost his virginity behind the bar when he was seventeen years old. Manish tells me with stars in his eyes about the legendary 'White Party' that he attended. According to Manish, the White Party, thrown by a Bombay industrialist, was even larger than a big Indian wedding, and featured a troupe of handsome foreign male strippers and barmen flown down from various parts of the world. Unfortunately the police raided the party and arrested most people there; Manish spent a night in jail, though he adds wistfully that jail time was worth that party. It is Manish's dream to organize an event as large as the White Party, and when homosexuality was decriminalized that might have been a distinct possibility but now things have started looking uncertain again.

I think back to Suri's article on being gay in India:

> The Bombay I grew up in during the 60s and 70s was quite incontestably unenlightened. Homosexuality was not mentioned, it didn't exist. I never once met anyone I knew to be gay. The only media input I remember was a single article in a women's magazine during my college years talking vaguely about far-away beaches where men supposedly found each other.[63]

At 3 a.m., I yank Kapil off the dance floor. It is time to go home. He has been dancing non-stop, unabashed and drenched with sweat, for four hours. In the car on the ride home, Kapil has stars in his eyes as he continues to hum the songs he has heard all night.

'Kapil, I'm sorry you didn't meet anyone,' I say to him apologetically. Finding a boyfriend for Kapil had been our original plan.

'No, Ira ma'am, why are you sorry? It was my first time in a disco, and it has been the best night of my whole life.'

◆

Kapil and I do not have the same taste in men. He likes thin, fair-skinned, nerdy men; I like dark, handsome, rakish bad boys. Kapil is probably wiser in this department. Kapil and I check out men at the 5th Annual Queer Pride Parade in Delhi. It is the first parade that Kapil has attended since coming out, and he has tied a rainbow scarf around his neck to show off his gay identity. He attended the parade last year, but with a mask on his face, afraid of being exposed. I too was at the parade last year for no other reason than that it was the biggest street party that Delhi had ever seen. I notice that this year there are fewer people shrouding their faces with colourful masks than last year. People are proudly preening their rainbow pride with banners, placards, hats, socks and scarves. The marchers are mostly men, but I see a fair number of women and small groups of flamboyantly dressed, attractive transsexuals showing off their perfectly muscled legs in tiny skirts.

The parade moves at snail's pace, like an Indian marriage baraat, stopping every few minutes to dance exuberantly to the drums of the dhol-wallahs who accompany the marchers. Kapil, too, dances along with the drums, fluttering his scarf in the air. The afternoon winter sun is harsh, and people crowd underneath rainbow umbrellas. People are proudly holding up placards that they have made: *'Be straight not narrow'*, *'Love is the law'*, *'Gay is Happy'* and the like. *'Meri chhatri ke neeche aja'* says one, held by a man underneath a rainbow umbrella. Others are more direct: *'If you want a straight son-in-law, support us'*. Another one held by a voluptuous transsexual, reads *'Kinky is queer'*. I, too, have made a placard, *'India in Love'* in rainbow colours, which Kapil and I hold together. Joints are being passed around, and everyone partakes in the fun.

After three hours of dancing and drumming, the parade finally ends, and the crowd slowly disperses for a picnic on the lawns of India Gate, a popular picnic spot where hundreds of people—families, couples and young lovers alike bask on the lawns. As Kapil and I walk towards the rainbow-coloured banner in the distance, Kapil tells me that he recently met the Director of IIT Delhi about starting an official LGBT club on the campus.

'What did the Director say?' I ask.

'He didn't know what LGBT meant. He thought that I was referring to a chemistry experiment,' says Kapil with an embarrassed look.

'Did you explain it to him?' I asked Kapil.

'I did. I told him that I was gay, but he seemed confused. I am doubtful that he understands anything.'

I wonder how it is possible that people could live in such utter ignorance. But then again, many of the Director's generation (and unfortunately many in this one too) are trained to reflexively block out anything that refers to sex—imagine that, in a 5,000-student-strong college in the middle of the city.

As the crowds swell at the gay parade picnic site hawkers flock the lawns. I see a group of hijra beggars amongst them, trying to finagle money from the crowd, as is their practice. The group approaches us, and they start grabbing at my bag. They tell me they will pray for a good husband for me if I give them some money. They see that I won't relent, so they target Kapil.

'We hope that you marry a beautiful girl, that your studies are good, and you stand first. Please give us some money,' they implore.

Kapil looks mortified and quickly runs away.

I ask one of the hijras if she knows why the picnic is being held.

She does not.

I try to explain to the group that this is a gay pride picnic, and that we are fighting for sexual rights, including theirs.

They stare at me utterly confused, and then one dressed in a colourful sari caked with dirt, puts her hands on her hips and asks me in a throaty voice, 'Are you giving us money or no?'

I really don't know what to say to them anymore, so I hand them ₹10 and walk away to locate Kapil.

The crowd at the picnic is mostly young. It is a sea of young faces, the average age probably being twenty-five. We sit amidst picnicking families and are accepted by everyone without the blink of an eyelid.

Kapil interrupts my thoughts, 'Ira ma'am, I told my mother I am gay.'

'Wow! Congrats, Kapil! That's a pretty big deal... what did she say?'

'Well, I told her I was gay...and then I told her I was kidding,' he says, blushing. 'I was just testing to see if she knew the meaning of gay.'

'Oh. Did she?' I ask curiously.

'Yes, she did. I was happy about that,' says Kapil.

'How did she react to the joke?' I ask.

Kapil looks at me sheepishly. 'She told me she is getting me married off as soon as I finish IIT.'

I am not surprised at the reaction. Kapil's stock in the marriage market is up considerably because of his IIT degree. The truth is that gays in India still find many reasons to remain closeted. There are no gay icons, no major Bollywood stars who have come out, no influential CEOs who have made their orientation public. The vast majority of gay men still get married: 70 per cent in Mumbai, 82 per cent in smaller cities, according to a 2009 survey by the Humsafar Trust[64].

'Never mind, Kapil. One day it will be the right day to tell her, and on that day, you will,' I say to him.

PIMPS AND HOES

'IT'S BEEN BUSINESS DOING PLEASURE WITH YOU'

It is the beginning of the auspicious Navratri, the nine days of fasting and worship during which Hindus pray to the Mother Goddess. A full moon blinks its way through a flurry of clouds as I make my way on a cycle rickshaw to GB Road (ironically renamed Swami Shradhanand Marg in 1965), Delhi's red-light district, and one of India's largest, with an estimated 5,000 sex workers residing in ninety-six brothels.

The British established GB Road in the 1930s by consolidating Delhi's five brothel areas, including the prosperous brothels of Chawri Bazar, which had once flourished under Mughal patronage, into one area. They sold the ground floors of the twenty buildings where the brothels were located to hardware merchants. Today, GB Road is famous for another reason—it is Asia's largest hardware market and India's largest market for sanitary ware. Nestled between the hardware stores are steep, vertiginous staircases that lead up to the kothas whose windows are boarded shut. Each kotha is distinguished by a number—the more prosperous kothas have their numbers inlaid in tiles, the less prosperous have theirs scribbled on a pillar in white chalk.

I sit on the floor of Kotha 36, the most famous kotha in Delhi for mujras. The room is bathed in the pale luminosity of artificial white lights. I am familiar with these lights from my investment-banking days; they are purposely bright to sting the eyes and keep workers awake. It is 11 p.m. on a Thursday night and it seems like I am the only customer here. The kotha isn't empty though; it is crowded with the women who live and work here; they're sitting around on plastic chairs waiting for customers to arrive. They wear refulgent saris in bright colours with tiny navel-exposing blouses, their generous stomachs exposed and spilling in all directions. They remind me of a set of matryoshka dolls, their faces plastered with white paint, abnormally pronounced red blotches on their cheeks, crimson lipstick, and dark eye shadow over long, sparkly fake eyelashes. They aspire to look beautiful, but look old and tired instead. They all clutch one or two mobile phones, not the inexpensive ubiquitous Nokias, but expensive smartphones with fancy displays and touch screens which they flaunt like diamond rings. As I am to discover, the mobile phone plays a critical role in this business; the nicer the phone, the more exalted the status of its owner. The small hall where we are all seated features a motley group of performers: a young boy playing the tabla, an old man with an orange beard playing the harmonium, and another clanging cymbals. A woman who looks distinctly different from this crowd, with an authoritative air about her, sits with them. She is dressed in a flowery salwaar-kameez, there is no make-up on her face, and her hair is tied back tightly. The hall abuts the living quarters of the women, and I can see a cluster of tiny, crowded rooms. This multi-purpose hall is also used as a bathroom and dressing room. A rusty sink is installed on the wall, next to which a plastic shelf holds a number of colourful toothbrushes; nightgowns and towels are untidily splayed on a row of hooks. Above the sink is a picture of the singer Lata Mangeshkar, a plastic garland around her neck. I had expected the brothels of GB Road to be a far cry from the luxurious bordellos of the past re-created in films like *Umrao Jaan*, but I had not imagined this sort of shabby decrepitude.

Everyone stares at me in bored silence. As I had guessed, the woman who sits with the band is the lady in charge. She throws me an angry glare.

'Are you from the media?' she asks.

'No, I am not,' I reply firmly.

'Are you sure?' she asks suspiciously.

'Yes! I am just here to see the famous mujras of Delhi!' I reply.

'Girls from good homes don't come here,' she says rudely.

I am unsure about how to respond to this so I say nothing. She considers me for a second more, then says, 'Just remember the lives of young children are at stake here,' and then she launches into a song from the movie *Umrao Jaan*. To my surprise, the woman sings well, and while the background music is poor, her voice is melodious and powerful.

As the show picks up pace, a few women rise and begin to dance, swaying gracelessly to the rising tempo. Brothels are hardly the place to expect tender things, but here amongst the women is a cute little girl who couldn't have been more than a year old. She has only recently learnt to walk and is waddling around on her chubby legs, chewing on the ear of a grimy teddy bear. It is not clear who this child's mother is as she is on friendly terms with all the women. She is picked up and cuddled freely, and then put down on the floor to waddle around some more. She goes over to the musicians, tapping on their instruments, and then at the beginning of an upbeat Hindi movie song, she squeals and breaks into a waddle-dance. This song, it seems, is not just familiar to her but also a favourite. I can't take my eyes off this child even though I feel rude staring like this. That said, half the women in this room have been glaring at me ever since I entered, so I probably shouldn't feel too diffident about staring. As the child totters around, someone hands her some masala chips, which she demands more of; she is given the entire packet, which she happily munches her way through. Another person gives her a sip from a soda can. It is 11.30 p.m., and I wonder why this child is still awake. She walks over to me and smiles. She hands me her teddy bear of indeterminate brown-grey colour in a gesture of friendship. She is a handsome child—fair, plump, with small, round features and a head of thick hair tied into two wispy ponytails. She is wearing a pair of frilly panties, discoloured but clean, a faded black tunic and a black thread around her neck to keep the evil eye at bay.

I can't help but wonder what her future will be. Will she, like her mother, become a sex worker? After all, 90 per cent of sex workers' daughters in India follow their mothers into prostitution.[65] As the tempo of the Bollywood song rises, two women begin dancing frenziedly. Their dance is just a series of bawdy pelvic thrusts, breasts and stomachs jiggling. The child, too, starts spinning in circles and then falls down on the hard floor. There are a few seconds of silence before she breaks into a shrill cry. Someone comes and scoops her up and takes her into one of the adjoining rooms. Finally, it is bedtime.

I have already given ₹100 as my entrance fee to the performance and a couple more ₹100 notes to the singer and musicians who demand it. There is one last note left in my wallet—it is my auto fare home. On my way out I bump into the child who, it appears, is having trouble sleeping and has found her way into the hall. She gives me a toothy smile and demands to be picked up. I take out my cab fare, fold it into a small square and place it in the child's palm. That was my last ₹100 and it leaves me stuck in a brothel at midnight without a ride home but I don't mind, for this child has stolen my heart.

◆

Prostitution in India has a long and storied past. From the verses of the *Mahabharata* to the renditions of the exquisite ganika in the time of Kautilya to the charm of Mughal bordellos, prostitutes have held an important place in Indian history. The first records of prostitution anywhere in the world were found in the ancient civilization of Sumer—the 'art of prostitution' and 'the cult of the prostitute' are two of the *'me'* (sacred treasures) given to the

Sumerian goddess Inanna by her father Enki, the god of wisdom. When Inanna takes the *me* back to the city of Uruk in the boat of heaven, the people turn out in droves to cheer in gratitude. The principal deities of the Egyptians were Osiris (Sun God) and Isis (Earth Goddess) and the cult of these gods gave rise to temple prostitution where young, prepubescent girls were donated to the temple to placate the gods, often in elaborate ceremonies.[66] Prostitution found its way from Egypt into India[67] sometime during the Brahmanic (Vedic) period when liberal marriage morals were being remodelled and virginal purity and an ideal of strict monogamist life was being established.[68]

The Devadasi, or temple prostitute culture in India has its roots in the Egyptian cults of Osiris and Isis. Temple sex workers were thought to have been an important part of religious and cultural life in India as early as 300 CE, and became an established institution by around 700 CE. Devadasis sang and danced for the temple god and provided sexual favours to temple priests and favoured male patrons. In time, Devadasis began to provide sexual favours to common visitors to the temple in exchange for money. Historically, these women came from tribal or lower caste communities such as the Nat, Bedia and Kanjars; daughters born to Devadasis were reared in the temple compound and initiated into the profession by their mothers.[69]

There were other strands of prostitution in ancient Indian society. One of these was concubinage in which women were traded, sold and offered as gifts or spoils of war. In ancient India prostitution was widely accepted by the government and the public. Prostitutes were not looked upon as socially and morally inferior beings as they are today, and several Hindu scriptures even extolled prostitutes as objects of good luck. For example, the *Matsya Purana,* the oldest of the Puranas, thought of the prostitute as a portent of good luck, and another religious text, the *Vishnu Samhita,* says that circumambulating a prostitute brought good luck. Though many of these practices have been forgotten, a rare few exist even today. In some parts of South India, for instance, the mangalsutra of a new bride is made by the hands of a prostitute, and in Northeast India, a handful of earth from the threshold of a prostitute's house is required to mould the statue of the Goddess during the Durga Puja festival.

One would imagine that the best time in Indian history to have been a courtesan was in the beginning of the third century BCE, during the prosperous rule of the Maurya dynasty, a time of great renaissance in art and literature. The prostitute or ganika as she was called in Sanskrit was a highly refined temptress adept in the arts of song, dance and seduction. The numerous discourses on prostitution during this time suggest a significant increase in the popularity of the trade. The ganikas were trained in the sixty-four kalas or arts forms that were prerequisites to be a ganika—these included song, dance, the art of seduction, and more scholarly pursuits such as the knowledge of warfare and literary recitations. Brothels were state-controlled, by the 'Superintendent of Prostitution', and the revenue from this institution went to the upkeep and teaching of the ganikas.

Ancient texts such as the *Arthashastra*, *Kamasutra* and *Buddhacharita* (Life of Buddha) are testament to the distinct, widely accepted position that courtesans held in Indian life. Kautilya's *Arthashastra*, the ancient and authoritative treatise on civics, lays out in elaborate detail the functions of the prostitute. It includes an entire chapter on the regulation of 'public women' and roles of retired prostitutes as cooks, midwives and nurses, or as maids of honour in royal households. In the *Kamasutra*, Vatsyayana devoted an entire section to ganikas, writing that it is the duty of a man to indulge the ganika who was an indispensable and estimable factor in public functions of the town and of the aristocracy. In the *Buddhacharita*, the author, Ashvaghosa, recounts a story. When the Buddha was travelling, he met Amrapali, a prostitute, who invited him for a meal, which he readily accepted. A little later, a Brahmin invited him too, but the Buddha said no as he had already accepted Amrapali's invitation. This act of the Buddha established equity between the highest caste of Brahmin and the prostitute.

Under the reign of the Mughals, the culture of the courtesan was enriched. They brought with them their own practices from Persia which integrated seamlessly into the practices of the ganikas.[70] The tawaifs were the courtesans of the Mughal times and were sponsored by rich and powerful nobles. They embodied luxurious and urbane living and were connoisseurs of song and dance specializing in vocal forms such as the dadra, ghazal, and thumri, and dance forms like kathak. Veena Oldenburg, a scholar who studied the lost tawaif culture of her hometown of Lucknow writes, 'Many of the musicians [in the kothas] belonged to famous lineages, and much of late-nineteenth-century Hindustani music was invented and transformed in these salons, to accommodate the new urban elite who filled the patronage vacuum in the colonial period'.[71]

It is said that during the reign of Emperor Akbar, courtesan culture was so popular, that Akbar had a separate space allocated to the courtesans of the time, known as the Shaitan Puta (or Devil's Ville).[72] Prostitution in those times was a seriously regulated affair and anyone who wanted to take the virginity of a woman had to formally apply for it by writing a letter to His Majesty the Emperor Akbar himself. During the reign of Emperor Shah Jahan, the tawaif culture continued to flourish. It only fell upon hard times during the reign of the last great Mughal, the puritanical Aurangzeb, who proclaimed that all prostitutes should get married or run the risk of banishment.[73]

A bizarre set of circumstances led to the downfall of the ancient tradition of the courtesan, cultivated through the centuries. At the time of the Indian Revolt of 1857, it was discovered that one in every four British soldiers was infected with venereal disease, and more British casualties occurred because of disease than combat. The battle to reduce European mortality rates had to be fought on the hygienic front to ensure a healthy European army for the strategic needs of empire. It became imperative that the courtesans and prostitutes of Lucknow, along with those in the other 110 cantonments in India (and in several towns in Britain) where European soldiers were stationed, be regulated, inspected, and controlled.[74]

To keep their army healthy, the British began regulating prostitution. The Indian Penal Code of 1860, drafted by Lord Macaulay, was the first legislative document that put prostitution under nationwide law. Though the law did not ban prostitution, it restricted it in such a way that it became virtually impossible to carry on the trade. According to the law, 'if a prostitute solicited customers in a public place or where a brothel is established and if this causes annoyance to the persons living in the vicinity, this would amount to public nuisance punishable by imprisonment'. In addition to this restrictive law, the provisions of Britain's Contagious Diseases Act of 1864 were incorporated into a comprehensive piece of legislation, requiring the registration and medical examination of all prostitutes in cantonment cities of the Indian empire. This act placed the wealthy tawaif and the common street prostitute in the same bracket making it mandatory for them to face medical examinations under similar conditions. With their aristocratic patrons slowly losing financial sway, and the British branding them as ordinary prostitutes by enforcing registration, the tawaif culture began dying out. The courtesans appeared in the civic tax ledgers of Lucknow in 1858-1877 where they were classed under the occupational category of 'dancing and singing girls', despite being the city's highest taxpayers with the largest individual incomes.[75]

Fortunately, the arts of the tawaifs did not die with them. By an ironic twist of fate, the bourgeoisie appropriated the song and dance forms of the tawaifs. Today, in India, classical dance is primarily a middle- and upper-middle-class phenomenon, and it is common practice for children from these households to grow up practicing these song and dance forms.[76]

Several memorable and heart-touching Bollywood films have been made featuring the downfall of the exquisite Mughal courtesan. The most famous of these films are *Pakeezah* (1972) and *Umrao Jaan* (1981). Both movies are set in the period immediately after the annexation of Awadh by the British, at a time when the courtesan played an important role in the cultural fabric of the city. These films bring to life the pitiable but prosperous lives of these tawaifs; beautiful women living in luxuriant boudoirs graced by well-to-do men, who with the deterioration of their culture have no option but to attempt to live a 'decent' life by marrying a man who will take care of them. As I was to discover, these nuptial desires have persisted.

THE PIMP AND THE PROSTITUTE

I am at Ramlila Maidan, a short walk away from GB Road, with my new friend Mohsin. On my maiden visit to GB Road, I had found Mohsin, smartly dressed in a crisp white shirt, smoking a cigarette at a paan shop, and he had helped me find my way to Kotha 36. Mohsin works as an AC repairman by day and as a pimp at night, and over the days he has helped me navigate my way through GB Road. Today, Mohsin has agreed to introduce me to his ex-girlfriend, Vimla, a sex worker at GB Road.

At the Maidan, Navratri festivities are in full swing and the grounds are packed with thousands of revellers. A rickety Ferris wheel is the prime attraction, along with other jerry-built theme-park rides, which add metallic shrieks and groans to the noise and confusion that surrounds me. A long procession of chariots is passing by; atop each chariot are people dressed as characters out of Indian mythology. On one sits a man painted blue—this is Shiva; on another chariot is a man carrying a large bow and arrow—this must be Arjun. The most joyous shrieks emerge from the crowd when a chariot carrying the quartet of Ram, Lakshman, Sita, and the monkey god Hanuman pass by. Even Mohsin, who is

Muslim, gives a hoot of delight. He tells me proudly that Hanuman is a friend of his. I assume he's referring to the man dressed as Hanuman. He also reveals that the woman dressed as Sita, who is meant to be the paragon of virtue in Hindu mythology, is a sex worker in real life.

Mohsin is insisting that we go for a ride on the dilapidated, dangerous Ferris wheel.

'No, Mohsin, I can't,' I say sternly after noticing that the Ferris wheel, which is run by a shuddering, squeaking generator, looks and sounds like it could break down any second.

'Iraji, if you don't go, I won't introduce you to Vimla.'

'Mohsin, I'm sorry, this Ferris wheel is not safe.'

'Iraji, if it was not safe, why would the police ride in it?'

Mohsin's observation is not unfounded, the Ferris wheel has many groups of gleeful khaki-clad policemen squeezed into its seats.

'Mohsin, I can't,' I say with trepidation.

'No story then,' he insists stubbornly, walking away from me.

'All right, let's do it,' I say running after him.

I am pretty desperate to meet Vimla. I have been visiting GB Road regularly over the past few weeks, but I have had no luck with the sex workers as they are all suspicious of me and refuse to open up. Mohsin is my last hope to try and get someone to share insights into what life as a sex worker on GB Road is like. On the Ferris wheel, we spin round and round, going much too fast, while all manner of nerve-wracking noises seem to suggest that the whole contraption is about to fall apart. Mohsin shrieks and giggles like a girl, while I clutch the handles and keep my eyes squeezed firmly shut. At one point, the daredevil Mohsin stands up on his seat, letting go of the railing. I nearly faint, thinking that this is the end for him, but he stays put and right before we halt, he jumps off and lands with a thud. No one protests, and he lies in the dirt whooping with delight. I get off the Ferris wheel with a spinning head, and promptly throw up all over my shoes.

As I steady myself, Mohsin announces Vimla's arrival.

Vimla is not beautiful. She is twenty-nine, about my age, but looks far older. Her face features a violent purple patch of acne and crooked, yellow teeth. Her lips are dry, scorched and papery. Despite these physical shortcomings, there is something attractive about her. I can't put my finger on it, but it has something to do with the confidence with which she carries herself and her easy manner of speaking. She is dressed conservatively in a polyester salwaar-kameez and is wearing minimal make-up.

At sixteen, Vimla ran away from her abusive husband and her hometown in Bengal. The first person she met when she got down from the train in New Delhi was a pimp who told her to take a walk with him to GB Road. It's been thirteen years since that day, and she still hasn't left. Vimla has a three-year-old daughter; she shows me a hazy picture on her cell phone. She doesn't know who the father is, but she says that some of her daughter's physiognomy—the fair skin, large nose and thick hair—points to a Punjabi father. But she has had sex with hundreds of Punjabis, so it's impossible to say which one.

Vimla tells me that the sex trade at GB Road is not what it used to be and neither is the clientele. She explains that Delhi is changing, as are its sexual needs. GB Road will never ever go out of business; it hasn't in the past two hundred years, and it isn't likely to in the next two hundred. There will always be men willing to pay for sex, and someone who will be willing to give it up for cash. But she has seen a transformation. In her early days, many men would come—rich men, handsome men, foreign men and powerful men—who left healthy tips. Now the clientele at GB Road consists of rickshaw drivers, coolies, druggies, and young boys whose 'dicks have barely gone hard, whose hair hasn't come, and who come in all of two minutes'. GB Road was once the only place for paid sex in this city; this is no longer the case. 'Everyone,' Vimla says, 'is a randi [prostitute] or a dalal

[pimp], and everywhere there exists a kotha [brothel]. Men,' she says, 'want polished young girls who speak English, whom they can have in posh hotel rooms, like they show in the movies.'

Vimla explains to me how GB Road is organized. Madams are generally former sex workers who have risen up the organizational hierarchy to secure a managerial position in the brothel. The madam, which is what Vimla hopes to be one day, looks after the upkeep and maintenance of the brothel, and maintains informal contracts with sex workers. Pimps, like Mohsin, take care of the outside world, soliciting clients. Everyone is apparently losing business with the decline of GB Road and the rise of a new breed of prostitution.

I ask Vimla how she felt about relaxing laws relating to sex work in India, a much-debated issue, and if this would help her business, or make her and her daughter's life better. Vimla considered the question for a moment, and then said to me with a shrug that it didn't really matter. When men wanted sex, no laws of any kind would stop them. Where there was money, there were always women, and since there was more money today, the quality of women had gone up. As for her life, even if she were a legal tax-paying resident like the prostitutes of yesteryears, she would always remain a prostitute, a randi, to the world. Men would still harass her; she would still be contained within the world of the brothel.

'Would legality give me izzat?' she asks me. 'No, so what is the point?' she says firmly.

Prostitution in India is in the peculiar position of being tolerated, despite not being entirely legal. The laws are nebulous—they do not abolish the trade nor do they legalize the profession, making the lives of women like Vimla difficult. The current legislation controls and regulates the trade in a way that conforms to the low social position of sex work rather than making the lives of sex workers better by giving them rights. The first national law dealing with sex work, the Suppression of Immoral Trafficking Act

(SITA), came into being in 1956. The name immediately became controversial because in Hindu mythology, Sita is the pure wife of Lord Ram who is kidnapped by the demon king Ravana. Like the Indian Penal Code developed by the British, SITA did not prohibit prostitution outright, but it did prohibit the commercial activities of the flesh trade like pimping and trafficking. One of the biggest drawbacks of SITA was that it covered only women, not children, men or transsexuals.

SITA was revamped in 1986 when the Immoral Traffic Prevention Act, or PITA, came into being. PITA (this time legislators changed the name so as to not offend people) worked off the framework of SITA but was more comprehensive, and included male workers, hijras and children. Like the previous law, PITA too maintains an ambiguous position towards sex work. It is not illegal, but a 'prostitute', defined as someone who is involved in sex work, is liable to be criminalized and the acts and conditions accompanying sex work are illegal. The law does not make prostitution illegal, but makes it illegal to practice sex work within a 200-meter radius of public places such as schools, temples, hospitals, nursing homes, or hotels. The law does not take a position on sex being exchanged for money, which is stated to be a 'private' affair but like SITA it does criminalize soliciting sex. It also makes it illegal for sex workers to live with their children (or other dependents) in a place where sex work is performed, making it difficult for a sex worker to find a house to rent. All these conditions make sex workers like Vimla dependent on other agents: pimps like Mohsin and madams. It also gives power to agents such as the police, leading to further exploitation of sex workers.

There is no easy answer when it comes to legislation regarding prostitution. Legalizing prostitution provides some benefits, but there are those who protest that it undermines so-called moral standards. Morality, though, cannot be legislated and immorality cannot be destroyed by legislation alone. Banning prostitution, arguably the oldest profession in the world, seems impractical and it is unrealistic to think that commerce and sex will cease to be intertwined. And trying to forcibly separate the two has often had unforeseen consequences. For example, many believe that the suppression of prostitution in Argentina in 1937 led to such an incredible spread of venereal disease, sexual perversion and crime that it was legitimized once again in 1954.

Organization of sex workers is a crucial dimension of the political economy of the market for sex work, and the unionization of sex workers could offer a partial solution to some of the legal problems that they currently face. In the red-light area of Sonagachi in Kolkata, sex workers have united under the NGO Durbar Mahila Samanwaya which has been able to increase the bargaining power of sex workers significantly by stopping trafficking and getting rid of pimps, middlemen, madams and policemen. A microfinance organization, USHA, has helped prostitutes shake off their financial dependence on madams and pimps. Though the model has been successful in Kolkata, the brothels of GB Road in New Delhi have not been able to unionize despite two NGOs being present in the area.

Vimla tells me that she doesn't care about organization, because she doesn't feel like it will help her.

What does she care about then?

She tells me that she cares about only herself and her daughter. She also cares about her marriage.

'There is a lack of good men and husbands,' she says glaring at Mohsin, who looks genuinely embarrassed.

'So if you were married, what would you do?'

'I would stay at home.' She adds, 'Obviously.'

Mohsin, who has been silent this entire time, grins at her and squeezes her breast. She yelps and slaps his hand.

There is no love lost between the ex-lovers. She reaches for his scrotum through his jeans and firmly squeezes and punches. He squeals and runs away.

Vimla has to leave now; she is meeting her new boyfriend, a man Mohsin only refers to as 'madarchod'. I buy Vimla a Thums-up and some fluorescent pink cotton candy. Mohsin helps me find a cab, opens the door for me, telling me that he worries about my wandering around Delhi like this. There is something ironic about a pimp worrying about my safety. I tell him I'll be okay and watch as he and Vimla drive away into the dusty, violet night on his motorcycle. She has her arms wrapped marsupial-like around him, her diaphanous dupatta unfurling behind them. The pimp and the prostitute, they zoom away, they could really be any couple in the world.

◆

According to a study by sociologists K. K. Mukherjee and Sutapa Mukherjee, in which they interviewed nearly 10,000 sex workers spread across thirty-one states and union territories, the number of prostitutes grew from 3 million to 5 million across the country over the course of their three-year study (from 2003-2006).[77] Their study states that earlier most sex workers were from scheduled castes, scheduled tribes and backward classes, and that poverty drove them to become sex workers. But today this is changing, as roughly 60 per cent of the commercial sex workers are in this 'low-end' category while 40 per cent of sex workers are from the upper classes operating as call girls, bar girls and high-class prostitutes. Whereas prostitutes like Vimla operating on the street and brothels earn between ₹2,000 to ₹24,000 per month, the 'new' Indian prostitute makes around ₹40,000 to ₹800,000 per month. These numbers don't mean that the low-end category is decreasing, only that one class of sex worker is increasing at a galloping pace to keep up with the growing sexual demands of an affluent demographic. There are several reasons why prostitution is increasing right across the spectrum—migration and urbanization, economic destitution, the erosion of traditional values, declining job opportunities for uneducated and unskilled youth, and a desire to earn easy and fast money.

A pan-India survey done by the Centre for Advocacy on Stigma and Marginalisation (CASAM)[78] in 2011 revealed that over 80 per cent of the women surveyed entered into the profession of their own volition as opposed to being forced or born into it. While poor family backgrounds and the need to look for incomes and livelihoods at an early age is what makes women enter the informal labour market, the possibility of earning higher incomes is what makes sex work today a more economically rewarding option.

◆

Ads for 'massage parlours' in the classified sections of newspapers are ubiquitous in any daily newspaper in any part of the country. These large ads in bold colours take up prime advertising space in the newspapers. They usually go like this:

> Hotel Guest Only, Royal Class Body Massage by Young, Educated, Decent Female Staff. J___ O___ 9871430390

Another:

> PRIYA Royal Escort. Luxury Call Only. Relaxable massage by Young, Educated, Decent Female Staff. Home/Hotel 24 Hrs

A third:

> Hotel Guest only. Body massage By Edu Decent Staff M/F H/H. 24 Hrs Service. All Credit Cards Acp. S____ S____ 9811068373.

I wondered if it would be as easy as calling up these telephone numbers to get access to sex workers. There was only one way to find out. I began by looking through the massage parlour ads and calling all the numbers in the newspaper, and asking for Jesika, Sophia, Priya and Nancy. Most of the women who picked up hung up on me, saying I had reached the wrong number. Maybe they smelled a rat when they heard a female voice on the phone. The sixth number that I tried, for 'Nita Escort Service', hit pay dirt. A man answered the phone, speaking in heavily accented English punctuated with Hindi words.

Me: Hello, is this, uh, Nita?
Man: Haan, haan, what do you want?
Me: I am looking for a massage service.
Man: Man or a woman? (He sounded suspicious.)
Me: Uh, woman. Home service please. (It seemed like they offered gigolos too.)
Man: Where do you live?
Me: Near Connaught Place.
Man: We can't do home service. But we can offer a five-star hotel.
Me: Which hotel?
Man: Where are you calling from? (Suspiciously.)
Me: Near CP, I found the ad in the newspaper.
Man: When do you want the girl?
Me: Now.

Suddenly, apropos of nothing, the man got nervous.

Man: Please don't call this number. (In a rush.)

He hung up the phone. I dialled again.

Me: Why did you hang up the phone? I just saw the ad in the newspaper and want service!
Man: Woman, right? (With hesitation.)
Me: Yes.
Man: You will have to come to (he mentioned the name of a five-star hotel). I have a girl there.
Me: What is the price?
Man: ₹10,000.
Me: Does this include the hotel room?
Man: Yes.
Me: Okay, I want a choice of girls though.

Man: I will give you a choice of girls, just reach the hotel and call me.
Me: I will reach in thirty minutes.
Man: Are you alone?
Me: No, there is a friend with me.
Pause.
Me: Hello?
Man: Boy or girl?
Me: Boy. (Pause.) He is my boyfriend.
Man: (Doubtfully.) Okay, reach (the hotel).

Thirty minutes later, outside the hotel, I SMSed the man. I did not receive a reply, so I called him.
Me: I am outside the hotel. Where should I meet you?

The man sounded nervous and hesitant. I heard a susurrus of sounds on the line.
Man: Come to (he mentions the name of another hotel), CP, Inner Circle.
Me: (I am beginning to get irritated.) Why didn't you tell me earlier? I have been waiting here.
Man: Just come to (the hotel).
Me: (Sigh.) I will be there in five minutes.

I get to the hotel in Connaught Place.
Me: I have reached the hotel.
Man: Where are you? Near the pharmacy?
Me: Yes.
Man: Are you alone?
Me: No, I have a friend with me.
Man: Only one friend, right?
Me: Yes.
Man: Go inside and wait on the first floor.
Me: Okay.

The largest commercial hub of New Delhi by day, at night, Connaught Place, the circular arcade that lies at the heart of Delhi linking the old city with the new, has a grimy, eerie air. The detritus of the millions of people who work here is evident—and peddlers, scavengers and beggars dominate the trash-filled alleys. I walk down a stained corridor lined with cramped shops that spill on to the footpaths and enter a lift to the hotel. The elevator opens up into a surprisingly spacious and well-appointed hotel lobby.

Vinayak has insisted on coming with me on this sting operation. I allow him to come because it adds more credibility to my story. After my experience in GB Road, I hope I will be looked upon with less suspicion if I present myself as one half of a couple. Single men walk in and out of the hotel freely, some taking a seat in the lobby area. A stout man dressed in office attire comes and sits next to me, popping open his laptop. Every time an inconspicuous, middle-aged Indian man emerges from the corridor, I can't help but wonder if these men are here for the 'massage service'. The hotel staff don't seem to wonder as much as I do; they don't give us, or anyone else, a second glance.

Five SMSs, four phone calls, and thirty minutes later, the pimp asks me to come to the second floor. We take the elevator up, and wait in the narrow second-floor lobby, across from a restaurant. I expect the pimp to emerge from the restaurant, after all it is dinnertime, but after keeping us waiting for another twenty minutes, the pimp sends me an SMS asking me to go to Room 240. The hour-long wait at the hotel has led to a build-up of anxiety, nervousness, and also excitement. Vinayak and I look at each other, hold hands, and ring the doorbell.

The door is opened by a petite girl with Mongoloid features, her long, greasy hair streaked with blond highlights. She has a charming, almost beatific face and smiles at us sweetly. She is wearing a cheap black dress with gaudy silver embellishments and a roughed up pair of high heels. She is clutching a high-tech mobile phone to her heart. This girl is as visibly discomposed as Vinayak and I.

We walk into the room, and realize that we are not the first visitors to Room 240 today. The room is in a mess, the bed unmade, the sheets twisted out of place and the pillows scattered on the floor. On the side table, two half-empty bottles of Kingfisher beer sit next to a bowl of peanuts. The smell of cigarettes and stale perfume pervades the room, and I spot, next to the sofa where Vinayak and I have taken a seat, a shiny used condom lying on the floor like the chrysalis of an insect.

I have asked Vinayak to do the talking, thinking it would appear more natural coming from a man, but the poor man has been rendered speechless by the entire scene, so I am compelled to take over. I am not sure how to broach the subject and, it seems, neither is she. We stare at each other, and then I break the awkward silence with a natural first question.

'What is your name?'

'Nita,' she says with a nervous smile.

'Hello, Nita, where are you from?'

'I am from Darjeeling.'

Nita's phone rings. The pimp is on the line. She hands the phone to me.

'Is she okay?' he asks.

'Uh, no, you had promised me a choice. Where are the other girls?' I ask.

'Hold on,' he says, before hanging up abruptly.

I hand the phone back to Nita.

Moments later, we hear a knock on the door. Two plump, fair-skinned girls walk in. One has a young face, though she looks older because she is dressed in a sari. She could easily be an office receptionist somewhere, with her neat, parted, shoulder-length hair, and a sari of subdued colours tied high on her waist, the sleeves of her blouse long. With her is another flinty-faced young woman wearing a colourful, expensive looking salwaar-kameez, which is tight around her large breasts. The three girls whisper amongst themselves, and then the one in the sari takes charge.

'You want group sex?' she asks in a commanding tone, speaking perfect English.

Vinayak and I look at each other, taken aback.

'Are you boyfriend and girlfriend?' she asks.

'Yes,' I say, snuggling close to Vinayak, wrapping my arms around him.

'Are you from Delhi?' she asks me.

'Yes, and you?' I ask.

'Yes, I am from Delhi. I am a computer engineer,' she says confidently.

'What's your name?' I ask.

'Nita. Yours?'

I think to myself that they are all named Nita, and then I remember from the newspaper ad that this is after all 'Nita Escort Service'.

'I am Ira, and he is Vinayak,' I say.

'You want sex with all of us?' she asks, pointing to the two other girls who stand in the corner.

Vinayak and I look at each other. He replies, finally finding his voice. 'No, just one.'

'Okay, you can pay in advance,' she says, placing her stylish black leather purse on the bed.

'How much do I have to pay you?' I ask.

'How much did you speak for?'

During my conversation, I observe that the first Nita has locked herself in the bathroom, and I hear her speaking frantically on the phone.

'₹10,000,' I reply.

Both girls look at each other. 'Okay, let me check,' she says.

Now there is mass confusion in the room. All three girls are speaking in hurried, frantic whispers to each other. They are walking around the room and bathroom, making calls from their cell phones. It looks like each girl has about three cell phones. I wonder if they suspect something. There have been a string of sting-operations by the media and police and the entire industry is enveloped in fear and suspicion.

Vinayak and I are frozen on the sofa. The original Nita spots the condom. She grabs a tissue from the bathroom, comes and picks it up. She goes back into the bathroom, and I hear the gurgling sound of the toilet flush. Without any warning, the two girls who had entered the room later leave, slamming the door shut behind them. The original Nita goes back into the bathroom. My phone rings; it is the pimp calling. 'Get out of there right now! Right now!' he yells, distraught. They are suspicious; I guess Vinayak and I are not their typical clientele.

'Why? What happened?' I ask.

'Now. You have to leave. Unless you want the first girl.'

'No,' I say, 'we want more choice.'

'Are you willing to pay?' he asks.

'Yes!' I say. 'We are willing to pay well.'

'Okay, do you want Russian?' he asks, now sounding avaricious.

'Okay, sure.'

'Then go to the first floor. I'll send you the room number… But leave this room,' he says.

Vinayak and I make our way out. Nita stands in the doorway. I ask her for her number.

She fidgets with her phone, clearly unwilling.

In the wisest move he has made all evening, Vinayak takes out a ₹1,000 note from his wallet and hands it to her.

She dictates her number. I note it down and give her a missed call, making sure that her phone rings.

We find ourselves waiting once again, this time at the bar. Vinayak desperately needs a drink. I call the pimp.

He tells me tersely, 'Russian left. You can come tomorrow,' and hangs up the phone.

As we walk out of the hotel, I wonder if the Russian on the first floor ever existed or if this had been a ploy to get us out of the room. Despite this setback I consider our mission successful now that I have Nita No. 1's number.

♦

After much persuasion and for the price of ₹3,000 'Nita' agrees to meet me for a coffee at Connaught Place. She arrives with a short Northeastern man with a Mohawk and messy stubble. He's wearing a Yankees baseball cap yanked sideways on his head. He takes a seat a safe distance away from us. Nita is beautiful. Her skin is a flawless gold, her nose a perfect little button, her eyes chocolate brown, accentuated with a 3D-effect because of the coloured contact lenses she wears. She looks fresh and pretty in a pink t-shirt and pink velour sweatpants. She carries a designer purse. She smiles, but I can tell she is nervous. I am not sure how to break the ice. I look at my outfit, my sartorial standard—unfashionable kurta with loose pajamas. Maybe it would be a good idea to dress less like a journalist for these meetings. I ask her to order something and she orders a cold coffee.

Conversation with Nita is painful, I feel like I am performing arduous surgery. Nita is not exactly forthcoming, and I know that if I probe aggressively, I will scare her away. Gently and patiently, with just the right amount of persuasion, I steer the conversation in the right direction. Nita's family lives in Darjeeling. Before she came to Delhi to study fashion, her life-long passion, Nita worked in her family's restaurant. She got into the sex trade when she was introduced to it by a fellow student. She likes the pulse of living in a big city, because living in Darjeeling 'got very boring'. She has quit fashion school, she doesn't say why, and at the moment she is looking for a job, hoping to find work in fashion. Nita doesn't mind sex work. It allows her to earn well and she says that sometimes it can even be fun. She has the right to choose her clients and also the right to say no. She gets paid ₹5,000 for one 'shot', plus the tips that her clients leave her. She lives in an apartment in South Delhi with her friend, the man she has brought along with her. He is also from Darjeeling and is looking for a job.

Girls from the Northeast make up a large part of the sex trade. This is partly because of the abominable economic situation and the soaring unemployment in these states, and because of the popularity of Northeastern girls in the sex trade. Indian men prefer Northeastern girls because they appear to them to be more 'exotic'. Nita tells me that many of the women in her trade have migrated from other states to the capital because their hometowns are 'boring'. Many of these women have other jobs, some of them even have families. She knows housewives who care for their husbands and families by day, but do sex work at night for the extra cash.

Nita tells me that she barely meets the lily-livered pimps like the one I spoke to on the phone, but she feels safer when she works with them, because they can step in if things go wrong. She collects the cash from the client (an amount fixed by the pimp) and a portion is collected from her by a courier and delivered to the pimp. The cut she receives depends on the type of arrangement she has with the pimp. If she is salaried, the entire amount is taken by the pimp. If she is a 'freelancer' then she keeps 50 per cent of the money received.

I ask her if she is afraid of getting caught. For a second she looks alarmed and, for the briefest moment, I see vulnerability on her face. She admits that sometimes she is. An infamous pimp has recently been arrested, and everyone in the industry is scared of a crackdown. She is careful about how she conducts her work, and services only regular clients. The pimps are also extra careful because they are the ones who suffer the most if caught. I ask her how long she will stay in the trade. She tells me, throwing a quick glance at the man she has walked in with, that she will do sex work only till she gets married.

When the promised hour of our chat is up, I place ₹3,000 on the table. Nita looks at the money and then shakes her head. 'It's okay,' she says, pushing the money towards me. I urge her to take the money. I tell her that it is part of our deal; it is what we had agreed on.

'It's okay,' she says and then adds, 'you are my friend.'

She gets up, motioning to her companion. Though it is a sunless, grey afternoon, she puts on a pair of sunglasses that cover most of her face, and walks quickly out of the coffee shop.

◆

Nita is the new face of the Indian sex industry, even as the old face—the destitute prostitute of GB Road persists. As the sexual landscape of India changes, prostitution is changing too, stimulated by economic growth, growing consumerism, and greater disposable income amongst the middle class. In a 2006 survey, 58 per cent of Delhi men (urban, middle-class) surveyed said that they had solicited sex workers.[79] These numbers are bolstered by a 2011 survey, in which 54 per cent of Delhi-ites in the same class segment said they had lost count of the number of times they had paid for sex.[80] Prostitution is just as widespread in other metros in India. According to police officials, things are going out of control in cities like Bangalore and Pune, where 54 per cent of male residents have said that they have had sex with prostitutes.[81] The takers for this 'new' kind of prostitution are men, typically middle-class and above, who are comfortable paying between ₹5000-₹10,000 for young, attractive and well-groomed prostitutes, girls like Nita, who have come to the city to find their fortunes. Some are runaways from conservative households, others are students, others have jobs in coffee shops and beauty parlours, and others are housewives moonlighting as prostitutes to supplement their income and their lifestyles.

Though the new form of prostitution is on the rise, the sex trade is not just an easy way for pretty young things to make money, for the older, squalid, exploitative version still exists. According to *New York Times* journalist Nicholas Kristof who investigated prostitution in Indian brothels, 'India probably has more modern slaves than any country in the world. It has millions of women and girls in its brothels, often held captive for their first few years until they grow resigned to their fate. India's brothels are also unusually violent, with ferocious beatings common and pimps sometimes even killing girls who are uncooperative.'[82]

Kristof's findings are further buttressed by findings of the Ministry of Women and Child Development—India has nearly 2.5 million prostitutes in nearly 300,000 brothels in 1,100 red-light areas across the country. Around 1.2 million children are involved in prostitution in India, and the trafficking of girls from Nepal to India is one of the busiest sex slave trafficking routes in the world, with anywhere from 5,000 to 10,000 Nepali women and girls trafficked to India every year.[83] Another survey conducted by the Indian Health Organization in a red light area of Mumbai shows *double* the government figure of 10,000 trafficked girls–with over 20,000 Nepali girls (between the ages of nine and twenty) in Mumbai brothels alone.[84] The situation *within* India is dire too, and there are increasing numbers of females from Northeastern states and Orissa who are trafficked and forced to marry men in states like Haryana and Punjab which have low female-to-male child sex ratios.[85]

SIN CITY

'In this city, anyone can be a prostitute—the girl next door, the married wife, even you,' says Kailash Chand, the fresh-faced sub-inspector responsible for the capture of two of Delhi's most notorious sex racketeers—Ichadhari Baba and Sonu Punjaban. I've been trying to get hold of Chand for days and have finally managed to track him down to his current posting at the Mehrauli Police Station. Till just a few years ago, Mehrauli, on the outskirts of Delhi, was a large village. Today, while traces of the village still exist, much of the area has been rezoned and developed into luxury malls, designer stores, posh nightclubs and bars. Mehrauli is also at the centre of a complex prostitution racket.

I meet Chand on the night of Dussehra, or Vijayadashami, the festival that celebrates the slaying of the demon Ravana by Lord Rama. Peeping at me through the window of the police station, against the silhouette of the historical Qutab Minar, is a giant fifty-foot-tall effigy of Ravana that has just been set on fire. Outside in the smoggy evening, there is a continuous eruption of fireworks that sound like gunshots. The crowds cheer rapturously as the flames crawl up Ravana's body; dark fumes creep in through the window.

'This mattress,' says Chand, proudly pointing to the grimy mattress that I sit on, 'is where Ichadhari Baba spent ten days. I became good friends with him and he told me his story.'

One foggy February morning, Kailash Chand was sent to recover an anonymous, unclaimed corpse—cause of death unknown. The post-mortem of the dead man revealed a ball of heroin lodged in his body. Using mules is a standard technique to smuggle heroin, but in this particular instance it had backfired, and the heroin had spilt into the man's organs, killing him. The cell phone of the dead man revealed Ichadhari Baba's number on the list of recently dialled calls, and it was suspected that the pimp may have been involved with this transaction.

The meteoric rise to wealth, and infamy of Shiv Murti Dwivedi alias Ram Murat Dwivedi alias Rajiv Ranjan Dwivedi, more popularly known as Ichadhari Sant Swami Bhimanandji Maharaj 'Chitrakoot waale' or simply 'Baba', was bewildering, to say the least. A Class X dropout, Baba hailed from a family of criminals. His father was named in five criminal cases including murder, dowry and theft, his elder brother was convicted for the murder of his wife, and his two younger brothers were convicted in cases of theft. After holding a variety of odd jobs in his hometown of Chitrakoot in southern Uttar Pradesh, Baba arrived in Delhi in early 2000, though at this time he was known by a number of simpler names like Shiva, Rajeev, Shiny or Swami. He began his career in Delhi as a rickshaw driver, but was later employed as a security guard at a five-star Delhi hotel because of his good looks and muscular body. At the hotel he was introduced to the flesh trade when he served as a delivery boy for payments. Observing the potential of the business, Baba became a gigolo. One of his first assignments was to have sex with a newly-wed couple from Punjab who paid him a handsome ₹1.5 lakh for a week of sex. It is unclear exactly when Baba gave up being a gigolo to become a pimp, but it is likely to have been in the mid-2000s. It is also unclear when Baba became a self-proclaimed swami, donning saffron robes, and preaching at a temple in South Delhi which he personally funded, but sources say that it was right around the time that he became a pimp.

During the day Baba gave impassioned religious discourses; handed out CDs, books, and pamphlets of his teachings; and lured female students away from colleges, private coaching institutes and hostels into his net through his spiritual humbug. At night he was a pimp with a network of over a hundred sub-pimps and a thousand prostitutes, eventually growing his business to become one of north India's most extensive prostitution rackets. Through his operations he had also amassed property in Mumbai, Noida, Kolkata and Varanasi. Baba was meticulous in his operations, keeping extensive records of his business, of the women he employed, their movements, clients and payments—one of the reasons he was able to avoid arrest for a long time. He also had multiple mobile phones and cars in which he transported the girls, and he was well connected politically and with the police.

In an interview for *Hard News* magazine, a woman claiming to be Ichadhari Baba's girlfriend revealed how he conducted his operations:

> [H]e used to lure drop-out college girls and girls working with BPOs with expensive gifts. Once these girls fell in his trap, he compulsively used them in the flesh trade. This was like a honey trap plus a vicious circle. A few days back, he

spoke to me about the CWG [Commonwealth Games]—
"how lucrative it could be for us". We could earn lakhs in
just one week and even get a chance to settle abroad. He
told the girls that lots of guests would come during the
games, from India and abroad, and that he has arranged
"facilitation jobs" for girls during the games in Delhi.[86]

On the night of his capture, Baba traded in his saffron robes for a pair of jeans and a stylish shirt, and tied his long hair in a ponytail. He brought six girls with him that evening, two foreigners and four Indians, all of whom were English-speaking, attractive and well turned out—dressed conservatively in jeans, long-sleeved shirts, and scarves. Of the girls on offer, two were airhostesses and the other four were students and foreign tourists. The two customers had spoken to Baba on the phone and asked him for fine girls, and were willing to pay a premium for the right ones. They settled on two Indian girls, offering to pay ₹20,000 for the whole night. The men finalized the girls of their choice, paid an advance, and agreed to meet at one of Baba's flats the next day. On the way out of the bar Baba was nabbed along with the six girls. The two customers were policemen in disguise, one of whom was Kailash Chand on the first sting operation of his career.

This was not the first time that Baba had been arrested. In 1997, he had been charged with being involved in the flesh trade under cover of running a massage parlour. Another time, he had been arrested for buying stolen items. His two arrests qualified him to be tried under the Maharashtra Control of Organized Crime (MCOCA)—a strict law used against terrorists, under which the accused is held under severe conditions, making it near impossible to get bail. The punishment for being charged with MCOCA is severe and life imprisonment is common. After his arrest Baba went back to jail, this time for a much longer period than he had anticipated.

Chand remembers a few things about the time that he spent with Baba. He remembers how handsome he was and how 'solid' his body was. He was also charming and personable, and Chand had found it easy to talk to him. Baba had been forthcoming with his information. Usually he had to beat criminals, but Baba happily regaled Chand with his life story. Baba told Chand that he felt that what he was doing was 'karma yoga', or selfless service; through his prostitution racket he was ridding society of rape, sexual assault and other crimes that could arise due to sexual frustration.

Baba has been in jail since 2010. He is yet to be convicted, but the endless trial goes on. Records reveal that he has a wife and daughter in his native village, though they are not in touch. Chand tells me that Baba has become quite a personality in jail where he continues to give daily spiritual discourses. As I prepare to leave Chand's office he turns philosophical. He points to the columns of smoke rising slowly into the clear night sky and tells me that he, like Lord Rama, burns evil—modern day Ravanas like Ichadhari Baba—to the ground.

THE QUEEN BEE

There are certain things that stand out about Sonu Punjaban from her case files. The first is her fetish for men with criminal minds. All three of her ex-husbands were gangsters who were killed in shootouts. Another is her extensive network and impeccable organization—impressive for a woman who hasn't studied beyond Class VII. Her phone book has more than 1,000 contacts: women are listed according to the prices they charge, pimps according to the area they serve. The third is her perspicaciousness. Though she owns flats and cars, and some estimate her daily income to be upwards of ₹1 lakh a day, nothing is registered in her name, a move that may end up saving her from a lifetime in jail.

After the arrest of Ichadhari Baba, Sonu Punjaban was the new kingpin of the flesh trade in Delhi. Like Baba, Geeta Arora alias Sonu Punjaban entered the flesh trade as a prostitute. Desperately in need of money after the death of her husband and the birth of her son, she was inducted into the trade by her colleague at a beauty parlour. Her husband, Vijay, had been a gangster who married a sixteen-year-old Sonu when he was out on parole. Vijay was killed in a shootout when she was pregnant, and his death was a turning point in Sonu's life. Her father was dead, her sister's husband was in jail, and her two younger brothers were school dropouts with no jobs. She was with child, and had no means of survival. This is when she turned to prostitution, and then quickly moved on to pimping.

According to Sonu's mother, who spoke to journalist Chinki Sinha when she was trying to piece together Sonu's story after her arrest, 'If Vijay hadn't died, Sonu wouldn't have become what she has. She wouldn't have destroyed herself.'[87] By the time her son Paras was born, Sonu was a drug addict and could not breastfeed her child. Sonu tried her best at motherhood, something that didn't come naturally to her, but eventually she left the upbringing of her son to her mother.[88]

Sonu may not have been a natural mother but she proved to be a natural Madam, and the timing of her business was just right, what with the growing consumerism and greater disposable incomes of the Indian middle class. Sonu married again—this time a car thief who helped her grow her business by acquiring flats to house her prostitutes and cars to transport them in. He was killed two years after they were married in a police encounter. Sonu's greatest love was her third husband, Hemant alias Sonu, a gangster whom she married in 2002. It seemed she had bad luck with men, for he too was killed in a police encounter in 2006.[89]

At the time of her third husband's death, Sonu's business was flourishing. She had identified her target market as middle-class men with limited disposable income who wanted a pleasant sexual experience that the brothels on GB Road could not offer. So she employed middle-class women who spoke English, were attractive and well dressed. She set up brothels in flats that she either owned or rented and appointed pimps who worked under her, in charge of specific areas.[90]

Prostitution is thought of as a soft crime by the police. Usually the police don't get involved with sex workers and leave them alone because they know that even if sex workers are arrested, they can afford bail and good lawyers, and they usually resume work almost immediately upon release. It is only when a pimp is involved in other criminal activities like drug trafficking or he/she becomes too powerful and their racket grows to threatening proportions that the police feel compelled to step in. By 2010, Sonu's network reached across the country, with an estimated monthly income of ₹50 lakh. Once again it was Kailash Chand who posed as the decoy customer to trap Sonu. Assuming that the baby-faced Chand was a customer of means, Raju Sharma, Sonu's right-hand man, led him straight into Sonu's den.

This is where Kailash first met Sonu—an attractive woman of medium height with sharp, hawkish features, fair skin and streaked blonde hair. The women that she offered were young and attractive, and as he negotiated the price with Sonu, Kailash remembers how the women titillated him, squeezing their breasts and groping their crotches through the short, polyester skirts that they wore. They licked their lips, fluttered their eyelashes, and blew him kisses. 'They acted drunk, or high, or maybe even both, though I could tell from the way they walked in their high heels that they weren't,' Chand tells me.

Sonu was nabbed and taken to the Saket Police Station, where she spent a week in jail, being interrogated by Chand. At that time, she was going through a rehab programme since she was addicted to cocaine. Without drugs or treatment, Sonu was fading, and she would smoke an endless number of cigarettes, almost a hundred a day, to get through the interrogation. 'The only time she cried,' says Chand, 'is when we put MCOCA on her.' She knew that there was no escape from this, and that she could be in jail for a long time.

Sonu has now been in Delhi's Tihar jail for three years. Her son is eight years old and lives with his grandmother. He hasn't seen his mother in two years. Even though Sonu is in jail, she has a boyfriend. Arun Thakral, a young man in his early twenties worked for Sonu as a driver and pimp, ferrying girls back and forth from their homes to clients. He was arrested with her but is now out on bail. He is hoping to marry Sonu when she is released from jail.

◆

Rashmi is sick. Her face is the colour of chalk, she has fiery red welts on her lips and face, and she is rake-thin, dressed in a pair of tight jeans and a kurta which hangs loosely on her skeletal frame. Rashmi is one of the fifty women who worked for Sonu on a monthly wage of ₹1.5 lakh. For this wage she was obliged to do five 'shots' a day, or have intercourse with up to five clients. She had one day off a week.

Rashmi joined the sex trade when she was nineteen years old. She was newly married and had moved to Delhi from Kolkata. Hers had been an arranged marriage to a man whom she had met only once, chosen on the basis of his Brahmin caste and a steady government job. He turned out to be a wife-beater and an alcoholic who raped her regularly. Rashmi left him, only discovering later that she was pregnant. Her parents would not take back a tainted daughter, and when she told her husband she was pregnant, he did not believe that the baby was his and threw her out of her house. Rashmi was forced to get a job, which she didn't have trouble finding as she was armed with a good education and could speak English well. A colleague of Rashmi's at the BPO she worked for introduced her to the easy cash of the sex trade, which she desperately needed now that she had a baby to care for.

At twenty-nine, Rashmi has now been a sex worker for a decade. She tells me that she has left the sex trade, and now works at a beauty parlour. From the look and feel of her soft-as-cotton, immaculately manicured hands, I do not see the evidence of hard beauty parlour work. Her comfortable, well-lit apartment strewn with bright children's toys and photographs of her pretty daughter suggests that she makes more money than a job at a beauty parlour would bring in, and there is only one way that Rashmi knows how to do that.

Over the five years that Rashmi worked for Sonu, she saw her grow from a lowly pimp into the kingpin of New Delhi, India's biggest market for prostitution. She attributed this to Sonu's business acumen and her connections with Delhi's gangster networks that could keep the police at bay. 'She was a mean, hard woman, with only one thing on her mind—money,' says Rashmi about Sonu. 'She was also a cheater and a scamster and was not willing to let even a rupee go.'

According to another employee who worked for Sonu as a pimp, Punjaban was an aggressive and domineering employer, interfering in his family life, and demanding absolute loyalty in return.[91] Sonu would systematically fleece the girls working for her. Sometimes she would send goons pretending to be police when the girls were with clients. When the girls called Sonu, she spoke to the men and offered them money to let the girls go. Sonu would then withhold this money from their salary, saying that she had used it to protect them. Rashmi had considered getting off Sonu's payroll many times, working only on contract, where she would get 50 per cent of the money that the client paid. But for this, the client usually chose the sex worker, and Rashmi felt she wasn't as attractive as she was when she was younger, and wouldn't be able to pull clients. She needed the regular income to maintain her household expenses.

Rashmi admits though that Sonu was occasionally kind. She says she would smile and act nice when she held Rashmi's daughter in her lap. 'She was kinder to women with children, maybe because she was a mother herself. She would occasionally give us small gifts and sometimes money. She was also nice to children, like she was to my daughter,' says Rashmi. Rashmi looks at a picture of her daughter and says with a sigh, 'I never imagined this to be my future when I was young, living in Kolkata with my parents. I was a very decent human being back then, but today, even though I am not decent, I am happier than when I was married to that demon. My daughter's future is not in my hands. I came from a good family but ended up like this. My daughter doesn't come from a good home but could end up with a good man. The only thing I can do is to pray for her.'

HIGH-CLASS HOOKER

'Our waitresses are beautiful, polished, and friendly. When you come to LAP [Lounge and Play] you feel like you've come home,' says the manager of LAP, the hippest nightclub in Delhi, promoted by Bollywood star Arjun Rampal. One of the unique offerings at LAP is foreign waitresses and hostesses. Every few months, a new batch of girls is brought in from various parts of the world, including Eastern Europe, South America and South Africa. According to a manager at the club which opened its doors in 2009, it is this concept of hiring foreigners as waitresses, hostesses and bartenders that has helped create a loyal member base for the club.

To Stephanie, a job at LAP sounded tremendously exciting. She was working at a resto-bar in Cape Town, South Africa, when a conversation with an agent, an Indian gentleman of silky refinement, led to the job offer. In her country, where unemployment was high, New Delhi seemed to be the centre of an alluring new world, so she signed a year-long contract, quickly packed her bags and moved. However, her experience at LAP had been disappointing. The nightclub itself wasn't bad, they paid her a decent salary, and the place, though gaudy, was fashionable. It was her experiences night after night that were unbearable. The nightclub seemed to her dominated by the worst kind of people—rude, tackily dressed men who would get too drunk too fast, and women who always looked bored, not caring what their boyfriends or husbands did. When she first arrived, she had thought about leaving the job and going back home, but she knew that with the current market scenario, it would be impossible to find a job, and she could not afford to stay unemployed.

While she was working at LAP, Stephanie met Sabrina, a French woman who ran an escort service in New Delhi and claimed to provide sophisticated entertainment to Delhi's most elite society. She offered Stephanie a job which included going to fine parties, hosting fancy dinners and providing companionship to lonely, wealthy, single people who wished for refined company. This was Stephanie's way out. She quickly quit her job at LAP and began working with Sabrina. Within a few months, it was clear to Stephanie that her elite clients wanted more than just refined company. In the beginning she only had sex with her steady clients, men she considered to be her boyfriends, and only because she wanted to, but soon she realized how lucrative this was, and began selling sex to whoever paid generously. She began making more money than she ever had in her life.

Stephanie's clients are mostly businessmen from Delhi and Mumbai. Her business is nation-wide and she travels frequently to the south, to Chennai and Hyderabad to service clients there. Recently there has been demand from smaller cities like Indore, Raipur and Ahmedabad as they explode with new money. She typically gets paid around $2,000 or ₹1 lakh per 'shot'. This is about twenty times more than what Nita gets paid, and 200 times more than Vimla. Stephanie's most gainful earnings were during the Commonwealth Games held in Delhi in 2010. She tells me that the pimps (many of them foreigners who flew in to reap the benefits of the Games) were very professional about the whole process. She was put through a series of medical tests and asked to show her reports before she was hired to service top athletes. She says that this was the first time that she actually felt like a hooker.

◆

The pioneer of the high-end professional escort business in the country was the 'Cadillac Pimp', aka Kanwaljit Singh who earned the nickname from his expensive taste in automobiles. The Cadillac Pimp's women of choice were from Russia and the CIS who came to India via Dubai. These women demanded a premium for their services (compared to their Indian and Nepali counterparts) and operated in five-star hotels, booking three to four clients a night: usually wealthy individuals—businessmen, politicians and visiting foreigners.

The Cadillac Pimp had an unremarkable past. He was born in Allahabad, his father was a government accounts officer and his mother a schoolteacher. He graduated with a degree in English from an obscure university in Kanpur. After graduating, he moved to Delhi to set up a small business supplying automotive parts which went bust after a while. His reasons for entering the sex trade are unclear, but some say that it was through a prostitute he met who also provided him with his initial stake.[92] Singh had first mover's advantage in a fledgling market; his business prospered and by the end of the decade, he ran India's most extensive prostitution ring which included top models, actresses, bar dancers, and his biggest money spinner—a bevy of foreign escorts. According to one police officer, 'He could get any girl… From Bollywood actors to top models, he had the best women.'[93] Singh had even managed to tap a growing international market, and supplied women to Hong Kong, Thailand and Singapore.

When he grew too big for his boots, the police raided his operation. At the time of his arrest in 2005, Singh had over 300 women working for him and was estimated to make over ₹10 lakh a month. He was charged and prosecuted under MCOCA, but after spending five years in prison, he was acquitted of all charges on the basis of insufficient evidence. Beyond confessions and a few cell phone and hotel bills found at his residence, there was no hard evidence against India's most infamous pimp.[94] After his release, Singh has gone underground. Some say that he moved to Dubai, others say he has changed his identity. Whatever the truth is, I am unable to trace him.

To get a better understanding of the high-end sex trade today, I speak with Mumbai's top pimp. Arif Khan is a well-oiled, well-spoken man who cuts a slightly menacing figure with his black-leather Armani jacket, gelled hair, and tattooed neck. He arrives for the interview in a luxury sedan accompanied by a personal security guard dressed in a smart navy blue safari suit. He claims to have thirty girls working for him full-time, personally hand-picked from across the globe. He has over a hundred girls who operate part-time. He also tells me that Indian men prefer girls from Eastern Europe.

Immigration officials estimate that of the 50,000-odd Indian tourist visas granted in the Central Asian countries of Ukraine, Kazakhstan, Uzbekistan, Azerbaijan, and Kyrgyzstan every year, nearly 5,000 visitors are part of the sex trade.[95] There has been such a surge of women from these countries to India that in 2011 the Indian government issued an official note to its embassies to carefully screen visa applications of women aged between fifteen and forty entering the country. This notice created such an uproar that it led to a protest in Kiev where women demonstrated topless in front of the Indian embassy.[96]

The prostitution racket involving foreign women, particularly from CIS countries began with the collapse of the Soviet Union. Young women looking for a quick buck ended up in Dubai as high-end hookers. Over the past five years, the racket has been diverted to India because of the financial crisis in Dubai and the flush of new money in India.

Eastern European women form the highest end of the sex trade, charging up to ₹10 lakh an hour for their services and an average of 40 per cent more than their Indian counterparts—a premium they can charge because of the colour of their skin, reflecting the Indian obsession with fair skin. According to Pramada Menon, a Delhi-based gender activist, 'Sex with light-skinned women is aspirational for some men.'[97]

Additional Deputy Police Commissioner Joy Tirkey, Delhi Crime Branch, says that the racket has become so professional that many pimps have begun to arrange paper marriages between foreign women and Indian nationals. 'In paper marriages, the husband is someone like a salesman at a local kirana shop. Once the visa issues are sorted, these women start living like normal people, they feel like they are free, and they go out to shops and malls without nervousness.'[98]

Just last year, Tirkey shut down three agencies that employed sixteen women from Uzbekistan, Kyrgyzstan, and Ukraine. To avoid suspicion, their handlers worked on rotation, bringing a girl for six months, then sending her back and replacing her with another.

Indian women find it difficult to counter the 'white cult' that is taking over the premium flesh trade. If it's an Indian woman, the advertisement reads: she is a 'Punjabi' (read intense and fair), 'model' (slim and beautiful), 'air hostess' (suave and smart), 'hygienic' (clean), 'broadminded', and 'sober'. Broadminded assures clients that the women will play out their fantasies, while 'sober' indicates that they will be professional about it.[99]

Arif Khan's clients include top politicians, businessmen, and a slew of foreigners who visit the city regularly and pay up to ₹10 lakh for his top girls. Khan's business has grown exponentially in the past five years. After the 2010 Commonwealth Games in Delhi, there was a crackdown on prostitution in Delhi, so many girls moved to Mumbai. Many of the girls harbour 'romantic Bollywood dreams' and hope that by servicing famous producers and actors they may land a role in one of their films. I ask Khan if any of his girls has managed to do this. He laughs loudly and says that a few of them have landed roles as extras on Bollywood sets. One of the girls, an exceptionally good dancer, became a back-up dancer, in the 'back row since she was so tall'. He adds that he could barely spot her during the film though he watched the song many times. He tells me that many of his girls stop their association with him when someone plants Bollywood dreams in their head.

With an ominous note of finality, Khan tells me, 'When they think they are going to become stars, they want to stop being prostitutes. But these women are not actresses, they are here to be fucked, and if they don't do what they have come here to do, they will be sent back to where they came from.' I ask Khan about the Cadillac Pimp. Khan looks awestruck as he talks about Singh and his operations. Khan was one of a kind, and no pimp has yet been able to take over his pedestal. Singh built a national, even international, network which would be unimaginable at this time. It is rumoured that Singh got into a tiff with a chief minister who then brought him down. The problem, Khan says, is that Singh got too big for his own shoes. 'You have to be smart to run a business like this. The people who get caught are the ones who become too big.'

◆

In Chennai, I speak to Ram, named after the virtuous Hindu God who is described in various Hindu scriptures as the perfect man. My Ram though is far from perfect, at least when it comes to the virtuous part. Ram has a face that is difficult to recall. The only distinctive thing about him is the look of caution that he bears. He works in his family business, a small leather goods import-export venture. Ram is dating Leela, whom he first met through an escort service. Leela is from Ukraine, where she tried unsuccessfully for many years to be a model. At the behest of Arif Khan, she moved to India, where she works as a model while moonlighting as an escort. In Chennai, Leela is a minor celebrity.

She is invited to all the hot and happening parties of the city, occasionally even gracing the society pages of the newspapers.

Though Leela's rise to fame is fascinating, I am here to speak with Ram and to explore the mentality of a client. Ram talks to me about the women he has dated, one of whom he loved and almost married. His family was dead-set against the marriage because she was Muslim and he Hindu. Succumbing to family pressure, he had to call it off. Since that horrible experience, he doesn't want to get involved in a serious affair that could end in marriage, or in the words of Ram, 'a life-long imprisonment'.

Ram opens up to me after a few drinks (he only drinks Black Label, on the rocks) at a trendy Chennai bar. He relaxes and speaks to me candidly about sex. Ram's first sexual experience was at eighteen with a prostitute in Mumbai. He had never had a girlfriend; he didn't even have many friends who were girls. The only women he knew were his cousins, who were strictly off limits. Since those early years, he has had girlfriends whom he has had sex with, but he continues to pay for sex. Today, though, Ram would never think about going to a brothel, and no one in his circle of friends would ever use down-market local or Nepali hookers who, 'you can bang for 300 bucks in a 200 rupee joint'. He 'only goes for white girls' whom he can afford due to his rising income and flourishing business.

As he continues tossing back glasses, Ram opens up about himself. 'In my teenage years, I was frustrated because there were no girls. They are kept in their houses with the single aim of marriage. That is why I went to that hooker on my eighteenth birthday. I was sick of being a virgin.'

I ask him why he continued to go to prostitutes even when he had girlfriends.

He considers, 'It's not the same with Indian girls. Most won't have sex with me, not till many months into the relationship when they feel it is "serious" or that I may marry them, so I am forced to go to hookers.'

Ram is not alone in his sexual pursuits: 49 per cent of young men in metro cities have had sex with sex workers.[100]

'Do your girlfriends know?' I ask curiously.

'I don't think so, but then shouldn't they expect it? I am a man and I have my needs.'

Ram tells me that he loves Leela, but that he could never marry her.

'She is not the sort of girl that I would marry, but I treat her like my queen, and she gives me the sort of pleasure that an Indian woman would never be able to give me.'

Does Leela, his present girlfriend, take clients on the side? How does he feel about that? I ask.

He replies in a reflective vein. 'She takes clients sometimes. It is her job, it is her need, and I don't want to stop her. It's like the time I was with my Indian girlfriend. I had my needs, so I went to hookers. Leela is a good girl, she is not the hooker type, but she too has her needs and I understand that.'

LOUNGE AND PLAY, LAP

At the bacchanalia that is meant to be New Delhi's hottest nightclub, the jeunesse dorée of the country guzzle astronomically priced bottles of vintage champagne—prices that would put the best nightclubs in Europe to shame. The cavernous nightclub is decorated in deep reds and luscious purples with heavy velvet curtains, outrageous chandeliers and blowzy Moroccan rococo festooning the walls.

Tonight Stephanie is stationed at the bar. She serves drinks expertly, occasionally glaring if someone gets too loud. Although she doesn't work full-time at LAP any longer, she sometimes comes in on a big night to do some bartending. I wait for her in a small room behind the bar, watching her work: she pours drinks swiftly, and never smiles, barely making eye contact with her customers. One man touches her arm, she moves away without a word. Another man leans over and taps her shoulder, she takes a step backward. She comes to take a break and lights up a cigarette. She looks angry and frustrated and pulls hard on her cigarette. She tells me that she's happy she doesn't do this any longer.

How does she maintain her cool, I ask. She shrugs and tells me that when she is on edge, on the verge of losing her cool and lashing out at these drunken demons, she remembers the much publicized case of Jessica Lal, the young model who was shot dead by a politician's son at a socialite's bar only because she refused to serve him a drink. What terrifies her most is that any of these men in this club could easily be that man. That case showed the dark side of India's nightlife. The sudden influx of money and unbridled hedonism into the country's once impoverished nightlife has led to sometimes unrestrained debauchery. Today nightclubs like LAP are an integral part of India's party culture and are filled with over the top and often obscene revelry. Brothels have always represented sensualism and a dissolute lifestyle, but this new form is often violent because it is too much too soon.

Stephanie takes me for a walk around the club. I am alarmed by how many foreign women there are in the club—at the door, at the bar, flitting around the tables. We pass by a large table on which many bottles of alcohol sit like proud trophies. There is a flurry of young, foreign girls mingling with the men and women at the table.

I ask tentatively, 'Are they...?'

'No, they are not. They are models who will eventually become,' she says with a small smile, 'like me.'

In many ways the girls at LAP are rather like Mughal tawaifs: beautiful seductresses. The courtesans of today are young foreign girls who may not be adept in the sixty-four kalas, but who have their own set of credentials. They look good, dress well, flirt expertly and titillate professionally. I ask her something that I have had on my mind for a while now. Why does she do this when she has other options?

'How can I go back to serving drinks?' she says wryly. 'I am addicted, I guess. Like an addict is to cocaine.'

It then becomes clear to me. Prostitution may have taken on a new look, but it remains a primeval game. Though a new form of prostitution was brewing where sex work took place in five-star hotels instead of brothels and girls solicited in nightclubs instead of on the streets, the mentality, the economics, the desperation, the addiction and the darkness too were as old as desire.

THE DARK SIDE*

Her violent death made headlines around the world. On 16 December 2012, a young woman the media called Nirbhaya (or fearless) was brutally gang-raped in a moving bus in New Delhi. The rapists were men between the ages of fifteen and thirty-four, new migrants from Bihar. The young woman too was from a migrant family from UP. Her father worked as a loader at the airport. While the woman epitomized an upward economic trajectory, and seemed set to enter the ranks of the great Indian middle class, her rapists—sex-starved, repressed and horrifically violent—were mired at the very bottom of Indian society and seemed doomed to enact the roles that had been waiting for them.

Beyond the barbarous bodily injuries that included broken ribs and limbs and acute damage to the abdomen, over three-fourths of Nirbhaya's intestines had been pulled out of her body through her vagina. The physicians on duty at AIIMS (The All India Institute of Medical Sciences) where she was first taken that night told me that they had never seen such brutal and horrific violence inflicted on a human body.

This time the rape struck home, more than any that had preceded it, because many of the nation's young people, many of its young women in particular, found it easy to identify with the young woman. She was young, she was bright; they admired her

---

*This chapter was contributed by Anjani Trivedi.

grit and determination to better herself, her free-spirited ways, the fact that she loved high heels and going to the mall with her boyfriend to watch movies. The truth was that Nirbhaya could have been any one of us, and any one of us could have been her, and perhaps this is what scared us all and finally brought us out on the streets.

Nirbhaya's brutal rape drew more attention to the status of women in India than any other event in the country's recent history. The Indian government promised justice, the capital would be safer they said, they would take action against these criminals and many others. The then chief minister of Delhi Sheila Dikshit broke down on national television after a visit to the hospital, the leader of the ruling party, Sonia Gandhi, cancelled her New Year's plans and mourned the death of this young woman who had done no wrong but board a bus.

Parents ordered their daughters to remain indoors for safety's sake, but that didn't stop the young from taking to the streets. The country rippled with anger and dissent as people poured out in droves, demanding the death of the rapists. I joined them, one of the thousands of young people who protested against antiquated legal systems, a lax police force, and the awful patriarchal mentality that has infested the nation from time immemorial.

Two weeks after the brutal rape, Nirbhaya died in Singapore where she had been flown for treatment. The nation mourned her death with silent vigils and in young hearts across the country a single resolution was made—the violence, the savagery would have to end.

◆

As we have seen in earlier chapters, India's rapid economic growth has been a mixed blessing to the country. While there is no doubt that it has had a profound impact on the personal lives of hundreds of millions—the 315 million[101] and growing youth demographic—the change that has resulted has often been for the worse. This is true of the sexual revolution as well.

Why this is so is not hard to see. It has happened too quickly with little or no time for the participants in the revolution to grasp what is going on, to settle down, to socialize, to internalize the change. The state has done little or nothing to help, and when it has tried it has been less than successful. The dark side then is a manifestation of what has gone wrong, what is going wrong and what will go wrong when people, who are not ready for it, have new ideas, visions and, above all, freedoms thrust upon their existing patrilineal, patrilocal and patriarchal thought processes.

Megamalls are erupting next to maize farms. A young woman buys a mojito at a bar; a young man, who has never seen a woman other than his sister or mother, is shaking up the cocktail for her. Young men and women are uprooted from their homes, and in the process, unknowingly at times, lose their social anchoring.

The uneven and unwieldy growth has also meant huge numbers of people moving across the country in search of work. According to a report by McKinsey, the geographic pattern of India's income and consumption growth is shifting too. In a decade, the Indian consumer market will 'largely be an urban story, with 62 per cent of consumption in urban areas versus 42 per cent today'.[102]

This great migration has meant layers of India's super-stratified society are forced to mix; people are intermingling like never before and are gentrifying the same spaces. All is seemingly healthy here, until the discrepancies and inequalities become apparent.

The resultant rapid urbanization is juxtaposed with an even faster influx of ideas. Bombarded with new ideas and sexualized content, generations are wrapped in chaos and confusion. This is India's challenge: aspirations gone sour, frustrations come alive.

AHEAD OF THE CURVE

Almost three years ago, *Tehelka*, the investigative website and magazine, found that 'age was more than just a number to several young people—it was a ticking stopwatch in the race to outdo each other in the bedroom'.[103]

Through interviews across the country the magazine's interviewers 'met terrifyingly sexual creatures of all shapes and sizes—nine-year-olds who distributed porn in class (spiral-bound and printed in booklets), 12-year-olds already visiting shrinks for relationships that had turned sour (because their parents discovered them having oral sex), 14-year-olds who had photographed themselves in the nude, made videos of their accomplishments and passed them around for classmates to cackle over and 16-year-olds who had impregnated 19-year-olds (and knew exactly "how to take care of it")'.

The revolution is apparent—through the eyes of those in it, those watching and those looking back.

Dr Shireen Jejeebhoy of the Population Council in India has been studying the situation and the needs of young people for three decades now, and has realized that addressing these needs is an integral part of addressing India's future and India's ability to reap what it sows. A survey of the literature and academic work makes it very clear that there isn't a comprehensive understanding of young people, particularly in a changing India.

From Dr Jejeebhoy's public health perspective, one thing is obvious: young people's sexual and reproductive health vulnerabilities are being ignored, the information and services for supportive socialization are being 'swept under the carpet' and a comprehensive discourse on addressing these concerns is non-existent.

Between November 2007 and December 2008, Dr Jejeebhoy and her team headed off to Bihar and Jharkhand to conduct a facility-based survey at abortion clinics across the states. Of their respondents, 78.3 per cent were residents of urban areas. Studies over the last few decades suggest that patterns in rural and urban areas are often similar when it comes to the proportion of young, unmarried women seeking abortions. Together with an NGO,

Janani, which performs most of the abortions across the two states, they surveyed 549 young women between the ages of fifteen and twenty-four at sixteen clinics. Young and naive, a lot of these unmarried women had never before spoken about their qualms about abortion and pregnancies out of wedlock.

Dr Jejeebhoy was pleasantly surprised by the enthusiastic response the team received. They were expecting to be stoned and thrown out of villages for prying into private lives. In fact, community members agreed that it was important to discuss sexual behaviour and violence. 'Of course, they denied that their children are sexually active...' Dr Jejeebhoy said.

She recalled that, initially, many women hid their marital status but the research team deployed a strategy to conceal the interviewees' identities and maintain that anonymity. After all, they were unmarried, young and pregnant—an unforgivable transgression in the eyes of the community.

The results of Dr Jejeebhoy's study couldn't have been more explicit—India's social infrastructure was 'devastatingly fractured'.[104]

Young, unmarried women were having sex and two thirds of the sample had wanted to have sex. Most of them had delayed realizations that they were pregnant. Then, they were having abortions in unsafe ways—from the foetus being beaten out of them to medical abortion pills to 'eating unripe papaya or drinking a brew made from peppercorn, papaya seeds and coffee'. These were unregistered abortions in unsanctioned places. What was interesting was that most of the women were either scared or anxious, but did not feel guilty.

Consensual encounters seemed to far outweigh non-consensual ones. And, as Jejeebhoy explained to me, the unintended and unwanted pregnancies were more likely to be a consequence of consensual encounters.[105]

That's a positive sign. However, scratching the surface exposes what is really happening under the sheets and behind closed doors; these affairs are largely driven by young men with a 'sense of experiment' in sexual relationships with young women who are usually coaxed into it under false pretences like marriage or a future together, Dr Jejeebhoy told me. Moreover, male manipulation was complemented by female naiveté.

Both the young woman and the young man were active participants in the act, yet the burden of honour was rooted in a woman's sexuality.[106] 'A "tainted" girl makes her family lose their reputation—it is very closely linked to girls, not to boys,' she said. Women were sexual capital and this had solidified the underpinnings of sexual stratification.[107] In India, this capital is the property of and transferrable by men; hence the entitlement.

Violence pervades this backdrop of male entitlement and female irrelevance—in homes, through workplaces, through lives visible and invisible.

Together, they make a potent concoction that engenders many forms of violence, and rape is only the tip of the iceberg. Dr Jejeebhoy says the women in Bihar saw only one possible alternative to the violence they endured everyday: death. 'When they talk about alternatives to sustain, they talk about suicide and taking pills, taking poison, burning themselves,' she told me.

Although Dr Jejeebhoy's sample was principally composed of girls in rural and semi-urban areas who could only be said to have been impacted by the sexual revolution that is taking place in India's cities at one remove, her findings do make an important point. For all the newfound freedom and sexual experimentation that girls seem to be engaging in, very little seems to have changed in the larger context, which has inevitably led to conflict and mayhem—the dark side.

'It's the culture we live in,' she said.

As is well known, women in Indian society are enshrined in religion or spirituality; there they are objectified as goddesses but they are otherwise never seen as harbingers of good luck or necessary to uphold a family's fortunes. Sons on the other hand are necessary to kindle the funeral pyre of their late parents and to assist in the onward journey of the soul. According to Manu, a man has to be reborn as a man in order to attain moksha (redemption). A man cannot attain moksha unless he has a son to light his funeral pyre. And only sons can till farms.

Indian society, like many societies the world over, is patrilineal, patriarchal, and patrilocal.

In the era of low technology, then, what was done with girls? They were crudely and systematically killed. This led to the much reported missing girls of India phenomenon and the severely skewed sex ratio which worsened over the last six decades.[108]

The entry of prenatal diagnostic technology in the 1970s changed the mode of killing young girls. Two techniques—amniocentesis and ultrasonography—flourished. Indians took to the latter, a cheaper and non-invasive technology, so much so that companies like General Electric had their heyday when they started selling ultrasound machines to India. No longer was it outright murder, it was now veiled in the womb.

'Ultrasound technology entered at the very time people wanted to have fewer kids and the fertility rate was on the decline,' says Mara Hvistendahl, author of *Unnatural Selection*, a book on how technology is skewing sex ratios and the Asian preference for boys. India's gender imbalance was exacerbated by technology.

In 1994, the Indian government came down hard with the Pre-Conception and Pre-Natal Diagnostic Techniques Act (PCPNDT Act) that made sex determination a criminal offence. But there hasn't been much of an uptick in the statistics. Instead, Indians are now fleeing abroad to have boys. Sex-selective fertilization is the latest trend. The advent of better technology means no killing, just choosing to have a boy. The number of Indians seeking sex-selective fertility outside the country has 'increased exponentially in the last ten years,' Dr Jeffrey Steinberg, one of the world's most high-profile sex selection doctors, told me a few months ago.

Amongst India's youngest populations,[109] the gender ratio continues to worsen.

'Everybody wants a son—whether wealthy or not wealthy. The idea is still not gone,' says a Delhi-based gynaecologist. She told me about disappointment-filled labour rooms every time she delivered a baby girl. Some superstitious patients go as far as to change their hospital for the next child.

The sex ratio is worse in wealthier areas. The more economically prosperous the place, the worse the decline in child sex ratios over the last two decades.[110] The economic cost-benefit analysis is no longer about tilling farms but about boys running the hundreds of family businesses that have cropped up during India's growth spurt. This is testament to India's access to technology, and the age-old obsession with male children.

The numbers, then, are hardly surprising. India's total sex ratio—defined as the number of females per 1,000 males—has become better over the past two decades, after dropping for the eighty years before that; but the statistic is still one of the worst in the world, alongside China. As of 2011, there were 940 Indian women for every 1,000 men, up from 933 in 2001.[111]

So, all told, India has 37 million more men than women, as of 2011 census data, and about 17 million excess men in the age group that commits most crimes, up from 7 million in 1991.[112]

TOO MANY MEN, TOO MUCH VIOLENCE

Gender imbalance in Asian countries has resulted in higher rates of crime, including rape, committed by young, unmarried men. The situation is worse (both in India and China) than it was ten years ago.[113] Violent crime against women increases as the deficit of women increases. This will constrain the life chances of females far into the future, according to social scientists.[114]

This violence is even proving to be economically perilous. Stories of women being harassed as they drive to work are frequent. One woman was shot dead as she was driving home from work in the evening, another gang-raped. As the International Labour Organisation (ILO) recently put it, the 'cultural attitudes and social norms about women in the work-place' in India shut women out. India's slowed economic growth is also attributed to a fall in female labour force participation.

Sexual harassment in India is an expression of the powerlessness of Indian men, not of their power, Shikha Dalmia of the Reason Foundation recently wrote. The 'real cause', as Dalmia put it, 'is free-floating male libido with no socially acceptable outlet.'[115] A broken social infrastructure that has not shown any signs of improvement is a harbinger of where India is headed.

LEFTOVER MEN

Other effects of the skewed sex ratio will be on marriage patterns in India. The probability of each and every man pairing up with a woman obviously drops as the number of men increases.

Christophe Z. Guilmoto noted that by 2025 the number of single men around twenty-five years of age 'will not only exceed the number of young women of corresponding age, but will also have to compete with a larger than expected number of older men who are still single'. He contended that many of these men will be left partnerless.[116]

Another consequence of too many men and the increasing deficit of potential female partners is likely to accelerate the trend toward marriage at later age and raise young men's risk of engaging in commercial sex. Experiences of young men in other parts of the world have proved this.

This has set the foundation for India's 'bare branches':[117] unmarried men from age fifteen to their mid-thirties who have limited prospects for employment. With India's youth unemployment rate hovering around double digits and labour trends showing young people withdrawing from the workforce, bare branches will flourish. Employment plays a pivotal role in shaping gender identities and gender relations. The employment status of a woman's partner affects her risk of spousal violence.[118]

These men are usually responsible for the majority of the

violence in societies. While a seemingly simplistic and causal allegation, just take look at the ages of all rapists in India, in fact, take a look at crime rates by age: the largest share is committed by men between the ages of fifteen and thirty-four. In the search for self-validation, they are prone to risky behaviour.

In such a fractured society, with a contorted demographic dynamic, the adverse effects of a sexual revolution are magnified. Hundreds of thousands of young people are falling through the cracks.

YOUNG, UNMARRIED AND...PREGNANT

I met Aasimah in a coffee shop in a busy neighbourhood in East Delhi. She stared out at the raucous streets and said dispiritedly: 'I never thought this was possible.'

A few weeks ago, Aasimah had felt something was off—she missed a menstrual cycle. Although she usually ignored such 'petty discomfort', a few days after her missed period she decided to stop by the 'ladies' doctor' or gynaecologist.

An uncomfortable examination and ultrasound later, she discovered she was four months pregnant. When the doctor told her she would have to be in the hospital for at least twenty-four hours, Aasimah insisted the procedure had to be fast—she knew she wouldn't be able to stay away from her conservative parents' home overnight.

When she walked out of the clinic, she headed to a cybercafe: she needed an education. She looked up 'abortions' and 'sexual intercourse' to figure out what had happened to her and what she needed to do.

Aasimah personifies the challenges that are increasingly plaguing India's young people. They are often sexually uneducated, practise unsafe sex, and then rush out to get unsafe abortions or are left with potentially lethal sexually transmitted diseases.

'This is the dark side of sexual liberation,' says Dr Rekha Khandelwal, Aasimah's gynaecologist. Dr Khandelwal, now in her late fifties, has seen the number of abortions skyrocket in the last decade.

A few years ago, the standard explanation for rising abortions would have been that women were killing off unwanted female foetuses. Today, however, according to Dr Khandelwal, the abortions that are being sought rarely have anything to do with gender. She gets ten to fifteen cases of pregnant, unmarried women between the ages of twenty to twenty-eight who want 'terminations' every month. And that's only half the story.

Women across the economic spectrum come to see Dr Khandelwal: some are young and callous, some are conservative, some are adulterous, some elite, some are on the cusp of urbanization; in other words it is impossible to typecast them.

Dr Khandelwal has evolved with the times as she has seen an increasing number of sexually active people walk through the doors of her clinic. For all the new lives she has brought into the world, for all the lives she has saved, she has also had to terminate a growing number.

She wishes young people would be more responsible, and she doesn't say this in a moralizing way, but simply wishes they would take better care of themselves. If they were more sexually aware, if they took more precautions, things wouldn't be as messy. There wouldn't need to be as many abortions.

The limited research in India attests to this—'first sex' is more often than not, 'unprotected for the majority of young people'.[119] Moreover, there is the huge risk of sexually transmitted infections.

A hospital-based study, done over a five-year period and published last year, reported a resurgence of syphilis in India and rising numbers of sexually transmitted diseases. The medical study noted that all the evidence pointed towards a change in the trends of sexual practices.

Aasimah had gotten pregnant out of wedlock; she had had sex with a man her age, in a closet in their college. She still doesn't understand how it happened, she says. The thought of a condom had presumably not occurred to either of them. Recent research has shown that more knowledge about contraceptives reduces risky sexual behaviour.[120]

'More and more young girls are becoming sexually active,' says Dr Khandelwal. A few years ago, she could tell whether young women who came to see her were married or not. She says the traditional symbols of married women—red sindoor in their parting, the beaded black and gold mangalsutra around their necks and 'general demeanour'—would be immediate clues about their virginity. Now, she can't rely on these symbols, signs of India's inherent transformation. Sometimes they come with men, who, until a few years ago, she could assume were their husbands. But today they are boyfriends, friends, or simply sexual partners.

There are two categories of unmarried girls, Dr Khandelwal explains, who are increasingly showing up at her clinic. The first is the 'advanced' ones who are seemingly liberal and come within the first few weeks, that is, within six to eight weeks of becoming pregnant. They come in, clueless yet unashamed, only knowing that they are possibly pregnant. And then there are those who are from generally conservative households, where sex is not only taboo but condemned as blasphemous and disastrous for the family's reputation. They are the ones, according to Dr Khandelwal, who arrive at the later stages of pregnancies and want 'quick' abortions.

In Aasimah's case though, a medical procedure to terminate the foetus never took place. The next day, when she turned up asking the doctor to 'complete the process',[121] Dr Khandelwal found out that she had self-induced an abortion (presumably violently) in the bathroom of her home.

Aborted pregnancies are now, more so than ever, those of young, unmarried women. In some cases, Dr Khandelwal says they attempt taking the morning-after pill but don't fully understand how to take it, when to take it and what it means for their young bodies.

Abortion has been legal in India for over forty years now.

India enacted the Medical Termination of Pregnancy Act in 1971 for cases of patients who have parental authorization, rape victims and foetal impairment, yet unsafe abortions persist. By law, women in India have the right to have an abortion if they are over the age of eighteen—they don't need permission from husbands and family members. Younger women, though, need a guardian's consent.

When India legalized abortion, it was seen as a pioneering act and lauded by pro-choice activists. Unfortunately, legalizing abortion hasn't translated into a comprehensive, safe system to take care of all the effects of the sexual revolution taking place in the country today.

The law only allows abortions if the pregnancy term hasn't passed the twelve-week mark or not aborting the foetus would be a threat to the woman's or the child's life. If the term is longer than twelve weeks but does not exceed twenty weeks, then two doctors have to be consulted. So what happens to all the young women who come to a doctor at a later stage? What happens in situations when two accredited doctors aren't available? Even worse, getting an abortion on the grounds of the contraception method failing is available only for married women. The wording of an explanation within the law makes this clear: 'Where any pregnancy occurs as a result of failure of any device or method used by any married woman or her husband for the purpose of limiting the number of children, the anguish caused by such unwanted pregnancy may be presumed to constitute a grave injury to the mental health of the pregnant woman'.[122]

Moreover, experts believe India's abortion policy is not based on good clinical practice. Today it is unofficially estimated that between 6.4 million and 6.7 million[123] abortions take place annually versus the reported numbers of 620,472 for 2012. And two-thirds of all abortions in India take place outside the authorized health facilities.[124] Approximately 63 per cent of all abortions in India have been found to be unsafe.[125]

'The official estimates are an underestimate. They refer only to those abortions undertaken in registered MTP centres [so exclude all those undertaken safely or unsafely elsewhere],' Dr Jejeebhoy told me.

This, even with the sketchy statistics, points to the increasing number of unsafe abortions and abortions in general, among young, unmarried women. What's worse is that findings from several available studies have highlighted the vulnerability of these unmarried young abortion-seekers: delayed abortions, lack of accessible support systems and the like.

India's public health system is restricted to cities. While on paper there is a vast network of primary health centres, community health centres and sub-centres in the rural areas, in reality, they aren't always there. And when they do exist, as I saw recently, they are skeletal structures with a tin roof often with sporadic electricity supply—less than 20 per cent of such centres provide abortion facilities.[126] So, when report says a woman in India dies every two hours because an abortion went wrong, it is believable.[127]

Tellingly, for a population of 1.2 billion, there are only 12,510 registered abortion facilities in India and their functionality is, at best, questionable.

◆

There is a fundamental disconnect between a rapidly evolving sexual and social landscape and the available social and physical infrastructure in India. Unsafe sex, pregnancies out of wedlock, thought-policing, unsafe abortions, sexual violence and an unstable society far outweigh available coping mechanisms. These agencies are an integral part of social infrastructure: sex education, health facilities and services, counsellors, support groups, policy dialogue. There is an unmet need; the gorge is getting deeper, the gap wider.

The void is filled by potentially erroneous sources of information and the case for peer communication is strong. Friends play a significant role in connecting young people with their partners, encouraging prenatal sex, informing each other about sexual intercourse and acting as their sex education teachers.

While peer communication is unquestionably a powerful tool to educate young people, the risk of incorrect information is pretty high, given the widespread inadequacy of sexual knowledge. Renuka Motihar, a sex education consultant, told me non-profits in India are now trying to tap into this social-network method to educate young Indians. Others like TARSHI have been hammering away about sex-ed with helplines and guides for almost a decade. For both men and women, television and films have been found to be the most popular source of information on issues related to sexual health.

Formal sex education as part of educational curricula is as good as absent in India. Without it, the media, internet, generally uncomfortable parents, or peers are makeshift ways to help young people get through the dangerous years until they are mature enough to take responsible decisions regarding their sexual lives.

In the 1990s, the government began to enhance some aspects of the country's social infrastructure as it began the whole process of liberalization. This marked the first serious attempt to initiate a formal sex education programme as part of the curriculum. In April 1993, the Ministry of Human Resource Development organized a national seminar and invited the who's who of academia, activists, curriculum developers, government bodies and whoever mattered to talk about sex-ed—actually 'adolescence education'.

Eventually they came out with a report in typical Indian bureaucratic fashion. The report decided that the three areas to focus on should be adolescence, education about diseases like HIV/AIDS and drugs. This, they boasted, would be a 'holistic' approach. They carefully named it the Adolescent Education Programme (AEP). The suggested module became a reality in 1999 and was sent around for approval to associated organizations. A few years went by as experts deliberated on what to include and what not to include, given these were 'sensitive elements related to sexual development in adolescents'. The chapters included basic information like the need for sex-ed, sex-related problems and so on. HIV/AIDS was not part of the curriculum yet.

Then, almost five years later, on 27 October 2004, a group of government departments met on HIV/AIDS prevention in India and there was a consensus that HIV/AIDS prevention education should be a part of the AEP. The following year, in 2005, together with the National AIDS Control Organization, another government body, the Human Resources Development Ministry, which oversees education in India, introduced the new and improved National Population Education Project. It was sent off to the state governments for implementation.

Of the educational materials developed for this savvy new programme, the most contentious was the flip chart. The flip chart, which would be placed on the teacher's desk, had a student page (with an image) and a reference guide page, which would face the teacher, seated at the front of the classroom. This flip chart instructed teachers to talk about how girls felt when going through puberty, menstrual hygiene, erections, wet dreams and masturbation as an alternative to sex, among many other issues. It was based on the acronym ABC: A for Abstinence, B for Be faithful and C for Correct and consistent condom usage, a commonly-used approach to HIV/AIDS prevention globally.

Students were also given blanket guidance: you should not indulge in sexual intercourse. Safe sex was defined as any sexual exercise which did not involve semen, vaginal fluids and blood entering another person's body or coming into contact with broken skin. Stimulating your own or your partner's genitals (masturbation), thigh sex, massage or kissing, using a condom for vaginal or anal sexual intercourse, oral sex (mouth contact with male or female genitals) is less risky than unprotected vaginal or anal sex and no sex (abstinence) is 100 per cent safe. It seemed to use the fear tactic to push people away from sex.

Teachers were given fact sheets, also a Q&A sheet on whether touching private parts, or a man and a woman sleeping next to each other could result in pregnancy. It instructed teachers to mention 'established methods' of a woman getting pregnant too. The fact sheets had been distributed and were being used for a while, when a sudden political uproar derailed the progress. One state banned it and then it all went downhill. Educators say no negative side effects or repercussions of any sort had been felt or seen as a result of the materials; nothing had provoked the ban. But a parochial political class started spinning stories in order to make the changing sexual landscape more explicable to themselves. The material 'allegedly featured offensive illustrations and classroom exercises', and the content on contraception and STDs vexed them, Renuka Motihar told me.

Politicians—those caught having sex in their offices, watching porn in Parliament, caught having sex on camera with midwives—vehemently went at it. This was the end of innocence for our children, they said. This material, deemed 'obnoxious', would ignite the curiosity of students about experimentation, resulting in teenage pregnancies and promiscuity. They didn't seem to know, or if they knew they didn't seem to care, that sexual behaviour in the country was already changing regardless of sex-ed.

Ms Motihar recalls how she went into a rural setting in Andhra Pradesh in the mid-2000s to speak to young women about the AEP. Ms Motihar says the thirty young women were 'so openly talking about having sex, about going out into the fields'. And then she went to speak to young women in a school in Vijayawada city in the same state where 'they were so inhibited and reserved, I remember reflecting: just look at the difference!' The landscape had been evolving for a while and India's government was ostensibly unaware.

By April 2007, some of the largest states of India—Gujarat, Madhya Pradesh, Maharashtra, Karnataka, Rajasthan, Kerala, Chhattisgarh and Goa—had banned sex education. 'Sex Education

Creates Storm in AIDS-Stricken India', the *Washington Post* reported, 'No Sex Education Please, we're Indian', other papers shrieked.

When the Indian state of Maharashtra—home to Mumbai city, unofficially India's most cosmopolitan city—banned the curriculum, an old politician Bashir Patel declared, 'We want our children to have good character. There is no need to give them sex education. It is done in the West and we don't need to follow that.' He intoned confidently, 'Sex education will ruin our society.' (NDTV, 2008)

Based on the bans, apparent witness interviews and field visits, the Rajya Sabha Committee on Petitions' report boldly concluded that 'there should be no sex education in schools' in India. Apparently, everyone consulted 'contended that the move to educate children about sex in the garb of HIV/AIDS prevention was quite reprehensible in view of our socio-cultural ethos'.

A few months later, two women (ironically, a teacher and a social activist) submitted a petition against this material to the Committee 'praying for national debate and evolving consensus' on whether or not the contentious sex-ed materials should be put into effect in central government-affiliated schools. They also wanted to stop further use of those materials till this 'debate' happened.

The Committee, with ten Members of Parliament from the Rajya Sabha and only one woman, examined this petition for a year-and-a-half. After deliberating on views and opinions from various stakeholders, it came out with a report with observations and prescriptive recommendations on what needed to be done about the AEP in 2009.

The exhaustive, seventy-seven-page report analysed the contentious material, what experts had to say and, apparently, what people were doing.

Amongst its various observations and recommendations, the Committee astonishingly concluded that sex before marriage was 'immoral, unethical and unhealthy', chapters on sexually transmitted diseases had to be removed from the curriculum, and the way ahead for India was through Naturopathy, Ayurveda, Unani and Yoga. And that was the end of the first round of debates on the sex-ed discourse.

Backward-looking, ill-informed, and retrogressive, it is instructive to let the report speak for itself. The reasons given revealed the backward and ill-informed sensibilities of those who had framed it. Here are a few lines from it:

> Once sex education is introduced, there would be peer pressure amongst growing children for its experimentation, which would increase rape in society as consent below the age of sixteen years is not considered as consent in the consensual sex. Again in consequential termination of teenage pregnancies would contribute to increase of crime graph of the society. Therefore, it would add more problem than solving those. (Rajya Sabha Committee on Petitions, 2009)

While India's central education board does prescribe an Adolescent Education Programme (AEP), a quick read through the teacher's manual exposes the limited scope. Not only is it shockingly superficial and ill crafted but it doesn't seem to address the real issues—what sex is and what consent means.

The sloppily written document I stumbled upon on the CBSE website bundles sex-ed with substance abuse and HIV, already framing the discourse in a negative arena. 'To develop healthy attitudes and responsible behaviour towards process of growing up, HIV/AIDS and Substance-Abuse' education is one of the objectives of the AEP. And not once in the document are the words 'sexual intercourse' mentioned, while there are activities titled '*Lets Celebrate Abstinence*' and '*How to Say No*'. (AEP Advocacy Manual).

Abstinence-focused sexual education doesn't change teenage

and adolescent sexual behaviour, nor does it delay the age of initiation of sexual activity.[128] In a policy review, the Guttmacher Institute, a fifty-year-old American organization that works on sexual and reproductive health and rights, noted that putting a negative connotation around this topic is counter-productive. Some may argue that empirical evidence (or rather the lack of it) from these studies don't apply to India—conservatives in India often tout its chastity and claim India is unlike the West. However, consider this: when you are told something is 'bad', you internalize that it is bad—like stealing, lying and being greedy.

Six years later, after the Delhi gang rape in December 2012, the Police Commissioner of Mumbai, Satyapal Singh said, 'Sex education needs to be carefully thought out. Look at America. It has sex education as part of its curriculum, but students are simply being taught about how to have intercourse,' speaking at a discussion on women's safety. 'According to a survey, rape is more common than smoking there. Countries with sex education in their curriculum only have an increased number of crimes against women.'[129]

Incidentally, the ABC approach and sex-ed tactics of the '90s were ideas that we took from President's Bush's era of sex education which propagated an abstinence-only outlook.

Mr Singh's view seems rather preposterous. But it is also widely accepted, as is Bashir Patel's. Singh is part of a system that administers information, quite literally. They choose what each young person in India should know. And while the Indian state has taken the onus of information dissemination upon itself, it has also withheld the rights of young adolescents: the right to information about their bodies and their sexual rights.

A distressed school principal from Mumbai, whose Class XII student committed suicide last year when she discovered she was pregnant, told me that even though he had tried initiating more rigorous sex-ed programmes after the unfortunate incident, many parents protested. They said they didn't want their children exposed to these Western evils. Sex a Western evil? Given the burgeoning population of this country, it definitely doesn't seem so.

There is no evidence from any studies or evaluations that exposing adolescents to comprehensive programmes on sexual and reproductive health leads to increased sexual risk-taking.[130] Yet, globally, sex-ed is contentious for varying and seemingly coherent reasons that are in line with other laws and policies of many countries.

For instance, Indonesia, where only 20 per cent of the youth is educated about HIV, is undergoing a sexual education revolution. Activists are mobilizing to make sex-ed a part of the national curriculum. But there is opposition from the Council of Ulema in the Muslim-majority country.

The Philippines is playing a game of Church versus State. In late 2013, the Supreme Court of the country blocked a bill which had been passed by the Congress a few months earlier— to provide free contraceptives to the poor. The main opposition comes from Catholic organizations that say the bill will promote promiscuity and 'offend the country's values and would lead to abortion, which remains illegal in the Philippines'.[131]

In 2013 religious conservatives of the United States were attacking Obama's healthcare rule that required health plans to cover birth control. Reports stated that many religious institutions filed lawsuits in twelve federal courts to challenge the President's legislation on employees receiving 'coverage for contraception in their health insurance policies'.[132]

Recently Mayor Bloomberg changed things for New York City. He overhauled twenty-year-old rules, and students in the city's public middle and high schools were required to take sex-education classes and not just HIV education which had been the norm until then. They would be taught about condom usage and the age at which sex is appropriate. Religious communities started protesting almost immediately. The same thing happened when HIV awareness and sex-ed was sought to be introduced over three decades ago.

So change is slow the world over, but the difference is women and children aren't getting raped every twenty minutes as in India.[133]

Sex talk of any kind usually gets flak from some sections of society. Elsewhere in the world, it is always on religious grounds whereas in India it is on 'cultural' grounds. Ironically, all this talk issues forth from the same culture that gave the world the *Kamasutra* and whose myths have celebrated sexuality over millennia.

Religious groups may interpret (or rather misinterpret) texts, but cultural opposition is baseless. Culture is sort of an overarching, all-inclusive term defined by traditions, language, art, food and various attributes of a particular group (be it a group of five or an entire country). India's culture has a purely ideological adherence to 'no sex'.

Over the years, sex-ed has been thoroughly researched and evaluated; there is now clear evidence that sex education programmes can actually help young people delay sexual activity by making informed choices and when they do start, to use contraceptives and practise safe sex.

Sex education does more than just reduce the risks of sexual activity like unintended pregnancy and sexually transmitted infections. Instead, it addresses their sexual and reproductive health and well-being 'more holistically', as Heather Boonstra of the Guttmacher Institute puts it.[134]

What works, what will work and what is appropriate for sex education will only be guided by experience and experiment. No scientific theory or formula will spit out a suitable, one-size-fits-all curriculum for a nation of 1.2 billion people, either pro-abstinence or pro-comprehensive sex-education. The social unevenness across India—the rural-urban divide, access to technology, access to the internet—makes it obvious that programme will have to be specifically designed if they are to be effective.

'The dream of constructing a programmes that's somehow

perfectly "neutral" on such a deeply fraught, inherently values-laden subject seems like a recipe for endless controversy, and little real progress,' Ross Douthat, the *New York Times*' op-ed columnist, wrote on the abstinence debate a couple years ago.[135] For India, these 'values' are steeped in hypocrisy.

Reproductive and sexual health rights of millions are being denied and millions are misinformed.[136] Sexuality education policies and programme should be rooted in human rights and, according to Boonstra, should 'respond to the interests, needs and experiences of young people themselves.'[137]

Unfortunately, if the gap is unbridged, the crack left unsealed and the needs of younger generations unaddressed, the dark side will only get darker.

◆

Over four decades ago India seemed to go through a moment of soul-searching when a young woman called Rameeza Bee was gang-raped by three cops. Activists and NGOs were on the streets, reports of rapes increased, people spoke of fast track courts and the need for a robust justice system.[138] A few years before Rameeza Bee's gang-rape, in 1972, a sixteen-year-old named Mathura[139] had been raped in the police station; her case was dismissed by India's apex court because the evidence—her body—showed no signs of rape. The laws were amended and new clauses on rape while in state custody were added. More recently, in December 2012, India had a passing moment of lucidity when Nirbhaya was gang-raped and murdered. All four of her murderers were sentenced to death in 2013.

In the aftermath of Nirbhaya's death, India was forced to take action and the Parliament passed a more stringent law by putting in place the Criminal Law (Amendment) Act of 2013 on 19 March 2013.

Rape was redefined with specific, physical detail. Under the law, death is the maximum penalty for rape if the victim dies or is left invalid. For the first time, stalking and voyeurism were introduced as offences and defined as crimes. Sexual harassment was added as an offence in the Indian Penal Code.

Although many proposals suggested lowering the minimum age for consensual sex to sixteen years, the government retained eighteen years as the minimum age after much opposition from political parties. Critics say the law falls short because it still does not include marital rape. The law states 'sexual intercourse or sexual acts by a man with his own wife, the wife not being under fifteen years of age, is not rape'. (Criminal Law [Amendment] Act, 2013)

There is no doubt that India is going through a sexual revolution. For the first time in centuries people are talking openly about sex. That is why there is more reporting of sexual violence—rape, assault and sexual harassment in the work place.

Though sex is edging out of the dark silence, the harsh truth is that until the majority, and more importantly, those in power, acknowledge and even embrace the sexual revolution, India's youth will be ignorant and mired in doubt, grappling to understand their bodies.

The potential of India's hundreds of millions of youth is immense—they are ambitious and aspirational, yet they face the threat of being left behind their global peers. For all the advances in education and technology which have manifested in economic growth, there are now hugely important cultural and social shifts that must be addressed to drive the next chapter in India's story, and properly managing the country's sexual revolution is one of these.

II
LOVE & MARRIAGE

LOVE REVOLUTION

My dadaji was a great one for aphorisms. I will never forget one he told me on my twenty-first birthday. He said I should get married quickly because 'women are like balls of dough. If they sit around for too long they harden and make deformed chapattis'. My grandfather believed that a good marriage was like a perfectly round chapatti and to achieve this perfection, the dough had to be supple, fresh and young. It has been nearly seven years since then, and now at twenty-eight, I am unequivocally, by Dadaji's standards, a hardened, deformed, inedible roti.

My marriage has been talked about since the day I turned eighteen. My first solo trip with my grandfather was to the Vishwanath (an avatar of Shiva) temple in Varanasi where I was made to perform a puja to acquire a good husband, with Dadaji supervising the proceedings. Of all the gods in the Hindu pantheon, Lord Shiva is the easiest to please as he is known to fulfil a supplicant's desires sooner than the rest of the gods. To appease my mother and to absolve myself of the consequences of any negative action in my past lives that could delay my marriage, I performed fasts for sixteen consecutive Mondays—the holy day of Lord Shiva.

Unfortunately the fasts did not work as my family had wished, and I remained unmarried. Ten years ago, I would have been considered way beyond my sell-by date, but today it is no longer unthinkable for an Indian woman to be single at twenty-eight.

I am stuck in the liminal space between the old and the new, the past and the present, the East and the West. I am a product of the hubris of this new India. When I was younger, ever since I could understand the concept of marriage, I was told that I must get married to a suitable boy: a Hindu, belonging to my Brahmin caste, preferably within the Kanyakubj sub-caste. Love, attraction, or even liking was not a priority. The first time that my grandfather saw my grandmother was on the day of their wedding. They were married for sixty-five years till my dadiji passed away two years ago. My parents saw each other in black-and-white photographs, and then met twice with their entire families present before they got married. As a kid, I listened confused and dumbfounded as I was bombarded with tales of the genetic superiority and mental purity of Brahmins. My uncle's inter-caste love marriage in the 1970s to my Punjabi aunt was narrated as a dark tale disguised as warning. All this was forgotten the day I left my parents' home to go to college in the US where I quickly, almost desperately, started dating all the wrong sorts of boys. Once that happened, it seemed weird to enter into an arranged marriage. Just like with my boyfriends, it seemed natural to want to get to know my husband-to-be intimately, to understand his mental make-up, his notions of love and hardship, his life before we met, what he liked to eat, what his preferred sleeping position was, and *only then* arrive at a decision for the commitment of a lifetime.

With the country's changing outlook on relationships, even my traditional family has begun to rethink their views on marriage. Just ten years ago, my elder sister, Ishani, was married at the age of twenty-one. A marriage broker would probably call her wedding an 'arranged-cum-love' or 'introduction marriage', a quaint hybrid of the traditional arranged marriage and a love match. In Ishani's case, my parents identified an appropriate boy—a well-educated, tall, fair boy of the same caste who was a doctor in the US. He was a perfect match for their twenty-one-year-old engineer daughter. Ishani had little option but to marry that suitable Brahmin boy; it would have been unacceptable for her to marry out of caste.

They remain happily married. A decade after Ishani's arranged marriage, my younger sister had a love marriage to Rahul, whom she met at work. My parents were thrilled that she had found a partner of her choice. Unlike in Ishani's case, Rahul's caste was a bonus, not the major criterion. Rahul *is* fortunately a Brahmin (though his family is from Kashmir, and speak a different language from ours, eat meat and have their own customs). My parents have changed with time as they see the children of their friends and family members marry out of caste, and even people of other nationalities; they have accepted that times are different, and caste no longer holds the supreme importance that it once did. Even people as traditional as my grandfather, the longest serving president of the Brahmin Samaja, known the world over for his prowess in getting young people married, is coming to terms with love and inter-caste marriage. On a recent visit to his native village, Etawah, he was overheard telling an old classmate from his college days how convenient it was that these days children found their own partners and parents/relatives no longer had to run door to door with their daughters' birth charts.

◆

For centuries, marriage has been the mainstay of Indian culture. In the institution of arranged marriage is embedded the idea of a lifetime of commitment—to each other and to family. Today, this is fast changing, and it is estimated that over 30 per cent of urban India chooses to marry for love.[140] Yet arranged marriage continues to be the preferred option in the country.

Let's look at why arranged marriage has remained so important.

A historical overview of arranged marriage suggests that it serves primarily as a means of solidifying alliances between families. Although this is a common feature of marriages across cultures, it takes specific valences in the socio-historical context of India. India's unique joint family social structure, in which men live with their parents, brothers, and wives, can be traced to the

Vedas.[141] Although urbanization and migration (both domestic and international) are changing Indian families, most families have adapted the joint family structure (for example, with one brother and his wife living with the parents, with children sharing finances with their families beyond marriage) rather than adopting nuclear family structures that characterize Euro-American unions.[142] Elderly parents continue to rely on sons for support, which also reinforces marriage as the concern of the extended family; only 1 per cent of the elderly population lives in old-age homes.[143] In this context, arranged marriages are particularly important because they ensure the well-being of the entire family rather than just of the individual, and elaborate wedding ceremonies again reflect this heightened significance. For example, in Mughal times, marriages fulfilled political alliances between different ruling lineages, including between Hindu rajas and Mughal rulers.[144]

Sources on Mughal marriages suggest that royal marriages were particularly important to the continuation of both family and political rule (which were united due to hereditary rule) and that rulers were most concerned with marriages in times of political instability.

The caste system too heightened the importance of arranged marriage. The Hindu caste system was traditionally based on employment categories and that demanded marrying within one's caste.[145] Throughout history marriage has been used to bolster caste and intra-caste cohesion. For example, the Hindu revival movement in the mid-twentieth century included caste conferences that called for endogamy in order to strengthen the caste system.[146]

British colonial rule saw the new rulers interfering with and moulding laws governing marriage as part of their drive to codify and regularize the 'personal laws' of the various religious and caste groups in the country. Some of this impulse sprang from a genuinely fair-minded desire to organize the plethora of confusing strictures that governed marriage and society in the country, and some of it was rooted in an attempt to perpetuate the divide and rule philosophy that the British followed. The British also codified Hindu marriage laws according to Brahminic customs, including dowry.[147] This resulted in the stringent adherence to endogamy within castes and religions, strengthening the system of the arranged marriage at the national level.

LOVE IN THE TIME OF BOLLYWOOD

Though arranged marriage may seem to be a totally retrograde concept to many in the West, the reality is that up until the late eighteenth century, most societiesaround the world had arranged marriages where love developed *after* getting married to a suitable life partner, not before. Marriage was considered to be an economic and political institution, much too important to be left to the whims and passions of two young and inexperienced individuals. It was only in the late eighteenth century that the idea of marrying for love, based on the free will of two people began gaining strength. Today, the idea of marrying for love is so deep-set in most of the West, and even a large part of the East, that we tend to forget that it has only been about 200 years since men and women began to wrest control of their marriage from their families and the church.

Historian Stephanie Coontz in her excellent book, *Marriage, a History: How Love Conquered Marriage,* studies the marital patterns in North America and Europe. She concludes that marriage has changed more in the Western world in the previous thirty years than it has in the past three thousand. The 'love revolution' began in the US in the eighteenth century when the development of a market-driven economy led to the erosion of traditional social systems. Young people began accepting the radical idea that love should be the primary reason for marriage, and that they should be free to choose their own partners. Yet marriage continued to be of paramount importance as men and women were seen as fundamentally different beings, sexually and otherwise—the man was the provider while the woman was the nurturer. By the 1970s, the love revolution culminated with marriage losing its centrality in society and people stopped believing that marriage was a necessary step to lead fulfilling lives. After extensive research, Coontz specified four criteria that led to the breakdown of traditional marriage.

These four criteria are:

1. The belief that men and women are different in terms of sensibility, lifestyle and sexuality.
2. The ability of society to regulate an individual's personal behaviour and punish them for nonconformity.
3. The combination of women's economic dependence on men and men's domestic dependence on women.
4. Unreliable birth control and fear of pregnancy.[148]

While Coontz's theory applies to the Indian scenario as much as it does to the US, the way it plays out is quite different. Though marriage in India continues to play an important role in people's lives, it is seeing a lot of change. The tradition of arranged marriage is breaking down as people choose to marry for love rather than for religious, caste, family or economic reasons. For the first time in thousands of years, India is going through a unique love revolution in which young people are taking the marriage decision into their own hands and choosing to marry for love. According to a study by the International Institute for Population Sciences and Population Council that conducted interviews with 51,000 married and unmarried young men and women from six states—Andhra Pradesh, Bihar, Jharkhand, Maharashtra, Rajasthan and Tamil Nadu—77 per cent of unmarried women think they should be able to take their own decisions about marriage.[149]

Let's look at India's love revolution more closely by applying each of Coontz's points to the Indian scenario.

1) *The belief that men and women are different in terms of sensibility, lifestyle and sexuality.*

The Victorian stipulations of the Raj-era that men and women are inherently different and should move in separate spheres are under attack. Till just a decade ago, single-sex Catholic convent schools were regarded as the height of educational excellence attended by the children of the elite. Today, many of the premier schools and colleges in India's urban centres are co-educational. Likewise, as Gita Aravamudan points out in her book, *Unbound: Indian Women at Work,* ever since Indian women began entering the workplace in significant numbers in the 1950s and 1960s, social attitudes towards them began changing in a number of ways. Men began wanting wives who were educated. After independence, new work opportunities came around which required men to move away from their hometowns and joint families. Without the support of a joint family, women were forced to leave their homes and undertake chores that their office-going husbands had no time for. As women left the confines of their homes, they discovered an attractive world and the advantages of economic freedom. A silent, almost unnoticed 'revolution' was occurring in the middle class and, suddenly, educated women were seen as financial assets by men. Women began entering the market force in large numbers as nurses, teachers, stenographers and bank clerks. These working women, exposed to industry, had higher aspirations for their daughters who grew up and took the work force by storm. By the 1970s women were working alongside their male counterparts in the corporate and public sectors.

With the opening up of the Indian economy in the 1990s, new avenues of employment presented themselves to women. These new opportunities were not segregated by sex and included positions in call centres, software companies, biotechnology and the new media. The autonomy of middle-class women transformed the traditional Indian family as girls were encouraged to get an education and a job. The Indian IT-BPO industry pioneered employment for women and, more than any other industry in the country, promoted the interests of women in the workplace. Today, the IT industry has a larger proportion of women employees as compared to other sectors. The coming together of men and women in the workplace, and their changing roles in society generally, has severely dented any existing notions that they are vastly different from each other.

2) *The ability of society to regulate an individual's personal behaviour and punish them for nonconformity.*

The ability of family, relatives, government and neighbours to regulate personal behaviour is eroding quickly in India. There is an increasing pattern of migration where young people are moving away from families to study and work, choosing to live alone in urban areas, free from family regulations and pressure. A 2010 McKinsey Global Institute study on 'India's Urban Awakening' predicts that 590 million people, about 40 per cent of the country's population will live in cities by 2030, and 70 per cent of net new employment will occur in cities; up from 340 million in 2008 (30 per cent of the population).

The pattern of urbanization and migration has allowed for far more anonymity in personal life, and less penalization for personal choices, as young people live and operate far from the watchful eyes of their families, relatives or communities. Age-old institutions such as the village councils or khap panchayats that regulate individual and societal behaviour are slowly losing favour, particularly amongst the youth, who would rather move away from small towns and villages than suffer these stifling regulations.

The economic boom in India has resulted in the rise of national and multi-national companies, banks and other impersonal institutions that do not hire based on sex, caste, religion or marital status, making it easier than ever before to lead anonymous lives free from the pressures of family and society. Anonymity also increases with the help of technology. Gone are the days of trunk calls and surreptitious love letters. Cell phones have greatly increased the ability of the individual to control his/her fate and be freed from societal restraints.

3) *The combination of women's economic dependence on men and men's domestic dependence on women.*

The dreams of the Indian woman are piercing through the walls of the kitchen and the living room, leaving behind rubble, glass and other debris. More women are working than ever before and becoming financially independent. The prevalence of women in the workplace is 30 per cent in metropolitan areas—with a 10 per cent increase in just the past year. According to a recent survey by the Centre for Work-Life Policy, more than 80 per cent of the women surveyed said they wanted top jobs and were prepared to work hard for them.

Women's income has also risen contributing to the 'girl power' economy. According to a recent survey by the Indian Market Research Bureau (IMRB) the average monthly income of women living and working in urban areas in India increased from ₹4,492 in 2001 to ₹9,457 in 2010. There has been a huge growth in savings accounts owned by women in the last few years—₹14 million in 2007 to ₹29 million in 2011, and also a 78 per cent growth in women credit card owners in the last four years.[150]

The effect of consumerism too has been a game-changer for women. The marketplace is flooded with gadgets like microwaves, washing machines, ovens, etc. that have decreased the time and labour spent on household chores. Most middle-class households have a fridge and, increasingly, washing machines. Day-care centres and pre-schools have increased options for child-care; this is particularly important for women in urban nuclear families. The freedom of Indian women to make their own decisions has also increased, shaping marketing and branding trends. It is estimated that 'the percentage of women who made decisions about buying household durables like washing machines, refrigerators, cars, etc. has gone up from 15 per cent to 20 per cent in the last few years.'[151]

Men too benefit from the easy availability of sophisticated white goods and are becoming less dependent on women. Bachelorhood has become easier than ever before, and even married men are beginning to take on more household responsibilities. A popular Indian chef, Sanjeev Kapoor, in an interview in *The Guardian* newspaper said, 'Twenty years ago if you said you cooked, people would ask what was wrong with you. Now it is the opposite.' Close to 49 per cent of the visitors to his website are male—a 20 per cent increase from just two years ago.[152]

I observe too that many of the young working men that I come across prefer to eat a lunch of fast food—pizzas, burgers and sandwiches—rather than a meal cooked by mothers or wives.

Couples marry (and stay married) when the gains of marriage exceed the gains of being single. In the past, these economic gains would allow advantages to both partners and traditionally centred around women having an economic advantage at home doing household work, and men generating income by going to work (or working in the field). Today, this has changed, and much of what was once produced at home by women can be purchased or produced by men. Women, like men, can do income-generating work. This decreases the gains from marriage. At the same time, increasing leisure time and disposable income, along with the changing landscape of sexual relationships potentially raises the opportunity cost of being single. All in all, marriage is not as economically viable as it once used to be. Changes in tastes, technology, and institutional and legal environments have decreased gains from marriage.[153]

4) *Unreliable birth control and fear of pregnancy.*
Various studies show that once the fear of pregnancy disappears, women's sexual conduct becomes unconstrained and sex, particularly premarital sex, becomes freer. In India, abortion

is legal and there are no social sanctions against the practice. Birth control is based on efforts largely sponsored by the Indian government as a measure for population control and contraceptive devices have been freely and openly available in India. Contraceptive usage has more than tripled—from being used by 13 per cent of married women in 1970 to 48 per cent in 2009.[154] Over-the-counter birth control pills are cheaply and widely available.

Nandan Nilekani, in his book *Imagining India*, delves into the history of birth control in India. He writes, 'As the global panic around population growth surged, the Indian and Chinese governments began executing white-knuckle measures of family planning in the 1960s'.[155] This reached its zenith in the mid-1970s with the announcement of the Emergency. Sanjay Gandhi made male sterilization his baby and the programmes he threw his weight behind were responsible for nearly eight million sterilizations, millions of them forced. A *New York Times* article from 1982 speaks about India's national birth control programmes launched by then Prime Minister Indira Gandhi:

> Prime Minister Indira Gandhi proclaimed February as 'family welfare month.' Billboards equating the 'small family, happy family,' were put up in every state, and radio programs advocated family planning.
> The major reason for the campaign is that India's census last year counted 684 million people, 12 million more than demographers had predicted. Subsidized birth control pills and condoms are being distributed, but most of the emphasis has been on sterilizations.
> Most of those turning up at the medical camps are women who receive $22 for submitting to a quick surgical closing of their Fallopian tubes. Men who get vasectomies are given $15. The difference in payments reflects the new emphasis on women as the key to family planning.[156]

In India, there is a fifth factor that has aided the love revolution: Bollywood. Bollywood has been a major influence and in certain sections of society, the Indian family has become far more tolerant to the idea of love marriages with the dramatic rise in movies that show inter-communal or inter-class love stories. This has also become a frequent theme on sitcoms and reality shows on cable television. Cable television, with a penetration of 200 million, has also had a significant impact. From two channels in 1991, Indian viewers were exposed to more than fifty channels in 1996 because of new economic policies. Foreign channels imported foreign cultures and norms, and Western concepts of dating and love were unleashed on Indian minds. The simplicity and prudishness of the national channel Doordarshan was replaced by Star TV, MTV and a host of others, and American culture was served on the go to an entire generation.

To find out more about how India's love revolution is unique, I speak with author Stephanie Coontz, author of *Marriage: A History: How Love Conquered Marriage*.

'For better or for worse, the love match is here to stay,' declares Coontz. 'Whatever our own personal opinions are and whatever the strengths of the arranged marriage system may be, arranged marriage is not going to exist indefinitely in today's globalized world.'

In the West, the love revolution happened in two distinct steps. First, there was the development of market driven, individualistic, nuclear families because of economic and social processes; as a consequence, the prevailing economic and social systems which were the means to exercise control over young people began to erode. This created an environment ripe for the love revolution to play out in its second stage—with rising female independence, new jobs, access to birth control, etc.

In India, though, everything is happening at the same time. The change in mindset that the family controls everything, the opening up of opportunities, the relaxation of social barriers, the creation of entertainment options, the easier mingling of sexes, access to birth control—everything is being churned together in one unholy mix.

The one key difference is that in the West, by the second stage of the revolution, the ability of parents to control their children had been wiped out. That has not yet happened in India. Even though there is a trend of young people wanting freedom from parents, and wanting Bollywood style romantic liaisons, they are also getting much more pushback than Western young women and men ever got. There are still many hangovers in rural and even urban parts of India of the old system of social production and reproduction, so the tensions that the love revolution creates are going to be much higher in India than they were in the West.

I wonder how much of a role religion and the caste system have played in the Indian love revolution. Coontz explains, 'Religion and the caste system are all intertwined. In the West, religion was intertwined with the development of marriage, but the religion there reflected more individualizing tendencies that led to the early development of the market economy. There was less cultural, religious, and socio-economic support for marriage in the West than there ever was in India.'

Since arranged marriage is rooted in the major religions of the subcontinent such as Hinduism, Islam, Jainism, Sikhism and even Indian versions of Christianity and Zoroastrianism, and religion is such an important force in India, how is this going to change? Coontz replies, 'Throughout history, societies have adapted to social and economic change. Religious structures in a religion like Hinduism reflect a society where control over the young was important to reproduction because of the caste system. But Hinduism has always been evolving, and as the tide gets strong enough to turn it, religion will adapt. It won't happen exactly like the Western model, but it will adjust to allow freedom in conjunction with its traditions.'

◆

Over the past decade or so, the biggest change to India's love story has been that romantic love has become a legitimate basis to wed. This has become a common experience amongst the urban, educated middle-class Indian. Essential to this love story is a Western-style consumerism and today in novels, films and television serials alike, young couples fall in love over coffee and movie dates, in malls and in exotic Western locales.

The Bollywood movie today is the most telling aspect of how modern India sees love. Very often the hero and heroine exchange an English 'I love you' even as they fight for their romantic love against the wishes of their families.

Displays of love too have seen an interesting journey in Bollywood films. Earlier, the kiss was considered to be a Western pollutant, and censor boards, filmmakers and even audiences saw the absence of kissing as upholding Indian culture and tradition. Over the last decade, this prudery is slowly disappearing and the kiss has become a common feature of Bollywood movies. For example, veteran filmmaker Yash Chopra depicts a long kiss in *Mohabbatein* (2000), when earlier he did not have a kiss even between an adulterous couple depicted naked in a bedroom sequence (*Silsila*, 1996). Most recently, in late 2012, Shahrukh Khan, India's leading film star, who never kissed on screen for moral reasons, succumbed to public pressure and shared his first on-screen kiss with his co-star in the blockbuster *Jab Tak Hai Jaan*.

India has had a rich, spectacular romantic past, and love, kama, ishq, pyaar, mohabbat, call it what you will, has always been an integral part of our cultural and historical past. Love in India may have taken on different names, forms and meanings, but it is the importance that Indian culture has given to love that has lent it richness. It is ironic then that a country like India that has recorded, celebrated and presented love in such a variety of forms shuns the concept of romantic love in modern times. Although the stigma associated with romance and love is decreasing, in many parts of India, there is still a grave threat to lovers and the love match.

THE LOVE COMMANDOS

When fiction bleeds into real life, the results are not as pretty, because as Kothari, Coontz, and numerous others point out, India is still far from ready to whole-heartedly embrace the concept of free love. This is where one of the unique by-products of this revolution has emerged: the Love Commandos.

I alight from an auto and traverse the narrow alleys of Paharganj, a central Delhi marketplace known for its cheap hotels and backpackers. 'Follow me' beckons the Commando who will show me the way to the central office of the Love Commandos. He walks slowly, but in the whirr of sounds, sights and people, I lose him. I struggle to find him in the maze-like ancient alleys of what was, in the eighteenth century, Delhi's principal grain market. Today, this is an urban marketplace, spilling over with people, automobiles and animals. I absorb the odours and bewildering sights and sounds as I walk past a shanty. I re-establish contact with my guide and follow him through a crowded market, past a shop featuring men's Lux Cozi underwear and another one where a pair of lime-green draw-string pajamas with an ice-cream-cone-print takes up prime display space. I walk past a stable, which holds twenty albino mares with fast-blinking pink eyes, some of them decked out in colourful wedding paraphernalia. These are wedding horses, traditionally meant to be white and female, on which the groom will ride on his wedding day. I cross a hole-in-the wall police station (so tiny that it has room only for one police officer, one chair, and a beat-up phone) which is in curious contrast to a 'Men's western saloon', a two-chair barber shop next door. The hulking Commando finally takes a left turn into a congested alley where an ancient woman with a shrivelled face is sitting on a cot peeling vegetables; another octogenarian next to her, wearing a pair of magnifying-glass-like spectacles is stringing together raakhis for the upcoming raksha bandhan festival—she gives me a toothless smile.

The Commando leads me into a decrepit one-room shanty, with uneven bruise-coloured walls, riddled with stains, scars and scribbles. He declares that this is the head office of the Love Commandos. The twenty-square-foot room is unventilated and has an unidentifiable odour. The floor is caked with dust and littered with several shoe-print-stamped loose papers. A stack of dirt-covered books lines the walls and wires sprout from many corners. The main points of interest in the room are a flat-screen monitor, a computer, a smut-covered printer and a blinking internet router. I am a little taken aback. The Love Commandos' website boasted a lot of media coverage, international and national, including the BBC, *The Guardian*, the *Times*, and a host of others. Most recently, they had been featured on the hugely popular television show, *Satyamev Jayate*, hosted by Bollywood celebrity Aamir Khan. I would have imagined that they would be operating with more resources.

Taking up most of the office space is a corpulent Harsh Malhotra, who introduces himself as the Chief Coordination Officer. Next to him is a petite Sanjoy Sachdev, the emerald-eyed Chairman of the Commandos. They are dressed for the interview in crisp starched white linen kurta pajamas. A grimy plastic stool is dragged forward for me to sit on. A noisy air-cooler makes it difficult for me to hear what they have to say, but the electricity promptly goes off and that problem is solved. Candles are lit in the dark, windowless room even though it is bright and sunny outside.

On the night of Valentine's Day, 14 February 2010, Sanjoy Sachdev and Harsh Malhotra spent the night in jail. They had been arrested for protecting lovers against the wrath of right-wing Hindu groups. That night they decided to dedicate their lives to helping lovers and took the fate of India's young lovebirds into their own hands. To deal with the inordinate number of honour killings that had been taking place, they started Love Commandos, an organization dedicated to helping lovebirds flee their pursuers. Their ultimate goal was to eliminate honour killings from the Indian landscape. Love Commandos is Chairman Sanjoy's brainchild, and he speaks passionately and poetically about how love must be unequivocally protected.

'People used to think we were mad. They captured us and threw us in jail. Do you know how many Valentine's Days I have spent in jail? More than you have seen in your life!'

◆

In a country with deep-seated traditions of patriarchy, casteism and family honour, falling in love across caste and community lines is difficult, and sometimes even life-threatening. Threats to the lives of lovers often come from their own families—families who believe they lose face in society by the romantic actions of their wayward kin and reports of honour killings of young lovers have become rather common in newspapers. These cases are often cloaked in obfuscation, with few legitimate sources and little evidence. In cases of inter-caste or inter-community romance, the risk of being killed is so great, especially in certain north Indian states, that the government has opened police shelters for runaway couples where they are offered protection against the brutality of their family members. 'The Punjab and Haryana High Court receives as many as 50 applications per day from couples seeking protection. This is a staggering tenfold rise from about five to six applications a day five years ago'.[157]

Despite the menacing odds, love and longing in the small towns of India is increasing like never before. Young men and women are braving centuries of social resistance and daring to fall in love across caste lines. '[A]nnually around 984 Dalits marrying non-Dalits get protection orders in runaway marriages'.[158] About eight to ten establishments in Chandigarh conduct marriage ceremonies to provide the required certificate of marriage to the couple and a marriage arranger in a temple claimed that a temple in Punjab had solemnized 1,500 marriages over the last five years.[159]

The Love Commandos' main agenda is to rescue endangered couples from the wrath of families and bring them to the safety of their shelter in Delhi where they offer protection. Once the couples arrive at the shelter, Harsh and Sanjoy act as mediators, speaking with their parents, community leaders and politicians, negotiating terms and conditions for the return of the lovebirds to their homes. Sometimes they even perform marriage ceremonies for runaway couples. They tell me about several life-threatening missions that they have embarked on, in most cases to rescue the girl, who is forcefully held by her parents. I ask if I can accompany them on their next mission. They refuse, saying that my life would be under serious threat if I were to go with them. They point to the Commando who has led me here.

'He is our Commando trainer. He is a black belt in martial arts! You have to train with him if you want to come!' declares Harsh.

I take a good look at the black belt Love Commando. He tries to look fierce, but he does not look particularly threatening, nor can he do much about his protruding stomach that spills several inches over his tight pants. I ask Harsh where the runaway couples stay and he points to the roof. I notice a rickety iron staircase near the entrance—it looks like this is the only way up. I ask if there are any couples in residence. He points to a pair of young women cooking in a kitchen attached to the office. Two other couples sit huddled around a black-and-white TV. They are not allowed to leave the cramped space without the permission of Harsh and Sanjoy.

I take a look around at the dismal conditions and ask them how they make enough money to sustain the organization. Suddenly Sanjoy looks gloomy and begins telling me his woes. They shot to fame after being featured in the media. Now they have hundreds of couples calling from across the country. They don't have the heart to deny them assistance, but they do not have the resources to house them either. They have had to sell their cars and houses to make ends meet. Sanjoy says that he has one piece of land left in his village which he will have to sell next if things don't work out. They receive some donations, but not enough. Sometimes lovers whom they have 'settled' send funds, but this is usually not the case. The ones who do give money are the journalists who come to interview them. Sanjoy takes out a carefully folded cheque from his pocket, and proudly shows it to me. He says that the $100 check is courtesy a Belgian journalist who has made a documentary on them. Harsh tells me with an eager smile that they are expecting something from me too.

As we are talking, a small man comes into the room with a box of white, milky sweets that he offers to us. Sanjoy tells me that this man had an inter-caste marriage against the wishes of his wife's parents, who kidnapped her after the marriage. The Love Commandos helped him get his wife back, so he has come to thank them.

Harsh has six cell phones, six different helpline numbers for lovers to call on. The phones ring continuously. Harsh picks up one phone and turns on the speaker for me to listen in.

The caller has a girlish, nasal voice. She is a student from Pune, called Pallavi.

'I am in love with the boy, what do I do?' she says squeakily.

Harsh: What is your age?

Pallavi: Nineteen.

Harsh: The boy's age?

Pallavi: Twenty-one.

Harsh: What does he do?

Pallavi: He works at a call centre.

Harsh: You want to get married?

Pallavi: Yes.

Harsh: Can you come to Delhi?

Pallavi: Uh…

Harsh: If you can come, tell me, if you can't come, tell me.

Pallavi: I want my parents to understand first.

Harsh: You want your parents to understand and then you want to get married? Or you want to get married anyways?

Pallavi: Uh…I don't know.

Harsh: How old is your love?

Pallavi: Seven years.

Harsh: When you first started your love, did you ask your parents? NO! The Indian Constitution says after eighteen the guardianship of your parents ends. You can do as you please.

Pallavi: My parents tell me they will commit suicide.

Harsh: Till date no parent has died, if anyone has died, then the lover has or the love dies. You have to raise your confidence, get married and come here. We will protect you from the problems.

Pallavi: My parents are asking me to come home but I am scared. My best friend was killed last month because she loved someone from outside her caste.

Harsh: Be confident. If your parents don't murder you, then they will do emotional atyachaar. When you want to get married, then you call us.

Harsh shakes his head in disgust when he puts down the phone. 'See, they killed her friend, they will kill her too. It's pretty standard. She has loved, so kill, that's the way the story always goes.'

Harsh and Sanjoy cite the example of the Manoj-Babli honour killing case. In June 2007, the killing of newly-weds Manoj and Babli was ordered by a khap panchayat in Kaithal district, Haryana, because they got married despite being from the same gotra or clan. Honour killings go both ways—for marrying outside the caste, or for marrying too deep within. The landmark case that followed convicted Babli's parents for the honour killing—a first in Indian history.

As in Manoj and Babli's case, often the killers are the lovers' families, in collusion with the khap panchayats of their village. Khap panchayats are kangaroo courts run by elderly men in villages and towns across India. These councils once dominated political life in villages across north India by exerting social control through edicts that governed everything from marriage to property disputes. Though several villages have grown into towns because of rapid urbanization and despite the fact that the Supreme Court has condemned these councils as illegal bodies, khap panchayats continue to thrive—a far from vestigial organ of the country's rural heritage.

A smattering of statements by various chaudharys or heads of the khap panchayats highlight their antediluvian views. The chaudhary of the Baliyan khap, Mahendra Singh Tikai, has gone on record saying, 'Love marriages are dirty, I don't even want to repeat the word, and only whores can choose their partners.' He further said, 'Same-gotra marriages are incestuous, incest violates maryada (honour) and villagers would kill or be killed to protect their maryada.' He scoffs at the laws of the Indian state, calling them 'the root of all problems'. 'That's your Constitution, ours is different.'[160]

Amongst many other retrograde suggestions, the khaps have advocated child marriage, saying that if it is instituted, the natural sexual desires arising when the child hits puberty will be avoided, while another has said that girls should be married at the age of sixteen as it will help young people satisfy their sexual needs and will also help reduce rape cases.[161] Some have suggested banning phones and jeans for women as a way to avoid titillation and rape, while another khap leader stated that chowmein caused hormonal imbalance which led to men raping women.[162]

To make matters even more difficult for lovers, the police are widely distrusted, especially in the cow belt of India, in states like Uttar Pradesh, Bihar, Haryana and Punjab. Despite orders directing the police 'to deal sternly with parents/relatives/other members of the society who threaten such couples', and to provide 'mediation/counselling cells' and 'to prevail upon resisting parents/relatives to reconcile with such couples',[163] people at large suspect the police to be in cahoots with the khap panchayats. This is where organizations like the Love Commandos are able to help. 'The Government is a fraud. They promised a bill against honour killings that has still not been passed. They know they will lose votes if they pass this. The khap panchayats control many votes. They even said they would get us [Love Commandos] involved, but we haven't gotten even one call!' exclaims Sanjoy in a fit of anger.

According to a 2006 survey, 'law enforcers as well as people (both rural and urban) in the affected states agreed that khaps were raising the right issues (81 per cent of the 300 police personnel interviewed and 46 per cent of the 600 residents'.[164] Even though young India is daring to fall in love, there is resistance from an older social order and this is why the awful khap panchayats have not been eradicated despite their terrible, misogynistic views.

Sanjoy sighs, suddenly looking tired after his burst of anger. He looks down at his shoes and says, 'It's sad, parents get so happy seeing filmi love stories, but when it comes to their own daughter's love, it's a different story.'

LOVE BIRDS

Over the coming weeks, I visit the Love Commandos more often than I need for the purpose of the book because I enjoy spending time there. Whenever I have a free moment, I hop into an auto and navigate the crowded alleys of Paharganj, the lime pajamas with the ice-cream motifs acting as a landmark to their decrepit little office. I help Sanjoy and Harsh, both of whom know little English, manage their popular Facebook page. Over time, I have come to admire these two men who spend their days helping young lovers with unparalleled optimism and always with a sense of humour. The stories that I come across here are so dismal and depressing, and the lovebirds-in-flight who arrive here are often in funereal spirits, but somehow Baba and Papa, as Sanjoy and Harsh are called by those they help, always manage to uplift their spirits. Baba and Papa, as I begin calling them too, take what they do seriously. They liaise relentlessly with politicians, police officials and lawyers to get their agenda noticed. They organize public meetings and fundraise aggressively. Naturally they bask in the media attention that they get, and give interviews with relish but I don't think anyone should grudge them that, considering all the good work they do. They are encouraged by the coverage that they receive and hope they will one day be a bona fide NGO.

The runaway couples spend most of their time in a cramped makeshift dormitory—a row of wooden beds with dirty sheets and a pile of mouldy newspapers in the corner. Perhaps the only clean place in the room is a little shelf which functions as an altar. Four small idols line the shelf, and a bunch of freshly picked flowers decorate the altar. Every evening the couples gather around the altar to pray. They aren't allowed to leave the shelter for fear of being discovered, so it is on a row of hard, wooden beds that we sit together drinking thimbles of sugar-laden tea as they tell me their stories.

Everyone here is young, in the age group of eighteen to twenty-five. All the women wear thick bunches of red and white plastic bangles and have red sindoor dotting their foreheads, proudly signifying their newly-wed status. The couples come from smaller towns where tight-knit patriarchal communities suffocate their love. In these towns, men and women do not interact freely and society still attempts to govern the behaviour of individuals. If people break boundaries, especially of caste and communities, they are often killed. In the course of the weeks that I have been visiting the office of the Love Commandos, I have begun to gain the trust of many of the runaways who have sought them out, and their stories are more often than not hair-raising examples of just how brutal this country's so-called guardians of morality can be when their notions of morality are flouted.

KAVITA AND PAVAN

This is not the first time that Kavita and Pavan have run away. They ran away three months ago from their hometown of Jaipur when their parents refused to accept their decision to get married.

Kavita's parents pleaded with her to return, and when she did, they told her that they had found someone else for her to marry, and if she refused, they threatened to kill Pavan. Undeterred, Kavita and Pavan ran away again. They got married in a hasty ceremony and then made their way to Delhi to get protection from the Love Commandoes because they knew that trouble, maybe even death, was at their heels.

'We have run away in support of each other,' Kavita says clutching Pavan's hand in a bold display of emotion. 'My parents don't want to listen to us, they just want to kill me, kill him, kill everyone,' she says matter-of-factly.

Kavita's parents live in Mahendragarh, a small agricultural village, but she is a student in Jaipur, completing a master's in computer science. Pavan is from Jaipur where he works at a computer institute. They are from different communities; she is a Gujjar and he a Kumawat. Though Kavita's family is threatening the couple, Pavan's family is supporting them. However, Kavita and Pavan have not asked for his family's help because they fear that under duress or violence from Kavita's family, they might disclose their location.

Kavita and Pavan's problems are common to many of the narratives that I hear. Two young people either across, or too far close within caste lines fall in love and want to get married. The boy's family is usually accepting of the alliance, but the girl's family is not, and they attempt to kill or intimidate the boy. The daughters are usually put under house arrest in the hope that the love or the lover will eventually die. In several instances, the boy or both lovers are killed by order of the khaps. According to reports, 94 per cent of the killings are carried out by the woman's family. At the heart of the problem is female virtue and chastity.[165] By falling in love the girl has disobeyed her parents and has defiled not only herself but also her clan. To reclaim their lost honour, the family kills.

The only time that Kavita seems joyful is when she speaks

of the past. She tells me about the Ganesh temple where Pavan and she met every day. 'This was our set place, Ganesh always protected us,' she says wistfully, toying with the Om pendant that she wears around her neck on a black thread. She continues with a grim smile, 'We have roamed around a lot, a lot of women wear scarves around their head in Jaipur and there is a lot of profit in this. We didn't know if we would live, so we wanted to make the most of our love story.'

Currently, Sanjoy is speaking with a Gujjar leader, hoping that he will help them arrive at a compromise with Kavita's parents. While they wait for a positive outcome, Kavita and Pavan will remain here—a dismal honeymoon if there ever was one.

On the face of it, honour killings seem to be a matter of caste but Arvind and Shikha's story made me realize that the issue went far beyond caste lines. Shikha has the face of a child, and she speaks in the lilting way of the young. She is stick thin—I can wrap my fingers twice around the circumference of her wrists. Arvind and Shikha are from the same caste, Kurmi, and were neighbours in Pilibhit in Uttar Pradesh. Their love story began seven years ago when Shikha was sixteen years old and Arvind had returned to his hometown on vacation from university. He fell ill and as he lay in his bed nursing a high fever he looked out the window straight into Shikha's living room at the doll-like young woman playing with her brother, cooking dinner, watching television, and tending to her parents. As his fever raged, he fell in love with her and decided he wanted to marry her.

Two years after Arvind fell in love, he finally mustered up the courage to speak with his dream girl. Shikha quickly reciprocated his love but hadn't anticipated the resistance she would face from her family. When Arvind asked her parents for her hand, he was thrown out of the house, but not before Shikha was brought before him and beaten with an iron rod. Arvind went back to Bareilly, where he was a university lecturer, wishing never to come back to Pilibhit, and determined to stay far away from Shikha.

He speaks with a pensive look on his face, 'I wanted to leave her alone because I didn't want to ruin her life. But I realized I couldn't stay away from her either, I loved her too much. I returned to Pilibhit and on 15 August 2010 I gave her a mobile phone.' On the occasion of India's Independence Day, she too got her independence.

'I always thought, I have love, I have everything. But this was just the beginning, our love would be tested,' says Arvind. Shikha is huddled next to Arvind in a pair of cotton pajamas and a long t-shirt. A cotton dupatta is flung across her neck. She musters the courage to speak.

'It was a sad day when my mobile phone was captured. My mother beat me, but Arvind got me another mobile phone. This too was discovered, and I was beaten again. This happened to us at least five or six times.' Since mobile phones seem to play such an integral part in the love stories that I hear, I ask the lovebirds what they would do if they didn't have mobile phones.

They look confused, because they cannot even imagine life without this lifeline. Then Shikha pipes up, 'The internet! We had to communicate for two months on the web when my mobile was discovered and Arvind was in Bareilly.'

'And without the internet?' I ask.

After a long pause, Arvind tentatively says, 'Letters,' and they nod their heads confidently. Yes, letters it seems would have done the trick—love letters, the way they show in the movies.

Why did Shikha's mother have a problem with her marrying Arvind, I wonder. They were after all from the same caste, and neighbours too. All in all, it seemed like a good match to me.

'We are of the same caste, but my mother doesn't like his family. Ever since I can remember our mothers have squabbled. I don't even know where the problem first began, but it was always something, the repair of the wall that joined our houses, water, electricity, there was always trouble,' says Shikha. She continues, 'When they realized that I wouldn't leave him my mother told me that he was using me. They told me that he had a wife in Bareilly. I didn't believe them. I had faith in my love.'

Shikha continues with a shrug, 'It's not a matter of caste, the issue is that of adhikar (right). Girls here are not meant to have any adhikar. And if they show it then they are thought to be disrespectful.'

It looks like honour killings go beyond just caste. It is essentially about patriarchy and control. If women stray or exercise their right, they are killed. Throughout the conversation Shika mentions her mother, never her father, and I ask her why. Both Arvind and Shikha laugh. 'Because her mother controls everything in the house, especially her father. Everything revolves around her.'

I find this bizarre. I would imagine that a matriarch would want to uplift her daughter instead of debasing her.

I ask about their future plans. Baba and Papa are negotiating with Shikha's parents to accept her marriage with Arvind. They will try their best, and eventually go back to Bareilly where Arvind's job awaits him. They both know that they can never return to Pilibhit. Even if their parents accept their marriage, their community never will. Arvind has a terrified look on his face. It is as if by voicing his plans to me he has just now realized the consequences of his actions. He says softly, looking at Shikha, 'This is our second birth, we feel reincarnated in just one lifetime.'

◆

Perhaps the most tragic of the tales that I heard at the Love Commandos is of Ankur and Arpita. He is a Dalit, and she a Rajput.

'She was in the eighth standard and I was in the eleventh. I saw her at the window, standing with her nose up. I kept on looking at her, day after day, through the window, and then I fell in love.'

Ankur continues, 'I fasted for her. I prayed that I could speak with her, if only for a minute. Five years after I had fallen in love with her, a friend of mine made us speak on the phone. I remember my body trembling, I couldn't believe that my dream had come true. We began talking, and we never stopped. We used to talk all the time, even during our exams. We never failed our exams, in fact we got the highest marks when we talked the most!'

I wonder if their parents suspected something, since they spoke on the phone all the time.

'We spoke at night mostly,' clarifies Ankur. 'This was the most exciting. We hid under the blankets and talked on the phone till our phones ran out of battery,' he says with a grin.

In the end, it was the cell phone that had incubated their love which finally gave the two lovers away. Arpita's cell phone with messages from Ankur was discovered, and she was sent to her brother's home where she was locked away till her family decided what to do with her. Arpita knew they would kill if her they came to know that Ankur was from a backward caste, so she escaped, fleeing with Ankur from her hometown in Haryana. Ankur and Arpita first went to Madhya Pradesh, where they got married, and after two months on the run, came to Delhi.

Harsh and Sanjoy know that Ankur and Arpita's is a lost case. A match between a Rajput and a Dalit will never be accepted in the world that they come from. They are just giving the lovebirds a place to breathe, to rest, and to plan for the future.

We talk of cities where Arpita and Ankur can run to. They don't want to stay in Delhi, they don't like it here. I tell them that there is more to Delhi than just the shelter and there are lots of opportunities for two young people like them. To me, it makes the most sense for them to stay here. They insist that if they stay in Delhi their families will find them. They cross their arms over their chest and stubbornly stare down at the floor. 'No, we can't stay here, we will go to Mumbai,' they say.

They tell me that even in the anonymity of a big city, staying invisible is close to impossible. But Mumbai is a difficult city, a city with so many people and little space. What about the countryside? Doesn't that seem like an attractive proposition?

There Arpita, armed with a degree in economics, can teach at a school. Perhaps Ankur who comes from a family of farmers can farm. I remember him telling me that he feels passionately about farming. They grimace in disgust. The countryside! Why would they go there? That is where they came from. It is a place of horror and atrocities, of khaps and of families who kill. But Mumbai is a place of hope—the city of dreams. And right now it seems like it is only dreams that keep these young lovers going.

◆

The young people who I met at the Love Commandos speak endlessly about the future. They don't talk about the bucolic past, about the families, relatives, and friends they have left behind. All they want to do is talk about tomorrow—of new cities, new lives and new plans. They are excited to make new beginnings in the new India they have heard about and watched on television. They appear to be in love, but at times I wonder—how much time have they actually spent with each other? They have shared stolen moments through windows and cell phones, but not much more. Now these young couples are taking on the world, with just themselves to rely upon. And if they have fallen so suddenly in love, what is to stop them from falling out of love? And what will happen then?

'YOU ARE BANGALORED'

After my exposure to the love revolution as seen at perhaps its bleakest, in the experiences of couples trapped in small towns and communities which are flailing around trying to reconcile traditional ways and the onrush of modernity, I decide it's time to see it at work in another setting—the hyper modern workplace of the IT and BPO sector. Bangalore, India's IT city, seems the place to see this side of the sexual revolution at work. Bangalore was once a sleepy town, remarkable only for its excellent weather and popular as a retirement town. Over the past few decades, it has seen a stark change, becoming India's IT hub, with its population increasing five-fold, as young people from across the country have flocked here to work.

When I get to the offices of the company where I am doing my interviews, I feel I could be in the grounds of a five-star resort—the office buildings are set amidst manicured lawns, fringed by palm trees, and new-age sculptures. Security is tight, there are at least ten uniformed guards checking credentials, but when I get past them, I'm suitably impressed by the hundreds, maybe even thousands of young men and women I see walking to work purposefully with their backpacks along the broad, spotlessly clean roads.

At the offices of the company, a BPO firm, senior manager Partha greets me warmly. He is tall and well-built, his sculpted body showing through his t-shirt. He is handsome too, with skin that glows with good health, and long black hair that he has gelled back—hardly the stereotype of a geeky engineer. Partha has been working at the company for the past three years, though he has been working in the IT sector for fifteen. The office is sparsely populated and Partha explains that the full work force of the office never arrives at any one time. They operate in various shifts, and employees have the freedom to choose their timings. The first shift begins at 7 a.m. the last at 7 p.m., and the guys who work this shift usually finish at 5 a.m. He, being a manager, works regular hours—9 a.m. to 6 p.m.

Partha and I go to his office to talk. There is a bicycle parked outside the office door, and a pair of sneakers under his desk. Iron Maiden and Pink Floyd posters festoon the walls, along with a picture of him completing a marathon. He tells me proudly that he is a fitness freak, and that he bikes ten kilometres to work and back home every day. 'Bangalore is an amorphous place. If you are young, you come here to get an IT job. You are paid well, you make friends, and most importantly, you have freedom. People come from all parts of India, they speak different languages, they look different and it is easy to assimilate here,' he says.

All through my days in Bangalore, I observe that what he says is true. Work spaces, like the company where he is employed, offer anonymity and the ability to lead a life free from family and societal pressures. In a place like Bangalore, all of Coontz's four factors are relevant, and this inchoate new culture is what makes Bangalore ideal for the love revolution to take root in.

I ask Partha about the culture of love and marriage in the world of IT. He explains to me that love is as much a part of the IT world as coding. Falling in love at work, then marrying that person with *or without* the approval of families is a common story here. In fact, love and marriage was almost part of the package deal in the IT world. Most young employees come here not only to get grand salaries, but also to find a boyfriend/girlfriend, have sex, hopefully followed by marriage.

But there was also another side to this IT culture. While on the one hand there were those who sought out the edgy lifestyle it offered, there were others who found it difficult to cope with. 'The culture here is difficult to handle, especially for people who come from traditional backgrounds, which is most of the crowd here. They are engineers, they have done nothing but study their whole lives, their mothers bringing food to their tables and their fathers disciplining them. They come here, and this open culture is at times too much for them.'

Suddenly he becomes serious and asks 'Did you see the news of the suicide this morning?'

I have indeed seen the news of a suicide in Whitefield, an IT Park area. A young IT professional, an employee of Hewlett Packard, was found dead in his car. Though the police have been vague about what happened, a suicide note was found in the car that indicated heartbreak.[166]

'This kind of thing happens here all the time.' says Partha. 'A lot of people can't deal with this sudden change in lifestyle.'

What Partha tells me is not far from the truth. The medical

journal *Lancet* declared in a 2012 report that suicide has become the second leading cause of death among young Indians, and that suicide rates were higher among well-educated young people from the more prosperous southern states. The study's lead author declared, 'young educated Indians from the richer states are killing themselves in numbers that are almost the highest in the world'.[167]

There are other instances of suicide that come to my mind. Last year, Amit Budhiraja, a thirty-year old software engineer working for Infosys in Bangalore smothered his twenty-eight-year-old wife, also an IT professional, and then killed himself. He left a suicide note, admitting to killing his wife because he suspected her of having an affair with a colleague. To make the situation worse, several people left comments on a Facebook page saying that death was an appropriate punishment for a cheating wife.

♦

What about the rumours of hedonistic sex in the IT world? More than one person had told me that so many employees have sex in the offices of an IT giant (with a holier than thou public image and pious utterances from its top management) that its plumbing regularly backs up because of all the condoms that are flushed down the toilets. I am curious to know if these rumours are true. Partha is hesitant to answer this question, and once again confirms that I am not recording this conversation, as requested. 'I can't tell you for sure,' he finally says. 'If you do a sex survey here, they'll be paavam kuttis (pure innocents). They'll pretend they don't watch porn, but they watch a lot of it, especially at night because people work 24/7 and have high-speed internet connections. People watch so much porn that I have to monitor it closely. We've had to put laws in place which say that people caught watching porn on company computers or on personal devices will be thrown out immediately.'

As Partha and I chat, Roshika, one of his colleagues, pops into the office. The gregarious Roshika is dressed fashionably in hip-hugging jeans, a tight t-shirt and a pair of trendy flats. She is carrying a fashionable pink Adidas backpack and has a pair of sunglasses propped up on her head. With Partha's permission, I quiz her about life in Bangalore. Roshika, who is twenty-eight, is happy to talk. She tells me she moved to Bangalore six years ago from Coorg, and that she loves it here, primarily because she is a shopaholic and the money she makes working in the IT industry allows her to indulge her addiction. She is single and lives in an apartment that she shares with two other girls. She speaks a lot about her friends, she tells me about her flatmates, both of whom work in IT and are single. They too, she says, love to shop.

She also likes to party, but as per government rules everything in Bangalore, including night clubs, pubs and restaurants, shuts at 11 p.m. The government gives 'moral' reasons for this curfew. In a fast-changing city, the government is desperately trying to hold on to the past. 'These stupid rules really suck,' grumbles Roshika. 'It wasn't like this before, but this new government is really silly. By the time we go out it is almost 10:30 p.m., so our party scene is lousy. The most exciting part for us is getting ready and wearing the clothes that we buy.'

Does she have a boyfriend?

'A boyfriend? No way,' she grimaces and then adds with a grin, 'I am single and ready to mingle. I don't want to be tied down with a boyfriend, especially not one of these jealous, possessive types. No way.'

What about her parents, are they pressuring her to get married?

'I don't want to get married right now, so my parents are going to have to deal with it. I'm independent, so it doesn't really matter what they think.'

I ask her how often she goes back to scenic Coorg. I imagine it must be pleasant to escape the city and visit family there. She just shrugs and looks away. 'I go sometimes, for festivals and stuff. But I don't really like to go back there. It's so boring, there isn't anything to do.'

From Roshika's reactions to my questions, it doesn't seem as if she is on good terms with her parents. According to a study on the lives of IT workers, 'The new youth subculture, with its supposed consumption-oriented and "fun-loving" lifestyle, is regarded as disreputable by the conventional middle class—giving rise to inter-generational and social tensions.'[168] I can imagine that Roshika is in a similar sort of situation.

When Partha leaves the office for a moment, Roshika opens up about work. 'I work in financial planning. I love my job, but the crowd is boring. It's okay in marketing and advertising but finance sucks. I do love my American counterparts though. I think they're cool.'

Roshika tells me about her recent trip to New York for a training session, her first time abroad. 'I'm a big *Sex and the City* fan, and I've *always* wanted to visit Manhattan. The first thing I did was to take the *Sex and the City* bus tour. I only had two days there but it was absolutely amazing.' She adds, 'The shopping was divine.' I ask her about dating in the office. She tells me that the company has a young crowd, lots of people are straight out of college, and the average age here is twenty-four.

'They just want to show off their love lives to everyone. You see people holding hands and cuddling during lunch breaks. They just try to be cool, but they are not really. If a girl wears a sleeveless shirt to work they give her a bad look,' says Roshika self-reflexively tugging at the sleeves of her own shirt.

Roshika is keen in her observation. According to statistics 51.7 per cent of urban men think girls who dress provocatively deserve to be teased. Surprisingly, 33.7 per cent urban women think so as well.[169]

'All the men wear jeans and sneakers and carry a backpack, and they think they are the coolest. That's the typical IT crowd.'

Partha takes me for lunch to the cafeteria upstairs. Just as Roshika had told me, there is a sartorial standard for the men—

they are all dressed in jeans, shirts and sneakers. The women display more variety, some wear 'western' attire—jeans, skirts, pants, others are in salwaar-kameez, no one wears saris. Over lunch Partha introduces me to a young woman named Priya. She is in her twenties, and is dressed in a plain salwaar-kameez. She is plump, plain-faced, and her most distinctive facial feature is a lazy eye. Partha bids me goodbye, and tells me that Priya has an interesting story to tell.

◆

When Priya moved to Bangalore for work there were some things that she vowed she would never do. She was never going to change her name to something more fashionable and easy to pronounce. She was never going to put on airs (her father used to call them *'city airs'*) and dress in pants and shirts, though her 5'9" slender frame allowed for that. She was never going to change her thick south Indian twang for an American one, not even when she was made fun of, not even when people had trouble understanding what she was saying. She was never going to forget her family and how much she loved them. And most of all, she was never going to have a 'romance' with the boys that she met. She was not interested in a love marriage and though she had studied in co-ed schools, she had never spoken to any boys.

After graduating from a small college in Tamil Nadu with a master's in Computer Science, Priya secured an internship with a multinational BPO in Bangalore. In her twenty-four years, Priya had never left her home state, and to live in Bangalore was a thrilling proposition. She had not expected to stay long though—she knew that her strict father would never allow it. An astrologer had told her father that Priya would not marry till she was twenty-six years old, and her father thought it best for Priya to get some work experience rather than to twiddle her thumbs at home. In his mind, a little bit of work experience could only improve Priya's prospects for marriage. Little did he know that life in the IT world of Bangalore would forever change the direction of Priya's life.

In Bangalore, Priya kept all her promises. Staying away from love though was harder than she had imagined, especially in the big, lonely city where everyone seemed to have a life outside the office. Priya had grown up in a large family, around lots of cousins and friends, and here she was desperately, painfully lonely.

Six months after she started work, Priya received a Facebook friend request from a colleague who worked on her floor. In his message he said that he liked her, thought she was very pretty and that he wanted to get to know her. This frightened Priya who had never been 'proposed to' by a guy. Men seldom paid much attention to her. She was dark-skinned and plain faced. Priya was curious about this man, but she had vowed to follow her father's rules that prohibited her from speaking to boys. Though she ignored her suitor, this incident confused her. Was she the type of girl who got proposed to, dated, and maybe even fell in love? Her father definitely didn't think so, but a small part of her did. She decided to resist the advances and blindly follow her father like she had done all her life. But her suitor kept pursuing her, on email, Facebook and through hand-written notes. He told her that he loved her, and that he wanted to marry her. Priya was deeply disturbed by this unsolicited attention, but she maintained her calm and told him that she could only be friends with him, because her father was looking for a husband for her.

The more she ignored him, the more he persisted. The Psycho, as she called him, followed her around, emailed her, and sent her notes, flowers, and chocolates. He got her mobile number, and called and SMSed her incessantly. Things got complicated when the Psycho's mother called Priya and asked her to marry her son. She told Priya that her son was frustrated and that he wasn't coming home to visit because of her. She even offered to call Priya's parents to arrange the marriage.

After the mother's phone call, Priya was greatly distressed, but she had been trained to be disciplined, to suffer quietly even when things were going badly. She would go into the bathroom and cry, and pray that it would all be over soon. Priya was afraid to tell her boss, because she thought he would think less of her; she was afraid to tell her parents because they would blame the entire incident on her. Finally, when she simply couldn't handle the harassment anymore she confided in a colleague, her older brother's friend who was working in the company. He immediately took her to HR.

HR told Priya that cases such as hers, of infatuation, were common. A study conducted in 2011 by the Centre for Transforming India found that a startling 88 per cent of female workers in the country's growing IT and outsourcing industry experienced sexual harassment on the job.

Her case was referred to the Standard Business Conduct (SBC) cell, which heard both sides of the case. The Psycho was fired immediately after the SBC concluded their case. Much to Priya's chagrin, even after the Psycho was fired from the Company on grounds of sexual harassment, he continued his emails and phone calls, which only ceased the day that Priya got married.

◆

On the sort of perfect evening that Bangalore seems to be able to produce on demand, Priya and I sit on the steps of her apartment building chatting. Priya's building is a mammoth, impersonal structure on the outskirts of Bangalore with small, cheap flats, where people from the neighbouring IT offices live. Priya seems calm as she looks through the window where the setting sun is warm and soothing. There is something lovely about Priya, a child-like innocence and an earnestness that is uncommon these days. Though Priya seems a bit lost at times, she is intensely aware of the world around her. Though her English is heavily accented, and at times broken, she is a perceptive conversationalist. With her the conversations are perhaps sad, but always without heaviness.

'I cried a lot that year,' Priya says speaking of the seven months of harassment. 'I'm still crying, but at least now I have someone who loves me.'

A few months after the Psycho was fired, Priya got another Facebook friend request, again from a colleague whom she had never met before. Priya didn't consider herself beautiful and she wondered why men were attracted to her. Like the Psycho (and like Priya herself) her suitor was Tamil so perhaps that explained the attraction.

Compared to their parents' generation, the social lives of IT professionals have become fragmented due to lack of time and the high level of mobility, but nonetheless a number of them cling to older middle-class social values and attempt to reproduce what they regard as the traditional Indian family structure. This may have prompted these Tamil men to pursue Priya, a fellow Tamil, in an attempt to structure a romance that vaguely resembled a marriage that might have been arranged for them by their parents.

Unlike what she felt for the Psycho, this time Priya was intrigued. His name was Kartikey, he was tall, handsome and had a kind, gentle face. Also, she felt so lonely in Bangalore. Her six-month internship at the company had been converted into a full-time job, and her father had not yet summoned her back to the village for her impending marriage. Kartikey seemed like such pleasant company, and slowly she began building a relationship with him. After three months of courtship on email, Facebook and phone, Priya too fell in love.

Priya thinks for a second, as if conjuring up Kartikey's image in her mind, and smiles tentatively. 'I somehow liked this character, and I wanted to be with him.' Unfortunately, her brother's friend, the same one who had encouraged her to take the Psycho to HR, stumbled upon her love interest and told her family about Kartikey.

She looks at me sadly and says, 'My father was very angry with me and told me to come home immediately. I knew that if I went back, they would just marry me off without even looking at the guy properly.'

Kartikey is from the Chettiar caste and Priya is from the Gounder caste, and Priya's father believes deeply in two things: caste and astrology. Priya tells me, 'My father thinks that inter-caste love marriage is worse than a disease. When I asked him why, he told me that love marriage was the reason why our society is falling apart. My parents cried when they found out about my love. They were sad before they got angry. But I knew that Kartikey was my first love, and I didn't want to leave him.'

Priya recalls what had happened to her cousin, who, like Priya, had fallen in love with a colleague. She was forced to quit her job, and was put under house arrest for four years. Priya told me that she got 'nice beatings' from her brother, and after waiting for three long years, her boyfriend eventually married someone else.

'My cousin is now thirty plus. She has crossed the age for marriage and now it is not possible for her to marry someone normal. Still they are searching. She can't sit at home and cry, so she will get married, though it will be a divorcee, or a widower with children. Everything got spoiled for her. I didn't want that to happen to me, so I didn't go back.'

On 7 March 2010, a year after they began their romance, Priya and Kartikey got married, against the wishes of her parents, in a simple temple ceremony in Bangalore. Kartikey's parents accepted the marriage, although grudgingly, and not before they put up a fight. Kartikey's mother wanted her son to marry her brother's daughter, something that is commonly done in the Chettiar caste but Kartikey was resolute and told his mother that if he didn't marry Priya, he would not marry anyone at all.

Priya told her parents that her decision had been the right one and wanted them to meet Kartikey, even if just once, to see this man for themselves. But they would have nothing to do with it. 'Throw away that mangalsutra,' they said. 'We'll find you someone else.' But Priya had made her decision.

When Priya married against her parents' wishes, there were

people she left behind and would never see again. There were things that she loved that she might not ever taste or touch or share again because she was hundreds of miles from all that she had known. From the moment she made up her mind she knew it would take effort and resilience to survive. There were moments when she regretted her decision, when she missed home so badly that it hurt physically. Udumalpet, Tamil Nadu, was still deep within Priya's heart, and the sight of some insignificant thing or a gesture would take her back and remind her of what she once was and where she had once been—it could be the sight of a boiled corncob, or slices of raw mango brushed with red spices being sold by street vendors.

'It's been a year-and-a-half now since I spoke with anyone from my family. They tell me that they don't want to see me till I die,' she says.

For Priya the consequences of her decision were felt a few months after she got married, when the flurry of first love calmed down and real life took over. Priya got pregnant and miscarried a few months later. Six months after her miscarriage, she was pregnant again, and this time around she got an abortion because of complications. After her abortion, Priya became severely anaemic and spent six months in and out of hospitals. Kartikey had to work to pay her hospital bills.

Priya looks away and she speaks impassively. 'Before my marriage, I had so many relations, so many people in my life, and now, staying alone like this, especially in the hospital, it was the worst time in my life. I told my sister about what happened, and I begged her to talk to me, but my sister told me that I took my decision alone and had to face the consequences alone. After this, I decided not to call my parents ever again. I told myself that I would have to live my life here with Kartikey.'

Priya tells me about Kartikey's family. He has two siblings. His sister is divorced; Kartikey supports her and her twelve-year-old daughter. When his sister had an arranged marriage, her husband was a manager at United Colours of Benetton. A year after marriage, he quit his job to become a professional astrologer, and moved to Jaipur. Priya says that he is a 'full-time drinker', and quips that it is ironic that he predicts futures when he doesn't have a grip on his own present. Every month Priya and Kartikey send money home to Kartikey's family, as is expected of the oldest son. They send a larger share then they can truly afford. Even with the double income, finances for the young couple are tight. Bangalore is getting increasingly expensive to live in.

Priya tells me, 'I used to get so many scoldings from my mother-in-law about cooking, about Kartikey's health, about my house. Now she likes me because I earn at my job, and I send money to them. I like working, but also I *have* to work. It's funny, first I came to work because I didn't want to sit at home. Now I have to work to survive.'

Now that night has fallen, we step inside Priya's apartment. Her home is extremely simple, but sparkling clean. The few pieces of furniture are comfortable, but old and unpretentious. Like a teenage girl, Priya has put up posters on the living room walls, of kittens, or puppies, of cartoon hearts. There are plastic dolls with blue eyes and frilly underwear and stuffed animals with beady glass eyes carefully preserved in a glass showcase.

Priya gives me her perspective on marriage. 'If you come to Bangalore, and earn ₹50,000–60,000 per month, you wonder why you should obey any man. This is the way that girls think. Girls are not "adjustable" like they were before.' She continues, 'See my mother, she was adjustable with her mother-in-law. I am not like that. Things are not like before. The older culture is gone.'

Over fluffy onion uttapams that Priya has made for us, I cautiously ask her about sex, unsure if this would be an uncomfortable subject for her to deal with. Priya though is forthright as always. 'In my apartment building we have so many love marriages. All these people are having *everything* before marriage. Those girls who are married have sex with some other guy who is married to some other girl. It happens like this only,' Priya says. 'According to me, though, marriage is not only for sex, it is for other things, and most of all to live happily. I told Karti that I don't want anything to happen between us after that last abortion. He is very understanding about it. He told me that he wants me to get well soon so I can be like before. Some of my friends tell me that their husbands hit them to have sex. My husband is not like that, he is very good to me.'

◆

Kartikey is tall and serious, with sloping shoulders and a relaxed gait. He is dressed casually in a pair of jeans and a shirt. An old habit not easily lost, he totes along his backpack, not the industrial-size backpack from work, but a small, green one for casual use. Priya is dressed in her weekend clothes—a decorative salwaar-kameez with lace and gold, and long golden earrings. Her face is sufficiently powdered, lending her a strangely dusty-white pallor, and her hair has been freshly washed, tied in a loose ponytail. I notice that she has beautiful hair.

We are lunching at Total Mall, one of the many new malls in Bangalore. Unlike his wife, Kartikey is shy and hesitant around me, and it is only after much probing that I am able to get him to tell me a little more about his side of their love story. 'When I saw her I just liked her, I don't know why. It took me a long time to propose. She had complained about another guy, and I was scared that she would complain against me, but I didn't give up. Initially she told me, let's be friends, but I told her, "No, I love you, I cannot be friends with you." After this the rest was history,' he says grinning at Priya.

I ask him about the love lives of his IT colleagues.

He tells me that a lot of people have 'relations'. 'Often you get lonely, far away from home, especially boys. And then there is freedom, no parents, no brothers, and no relatives. You earn a lot of money, and you don't have to ask anyone for permission.

Some people hook up on site, then break up, some stay together. Most people in IT are having love marriages. It is easier that way, because the lifestyle is similar.'

I have heard this before, my grandfather used to make a case for arranged marriage within the caste, saying that 'similar lifestyles and culture' made it easier for the marriages to work out. Economic growth and industry are helping bring down some of the age-old social barriers. For Priya and Kartikey and so many others, it seemed to me IT was a sort of new caste system.

Priya and Kartikey seem very much in love. Like high school lovers, they joke with each other, hold hands, and gaze at each other shyly. Priya tells me that they are going to visit a friend who has recently had a baby. Her voice is soft, with a tentative edge to it. They are overjoyed by the birth of this baby, because before the birth of this child, that couple too had to deal with a miscarriage. I know Priya is desperate to have children so she can quickly fill the blank spaces within her heart.

We take pictures together in the mall, Priya, Kartikey and me. Priya hugs me tight and thanks me for the time that I spent with her. She says she has had more fun than she has had in a long time because I am someone who listens to her carefully, without interrupting her or judging her. I remember a walk that we took, through the office complex one afternoon. Suddenly, apropos of nothing, she turned towards me, and gave me a tight hug, taking me by surprise. She told me that this was the happiest that she had been in days and that she was thrilled to have a friend like me.

◆

'Bangalore has changed more in ten years than in the past hundred. It has seen the most revolutionary cultural change in the recent past since the days of the British,' says Dr Shyam Bhatt, a Bangalore-based psychiatrist who also hosts a popular radio chat show on love, sex and relationships.

Migration and urbanization, and perhaps the most important—a changing culture of love and marriage—have lent the sleepy, south Indian city of his youth a brand new identity.

I meet Shyam Bhatt at a Cafe Coffee Day outlet, the ubiquitous nationwide chain of coffee shops started in Bangalore with the suggestive tag line: 'A lot can happen over coffee'. Its credo seems apposite this morning as the coffee shop is full of amorous couples sipping cappuccinos and sharing dessert.

After spending fifteen years in the US, Dr Bhatt moved to Bangalore, his hometown, to capitalize on the numerous business opportunities available here. His business is burgeoning because of increasing relationship problems, particularly amongst IT professionals.

'Love marriages,' he says, 'are on the rise.' The bulk of his patients are from the IT sector. Typically two young people meet in Bangalore at their work place, marry, and set up permanent base in city. The office atmosphere is like a hothouse because men and women from traditional, conservative families are thrown together suddenly. They experience a sense of freedom, and romance blooms. But with this romance comes a series of problems.

'When they are young, in their twenties, they can handle it. In their thirties, they begin to feel the impact of this new way of life.'

Inexperienced with romance and relationships, they don't know how to deal with the problems that come along with it. As they have often pursued their romance without their parents' knowledge and against their wishes, they have no emotional support network when they hit a rough patch. They look for answers in Western media and other foreign, inappropriate sources and this simply exacerbates the problem.

Shyam worries about the future, he feels that India's love revolution is creating widespread emotional havoc and isn't sustainable. There is too much change too fast. People are now beginning to search for an anchor and for some stability. Many of them have turned to religion and spirituality, and this has led to the mushrooming of spiritual organizations in the city, among them a mammoth Art of Living centre, a New Age spiritual sect, on the outskirts of the city, which propagates a set of meditative breathing techniques for well-being. And there are many spin-offs of this organisation dotting the city.

◆

During my last few days in Bangalore, I move from the centre of the city to my cousin's home in the suburbs. My cousin resides in a lavish colony complete with palm trees, manicured lawns, smooth driveways, a swimming pool and squash courts. I feel like I am in an American suburb, except that everything here feels smaller—compact town houses instead of sprawling mansions, dinky Tata Nanos instead of hulking SUVs, narrow streets instead of mile-wide ones. This housing complex is tastefully done, and well planned, in contrast to the world outside this gated community, where the road is yet to be built, and the stench of sewage is so strong that several of the security guards wear gas masks. Outside the gates of the compound, remnants of village life are still visible. Coconut trees sprout next to dumpsters, a verdant hillock sits next to a two-storey supermarket, mud-coloured houses and walls plastered with cow dung stand warily next to shops selling internet connections and SIM cards. Cows, chickens and other livestock amble around the trucks carrying construction materials for buildings to house the growing population of IT employees.

Here, in this housing complex called Palm Springs, I am protected from the village life outside. I wake up to the sounds of young American voices and cricket games, instead of the sounds of Bangalore that I have gotten used to—clanging temple bells and the raucous sound of traffic. I look out the window into the watery monsoon sunlight and a see a group of boys, mostly South Indian it seems from their dark skin and small frames. They speak and dress like American boys, except that they play cricket instead of baseball. In the years of the brain drain, their parents left India, armed with engineering degrees, to mint their fortunes in the land of dreams, but now India is where the future is, so they have come back—returned to their roots in Bangalore, but with American ideals. Here they seem to have the best of both worlds—maid-servants, drivers, steaming cups of morning chai and elaborate South Indian breakfasts, but also the infrastructure: manicured lawns, communal swimming pools and IT firms where they interact with more Americans than Indians. They vow to raise their children the way that they grew up, with Gandhian values of austerity, discipline, and hard work. Looking around at kids wearing the latest Nike sneakers and sipping from bottles of mineral water I am not sure how this will happen or what this new breed of children will be like. They bring with them American sensibilities, but will grow up in India, they will create their own unique value system—taking a bit of both cultures.

I have promised to go for an evening walk with Tanisha, my cousin's sweet teenage daughter. I go look for her and as I suspect she is on her computer, on Facebook, listening to Rihanna, and looking at photos of the Irish boy band One Direction. Like her father, a talented engineer, thirteen-year-old Tanisha is being trained to solve mathematical problems that would boggle an eighteen-year-old's mind and is expected to attend a top college. She is one of the nicest thirteen-year-olds that I have met. In India, children are always younger than their age, and more innocent. She doesn't demand her privacy, she is very obedient, and listens to her parents, following their orders without any friction.

Her mom, my cousin Ritu, is a successful fashion designer who had an arranged marriage to Anand fifteen years ago. Theirs is a happy, peaceful marriage, though their personalities are so different—my cousin gregarious and social, while Anand is a quiet banker who prefers to spend his free time with his family. Ritu and Anand connect on something more basal: a shared sense of values, similar family and community beliefs.

That weekend, Anand's seventy-five-year-old aunt and uncle have come to visit. They are celebrating their sixty-first marriage anniversary. They live amicably with three generations in one home—each one raised in the same country but in different worlds. The septuagenarian aunt and uncle peacefully accept the world as it changes. They have seen so much change in their lifetimes that nothing surprises them anymore. My cousin Ritu, in her forties, stands on the cusp, grappling with both worlds expertly—the India that buys her fashionable slinky dresses and also the world of arranged marriage. Tanisha goes to an international school in Bangalore and has Korean, Irish, German kids in her class—all of whom live here because their parents work in IT. Tanisha is exposed to world-views of love, dating and romance. When she grows up, arranged marriage will seem bizarre to her, a primitive thing, a vestigial organ of the past. As for me, I am probably the most confused of the lot. Ritu escaped the madness; she came of age before many of the influences that my generation has seen arrived. That said, many women her age have been influenced by this cultural shift, and are getting divorced or having affairs. As for me, I belong to *une génération perdue*—a generation lost. My generation does not have the choice to look back and reclaim the past because we have moved too far ahead. The only thing that we can do is to prepare ourselves for the battle ahead with the sparse resources that we have. I don't know what the future will bring and like Dr Bhatt and Partha, I too am wary of how things will turn out. All I can do is wonder: how long will it take us to find ourselves again?

MATCHMAKER, MATCHMAKER

THE MARRIAGE BROKER
At the South Extension, New Delhi, offices of A to Z Matchmaking Management it is an unusually busy day. A set of parents who have arrived on the morning train from Lucknow wait their turn to register their daughter for marriage. Another anxious pair is scouring biodatas on the A to Z database. Three weddings that the company has brokered are taking place and as part of the service agreement, representatives of the company have to be present at all of them. The auspicious wedding period has begun and there are thousands of weddings taking place every day. There is nothing like a wedding to make people feel anxious about marriage, so clients are pouring in.

Gopal Suri, the founder and man in charge of the most popular marriage bureau in South Delhi, is a small but aggressive man, abrasive in a way that at first is off-putting, but over time becomes endearing. He always wears tight shirts and black jeans, combining his standard outfit with shiny, black, pointed shoes in the summer and a pair of cowboy boots in the winter. He has weaselly eyes and reading glasses dangling from a long golden chain around his thick neck. He is bald, the gleam of his cranium matching that of his shoes. He works out daily, and his chest stretches his shirt impressively. He has a staccato manner of speaking, and his hooded gaze is direct, almost fierce. He is an unlikely marriage broker. I could easily imagine him as a gangster or the operator of a rather shady import-export business. The first time I called, asking if I could interview him, he became extremely defensive, inquiring if I was a private detective, and if his wife had sent me. A year-and-a-half later, I am a regular at the firm. I know most of the cases on file, I have edited biodatas, I have posed as Gopal Suri's assistant in over fifty meetings, I have been set up on dates with prospective husbands, I have even taken charge when Gopalji (as I call him) was indisposed, matched prospective candidates and made marriages happen.

Gopal Suri entered the marriage business by sheer luck. He began his career working with his father in the property business. He then started a guesthouse, Swisston Palace in Karol Bagh—a congested residential area in Delhi. In 2000, a guest from the US stayed at Swisston Palace for over a month, an inordinately long time even at the low rates offered by Gopalji. At this time, there was a rash of terrorist attacks taking place in the country and Gopalji grew suspicious about his foreign guest, Mr Singh. When he eventually confronted him about the unnatural length of his stay, and asked him what he did in his room all day, Mr Singh looked sheepish and said he had been trying to arrange the marriage of his daughter, without any luck. She was thirty and her time was running out; he could not go back to Chicago until he had found her a groom. His last hope was to find a match through the matrimonial ads he had placed in several newspapers. Gopal commiserated with Mr Singh because of his own experience looking for brides through matrimonial columns. He had met eighty girls before he found his wife, the eighty-first.

After a cursory glance at Mr Singh's elegant advertisement for his daughter, Gopal spotted the problem—the trouble was with the wording of his ad, there was nothing wrong with the girl. Mr Singh was simply doing a poor job advertising his daughter. Gopal was an excellent scribe, and the advertisement he drafted for Mr Singh's daughter attracted an unprecedented number of prospective grooms. The boys queued up to meet the 'fair, homely, conservative yet modern US citizen'. In yet another creative stroke, Gopal opened up what he liked to think of as the presidential suite of his guesthouse as a venue for Mr Singh to meet aspiring suitors for his daughter. An ecstatic Mr Singh found the son-in-law of his dreams and decided to book all the rooms at Swisston Palace for the ensuing ten-day-long wedding. In the weeks following Mr Singh's daughter's wedding engagement, Gopalji found many aggrieved parents at his doorstep. They begged him to draft matrimonial ads for their own unwed progeny. Gopalji was only too happy to oblige and had only one condition for anyone who wanted to use his service as a matchmaker—the wedding would have to take place at his guesthouse. Due to burgeoning demand and his enormous success, Gopalji decided that it was time to commercialize his largesse, and he set up A to Z Matchmaking. Today, the annual income from his matrimonial business is ₹1 crore.

◆

Before matrimonial advertisements began appearing in newspapers and periodicals in large numbers from the early years of the twentieth century, the task of finding and negotiating marriages primarily belonged to the traditional matchmakers, the ghatak (male) and the ghataki (female) as they were called in Bengal.[170] The main functions of the ghataks were to select appropriate matches, keep registers and records of marriage and important social events and also to decide the social status of the kulas (families).[171]

George Johnson remarked in a travelogue published in 1843 that ghataks were 'men of a fawning and flattering disposition' who in the 'assemblies of the Hindoos' would 'often panegyrize some individual as much for his giving them a few rupees, as they would satirize him for not listening to their adulation'. He goes on to say: 'They sometimes involved parties in difficulties by getting up matches of a disreputable character; yet nuisances as they are, their services cannot be dispensed with so long as the present system of Hindoo marriage continues, which does not admit of an interview between the bride and bridegroom before the wedding night.'[172]

The occupation of matchmaking by ghataks was compared to horse breeders in an article published in 1886 in the popular Calcutta-based journal, *Prachar*. 'If you go to breeders in these countries,' wrote the author, 'they can trace the lineage of a particular horse. We need professionals who can supply the same information about human beings.'[173] These pandits of yesteryears were trumped first by newspaper matrimonial ads, and later by online matrimonial portals. Today, the pandit has emerged in a new form. Marriage brokers are no dhoti-clad pandits, they are shrewd businessmen (and women) taking advantage of the global ₹25 billion-marriage market of Indian weddings.

A BRIEF HISTORY OF MARRIAGE

Though the love match is gaining popularity in much of urban India, in many parts, arranged marriages are still the norm. It was not always this way. To get a broad view of how the system of arranged marriage evolved into its present form within the Hindu community (this is followed with some cosmetic variations in the Sikh and Jain communities and to a surprisingly recognizable degree in many sections of the Christian community; the Islamic community, the Jewish community and the Zoroastrian community have different methods of arranging marriages), let's take a look at the main texts written during important historical periods to paint a picture of the popular ideologies that existed then.

The *Rig Veda* composed in the latter half of the second millennium BCE tells us that the status of women was equal to that of men; they received an equal education and were taught to recite the Vedas. Even more liberating were the *Rig Veda*'s views on marriage. Women were allowed to marry at a mature age and were free to select their husband.[174]

In the Vedic age, the life of a girl was described to be easy, gay and free.[175] The *Rig Veda* and *Atharva Veda* both mention the Samana festival, during which men and women could meet and choose their partners. It was not uncommon for women to engage in premarital sex or to remain unmarried.[176]

There were eight types of marriage during the Vedic age including the Gandharva and Swayamvara marriages, based on mutual love and attraction. The story of Shakuntala and Dushyanta in the *Rig Veda* is an example of the Gandharva form of marriage—Shakuntala, the beautiful adopted daughter of the sage, marries the handsome king Dushyanta when they fall in love. In the Swayamvara tradition, girls of royal families chose their husbands from among eligible bachelors invited to their houses.

The next stage in the history of marriage is described in the *Mahabharata*, the earliest portions of which date to about 900 BC.[177] It appears that marriage in the age of the *Mahabharata* generally took place within the caste, though marriage outside the caste was not rare. Polygamy or marriage to two or more women by a man was widely practiced and even polyandry, where a woman had multiple husbands was accepted as we see in the case of Draupadi. Premarital and extramarital relationships occurred too, and there are numerous direct and indirect examples in the *Mahabharata*.[178]

According to scholar George Monger, the *Mahabharata* explains the origin of stricter marriage norms by stating that women were once independent and could go astray from husbands, until Svetaketu, the son of Rishi Uddalaka, ruled that husbands and wives should be faithful to each other.

Around 100 CE, the authority of the Smritis and the Puranas replaced that of the Vedic scriptures. Sex and marriage as depicted in the age of the *Mahabharata* came to be inhibited by further taboos and restrictions. The Smritis or *Dharmashastras* were written by multiple authors, of which the best known was the *Manusmriti*,[179] which we have already run into in the course of this book.

The Laws of Manu declared that four of the eight forms of marriage described in the Vedas were invalid. In all four that were considered blessed, fathers found grooms for their daughters; it was said that only these marriages would result in sons who would understand the Vedas. The four others were called 'blameable unions', and included the Gandharva marriage which was a voluntary union in which the daughter chose her own spouse.[180]

There was a distinct shift in attitudes in society as the liberal marital traditions of the Vedic period were dismissed and arranged marriage placed women under male control through a hierarchical and strict system. Society became patriarchal and caste-based, and the union of a man and a woman became intertwined with maintaining social, political and economic status within society. Members of the upper castes arranged marriages between themselves to prevent defilement of their castes.

Chapter 1 of the *Manusmriti* explains the caste system in terms of the birth of each caste from a different body part of Lord Brahma—the Brahmins, Kshatriyas, Vaishnavas and Shudras.

The Laws of Manu dictated that marriage should take place within the caste, and also set out the consequences for breaking the law. For example: 'A Brahmana who takes a Shudra wife to his bed, will (after death) sink into hell; if he begets a child by her, he will lose the rank of a Brahmana.' (V.3.17)

In the Smritis, extramarital affairs were treated as adultery. According to Apastambha, 'in adultery a man's penis and testicles are to be cut off, in evil-doing with a maiden his property shall be seized, and he be banished from the land'.[181]

Child marriage too became the norm rather than the exception.

The rules below constituted the now orthodox marital practices of the Hindus.[182]

1. Marriage must be completed by the recitation of mantras, performance of yagna, and pacing of the seven steps.

2. Marriage must be within the caste and the daughter must be married before puberty.
3. In marriage one is to avoid strictly one's gotra, pravara and sapinda.
4. A married woman must observe the strictest rules of chastity and remain a pativrata.

Among the many strange laws that were framed in ancient times was one that set out the strict order in which siblings were to marry. It was unlawful for the younger sister to marry before the elder one. Further, in the case of such a marriage, 'the husband of the younger but first married sister, and the husband of the later married elder sister must be expelled from the caste and not to be invited to the *shrad* ceremony'.[183]

I wonder what my younger sister and her husband, who married before I did, would make of these laws!

The third chapter of Kautilya's important text, the *Arthashastra* gives us a very detailed account of the state of marriage during the time of its composition. (200 CE, though this year varies across texts. The *Arthashastra* was important roughly during the age of the Smritis.) In the *Arthashastra*, women were granted considerable independence and they had the right to own property. Both women and men were allowed to remarry, a form of restricted polygamy prevailed and inter-caste marriages and divorce (in some circumstances) too was permitted.[184]

THE ARTHASHASTRA SAYS:

If the woman engaged herself in amorous intrigues, or drinking in spite of the order of her husband, she was punished with three pana. If she went out to see another man, she was fined twelve panas. If she committed the same offences during nighttime she was fined double.

For more serious punishment, like holding a conversation with a man in a suspicious way, whipping was prescribed.

With *The Laws of Manu* began a gradual decline of the social status of women; marital practices grew steadily illiberal, and this worsened under colonial rule.

The British often interfered with the social customs of their subjects as a means of strengthening their rule. By creating divisive personal laws, and politicizing marriage and community laws, they were able to control and keep communities apart, and ostensibly provide better administration and law and order. Under the British, there were separate marriage laws for Hindus and Muslims. Colonial laws defined property as belonging to the joint family, and individual shares were calculated on marriage and death, escalating the importance of marriage. Colonial law outlined different forms of ownership for women, including the times when women could receive gifts from their families. For example, women could only receive inheritances from their family during marriage, which made it critical that women marry with the approval of their family, or risk losing everything.

British rule played a crucial role in strengthening arranged marriage amongst their subjects at a time when love matches were becoming common in many parts of the world. Marriage and the family at the end of the nineteenth century and the beginning of the twentieth century were a hybrid product of Indian society's encounter with colonial rule, as well as struggles internal to that society.[185]

Despite colonial repression, some social changes helped improve the status of women. Raja Rammohan Roy led the movement to eradicate sati, which led to the Bengal Sati Regulation Act in 1829, and then the Widow Remarriage Act in 1856. Other significant legislation to be enacted at the time was the Child Marriage Restraint Act of 1929, which stipulated that the minimum age of marriage be fourteen, when the mean age at marriage for females at the time was just thirteen as calculated from the 1901-1931 census data.[186] Ironically, it was the same Raja Rammohan Roy who made marriage more liberal who held on to retrograde views on sex.

Post-independence, there has been a progress in marriage legislation which has weakened the caste system, democratized marriage, and given women more rights, justice and freedom. There has also been a slow but steady rise in the age of marriage, though child marriages continue to take place in many parts of the country. It was only in 2006 that a new law banning child marriage was passed.

The most important legislation on marriage has been the Hindu Marriage Act of 1955, which allowed for divorce. The Special Marriage Act (reformed 1954) allowed for inter-caste marriage, and was followed by the Foreign Marriage Act, 1969, where Indians could marry other nationalities. The Hindu Married Women's Right to Separate Residence and Maintenance Act of 1946 declared that a Hindu married woman would be entitled to a separate residence and maintenance under certain circumstances.

LONELY HEARTS

British rule not only brought with it an oppressive view of marriage, but also a modern way of partner hunting. Personal ads have been a popular way of finding partners for over 300 years in this country. Marriage advertisements came to India with the British. British Civil Service officers posted in remote places in the subcontinent had little hope of meeting young English women, so ads were placed in newspapers to reach the eyes of single ladies and their families.

Indians quickly adopted this practice, and in India in the second half of the nineteenth century the methods of spouse selection through matrimonial advertisements gave a fillip to the marriage market and escalated practices such as dowry.[187]

As traditional social networks weaken, the matrimonial ad is once again in vogue. It is estimated that about ₹2,450 crores is spent annually on newspaper matrimonial ads, and an astounding 7.5 million Indians use the internet to find partners.[188]

◆

Ever since I can remember, I have loved reading the matrimonial pull-out of the Sunday papers. This was a favourite activity of mine when I lived in India, and when I did not, it was one of the reasons I looked forward to coming back. What I found in these pages never failed to amuse, astound, and at times disturb me. Year by year, I have noticed the matrimonial sections getting leaner, and today most matrimonial sections of popular English newspapers are terribly lean—just two to four pages long—a considerable contraction from the previous twenty to fifty page deck, possibly because seekers of marriage are moving to new platforms like e-portals and marriage bureaus. However, the range of ads has widened. And, as people move past caste lines, new categories have emerged such as 'Doctor', 'MBA', 'Second Marriage', 'Cosmopolitan', and 'No Dowry/ Spiritual'. Featured at the bottom of many ads, 'Caste No Bar' too appears more often, heralding a welcome change from the past.

A typical matrimonial posting for a bride would ask that candidates be: fair, beautiful, god-fearing, homely, quiet, respectful, innocent, humble, and cultured. 'Homeliness' is omnipresent in matrimonial ads. As per the dictionary, the definition of homely is *'lacking in physical attractiveness, not beautiful, unattractive'*. Who wants a homely wife? On enquiry, I discovered that in the context of Indian matrimonial ads, 'homely' simply means that the girl should like to 'stay at home'.

Skin colour remains an important marker of physical attractiveness especially where women are concerned. Research has shown that in matrimonial ads, more women than men announced skin colour, and men indicated a preference for fair-skinned brides. I notice an advertisement in the Muslim Sunni column:

Vitiligo/ Leucoderma Girl. Beautiful, V fair. 26/5'2". Living in Gorakhpur.

A person with leucoderma actually suffers a loss of pigmentation but this appears to be a plus in the Indian matrimonial market.

Since we are in the middle of massive societal change, it is not uncommon to see confused ads with descriptions like 'traditional girl with modern qualities', 'homely working girl', 'fair, educated beautiful, slim outgoing yet conservative', or 'MBA workaholic, teetotaller, 29, 5'9" well settled IT boy seeking fair homely but active girl'.

As divorce rates skyrocket, there are an increasing number of divorce advertisements:

GUPTA 39/5'7.5" LOOKS LIKE 35 ONLY. Divorced with 1 male child, well-settled business at Lucknow seeks soft-spoken fair I'less girl from decent family. Mail complete biodata with RECENT coloured photo.

I'less here means 'issueless', and an issue is a child. Indian men may have several 'issues', but a woman with an 'issue' is a serious issue. An ad for a woman divorcee typically looks like this:

KHATRI pnjbi sawhney girl 5'1"/30 fair own aerobic centre 2 day divorcee, no issue

A '2 day divorcee', 'early marriage' or 'very short marriage' are common in advertisements from women divorcees since divorce is still considered by many to be taboo.

Sometimes in addition to the usual, caste, skin colour, weight, height traits one does notice some strange personal qualities advertised. For example, one centre page, large boxed ad goes like this:

> A Jat Sikh professional and business family well settled in London, England since 1960s seek a bride for their 30 year old Doctor son. He wears turban and uncut beard, which he ties very neatly. He is Non-vegetarian, 5'9", tall, slim, athletic and fair.

Their description for their well-endowed son is specific, as is the criteria for their daughter-in-law to be:

> We are looking for a Sikh girl who is a Medical Doctor with MBBS or MB or BDS or MDS between the age of 25 & 28 yrs slim, fair and pretty between 5'3" and 5'6".

A report that I recently read said that among those who responded to a series of advertisements seeking HIV-positive partners for HIV-positive men, eight prospective brides thought HIV-positive was an educational qualification.

My all-time favourite ad is perhaps this one: 'Family seeks homely, convent-educated girl for son. Caste no bar. But must be able to drive tractor. Photo of tractor appreciated.'

While reading the matrimonial section made my Sunday morning more enjoyable, as I've noted, there is a strong move away from print ads to online matrimonial ads.

When matrimonial websites were first launched in the early 2000s, they were thought of as the last, desperate effort to get married. Today, the 120 per cent growth rate for the US$1.4 billion (₹8,719 crore) online matrimony industry indicates that there has been a paradigm shift in market sentiment.[189] There are more than 20 million users on over 150 matrimonial websites and an astonishing 48 per cent of internet users in India use matrimonial sites.[190] As of 2009, Shaadi.com, a popular matrimonial website, claimed to have over 8,22,073 matches to their credit.[191] E-portals are now expanding to tap into regional and vernacular markets by launching sites that are tailored specifically to the requirements of India's various states and their regional needs. They are also beginning to harness the potential in television and mobile markets. Recently, Shaadi.com produced a television reality show that traced the journey of participants from finding a suitable match online to getting married and living as a nuclear family. Bharatmatrimony.com, a large online portal, has partnered with Idea Cellular to launch customized matrimony services to tap into the fast-growing mobile market.

Matrimonial sites have also evolved to cater to niche markets with portals like Overweightshaadi.com for overweight people, Positiveshaadi.com for people who are HIV-positive and, with the skyrocketing divorce rates, Secondshaadi.com, a website catering only to divorcees.

Matrimonial websites present certain advantages over traditional newspaper websites and this has led to the shift from newspaper to the internet for the urban, educated, middle-class population. The popularity of E-portals shows an interesting change in the role of the family in marriage as partner selection is gradually moving away from parents to the prospective brides and grooms as a trend of online courtship emerges.

E-portals have also reflected the decreasing role of caste in marriage. For example, on Shaadi.com, users need to select their caste from a dropdown menu with more than 400 choices when creating a profile. But just below this, the portal has introduced a little box to ask if the person is open to inter-caste marriage. The company has found that many are choosing to tick this box.

'The heads of some of India's most successful matrimonial websites agree that there is a rising stated preference for partners outside the applicant's own caste. "The majority of our users now state 'caste no bar' in their profiles. It would be around 60%, I think," [says] Gourav Rakshit, Chief Operating Officer of Shaadi.com.'[192]

Marriage portals though do come with their fair share of trouble. Many parents complain that online matrimonial sites are more 'dating sites' and young people use these websites to meet people though they aren't interested in marriage. In a country where access to women is still difficult, matrimonial websites present a new universe of opportunity to men.

Another problem is fake profiles. Matrimonial portals went under the scanner in 2007, after the arrest of Liaquat Ali Khan who advertised himself as a UK-based Indian engineer with two homes.

Khan allegedly tricked many women from India into marriage. In their enthusiasm for a 'groom from abroad' these women did not check the veracity of his claims. He fleeced them of money, telling them that he needed it for wedding arrangements—passports, visas to the UK and the honeymoon. After forty-two engagements and eight marriages, Khan's exploits were discovered when computer studies student Sangeetha Dineshan filed a police complaint. It was discovered that Khan was married, had a daughter, and lived in India, where he ran an internet café.

It is not only customers who are realizing the risks of finding spouses online. The lack of transparency and insecurity in the e-matrimony market is leading to the revival of the age-old matchmaker. Even matrimonial sites have diversified into the offline world with brick and mortar structures or marriage bureaus. Recently Shaadi.com started Shaadi Centres or offline, brick and mortar matchmaking outlets. Today, almost every residential colony in every urban neighbourhood has its local marriage bureau. Here sit marriage brokers, professionals who realize that in India marriage is often as much of a business transaction as an affair of the heart. It is here that the marriage brokers conduct their business—the twenty-first-century version of the old style matchmakers.

◆

Since its inception a decade ago, A to Z Matchmaking has arranged over a thousand marriages worldwide. I am enchanted by the efficiency of this organization, which is run like a boutique investment bank. Teams of young women in their early twenties are dedicated to different segments of society ranging from the middle class to the elite. An in-house astrology team pulls up birth charts on laptops, and a detective team, headed by a cranky retired colonel, performs background checks on listed clients. A to Z has an extensive menu of services and various matrimonial packages for different sections of society—middle class, upper-middle, elite and a super elite category. Registration in a higher bracket gives access to people with more wealth, and there is an option to upgrade for a fee at any point during the process of finding a spouse. The colourful brochure, filled with pictures of happy couples (including one non-Indian, blonde, blue-eyed couple) advertises a full range of services that include 'showing' the girl, relaying messages between the two families, supervising boy-girl meetings, negotiating wedding budgets, and being present at all wedding functions from the engagement to the wedding reception. These investment bankers of love specialize in organizing 'live deals'—making marriages sound like something from the Goldman Sachs mergers and acquisitions department.

'This is a very good business,' Gopalji tells me. 'There is never a down cycle. Whether the economy is good or bad, people are always getting married. If you think about it, it is probably the most stable business in the world.'

According to eminent psychoanalyst Sudhir Kakar, who has studied the Indian psyche for decades, especially in the realm of relationships, 'Perhaps the greatest attraction of an arranged marriage is that it takes away the young person's anxiety around finding a mate. Whether you are plain or good-looking, fat or thin, you can be reasonably sure that a suitable mate will be found for you.'[193] What Kakar says is true. In India, everyone is matched, from the mentally impaired to the physically handicapped. Marriage is something that must be done and is regarded as the first step into adulthood.

Apparently the marriage brokerage business has flourished in the past ten years, mostly because of Indian parents' perennial anxiety around the marriage of their children. Traditionally, family members used to bring rishtas (matches) and guide parents but now people are worried that if the boy or the girl turns out to be 'defective', implying badly behaved, impotent, or with 'bad habits' like alcohol or drug abuse, then they will be blamed. Gopalji says this is compounded by the ever-increasing rate of divorce which has made families paranoid, so they begin to look for someone reliable to help them navigate the marriage process and find a stable match for their son or daughter. In fact, the high divorce rates have compelled Gopalji to add a small disclaimer to his registration form, 'Marriage will be done at the risk of the couple only'.

Gopal Suri's language has its own idiosyncrasies, its own syntax, its own vocabulary, and its own rules of grammar: the genesis of his language is newspaper matrimonial ads. Here is a sampling of his (and other brokers') 'vernacular':

- No matter how old the to-be-wedded are, they are called 'children' or 'kids'. In the world of Indian matrimonial ads unless you are married you never really grow up.
- The to-be-married are simply referred to as 'those in question'. The girl's family is referred to as 'girl's side', and the boy's as 'boy's side', or as 'the party' or 'interested party'. For example, Gopalji would tell me that 'a party' called him today to discuss negotiations.
- Age is relayed not by numbers but by year of birth. I am '84-born' instead of twenty-eight, a thirty-year-old is '81-born'.
- The 'budget' is the amount of money the girl's side is willing to spend on the wedding.

An arranged marriage is a ponderous mating dance between two families. It is the parents of the singleton 'in question' who are usually in touch with Gopal Suri, almost never those who want to get married, as this is seen as a sign of desperation. Occasionally the 'ones in question' who do show up are the thirty-plus girls who are so desperate to be married that they spend endless hours at the office, almost as long as I do. Siblings too, are often intensively involved in the matrimonial process, especially brothers. Usually parents or a mother-brother duo or a mother-father-brother trio will come to meet Gopalji and scour his database to find a good match.

The first step towards a successful match is to have an

impressive biodata. A biodata is essentially a resume that includes a large colour photograph, birth date and time (for astrological purposes), height and weight, and also details of the family members including their income. Gopalji is a master editor and can add sheen to even the dullest of biodatas.

For example, take Amar Prashant Khaitan Dhingra below:

Name: Prashant Amar Dhingra

> Date, Time & Place of Birth:
> 21 January 1981 13:42 Delhi
> *(Most parents insist on matching horoscopes, and if the time of birth used to make a birth-chart does not match with a prospective biodata, then Gopalji has no scruples in changing the time by a few minutes.)*
>
> Height 5'11"
> *(Amar's height is 5'8" but Gopalji has added three inches. He tells him to wear shoes with heels when meeting girls.)*
>
> Family : Presently working for Nine 'O' Nine Exports as financial consultant. Has worked with a renowned export firm as senior financial consultant for 9 years. Earlier worked with SBI on a managerial position.
>
> Amar Prashant is our only Son.
> *(This is an important point. Being an only son or the eldest son ensures an inheritance.)*
>
> My wife has earlier worked with SBI as a branch manager and is now a practicing home loan counsellor with SBI.
> My daughter is an MBA (finance) working as a Lecturer with a Management Institute & is also pursuing a PhD (International Finance) from DU.
> *(The more educated the family, the better. Since the family is well-educated, Gopalji thinks it wise to include everyone's education.)*

Education : Engineering from Amity school of Engineering & Technology Affiliated to IP University. Also pursuing Executive MBA (IB) from IIFT (Indian Institute of Foreign Trade).

Occupation : My Son is working as Module Leader with a renowned MNC in Noida. He has travelled abroad twice.
(Travel abroad shows international exposure.)

Assets & Status : Ours is a very affluent outgoing family with values & ethics & assets around Delhi.

ANNUAL INCOME (boy) : 5.60 lakhs.
(His actual income is 4 lakhs but Gopalji feels that an extra 1.60 lakhs would attract considerably better matches.)

Let's now take a look at the biodata of one of the prospective brides that Gopalji has in his database.

Name: Namita Aurora
Namita is very soft spoken, sweet natured and down to earth girl. She is smart and confident as well. She has very good small-town values.
(Being 'soft-spoken' is seen as a very positive trait in the matrimonial market, as it usually implies that the girl will be 'adjustable'. Also small-town values are often an asset—though it is clarified that she is smart and confident—especially in the metro cities, where conservative families feel girls are becoming too liberal.)

Date of Birth : 13 June 1979
Time of Birth : 09 42 Hrs.
Place of Birth : Jammu
Religion : Hindu
Height : 5 Feet 04 Inches
Complexion : Fair
(Namita is not exactly fair. In matrimonial terms, she would be

'wheatish', but Gopalji has photoshopped her photographs, and asked her to wear make-up on visits.)

Hobbies : Gymming
(When the candidate has no considerable hobbies, Gopalji, invariably lists 'gymming' because it suggests that the person takes their body seriously and will remain in good shape.)

Astrologically : **NOT A MANGLIK**
(Gopalji has made this bold, because, as I will discuss later, being a manglik is no good.)

Smoking Habits : Non Smoker
Drinking Habits : Non Consumer
(No virtuous Indian girl in the matrimonial market will smoke or drink.)

Monthly Income : ₹3.4 Lacs PA
Special Achievement : Won Four Appreciation Awards & Certificates In Airtel.
Education : Schooling Tiger Army Public School, Satvari, JAMMU 1997
B.Sc G.G.M. Sc. College, JAMMU 2000
MBA (Finance & Marketing), JAMMU UNIVERSITY 2002
(Namita's education from Jammu, a small town, is highlighted to exemplify her small-town values.)

Occupation : Pvt. Sector Officer R.I.L Communications, Assistant Manager, 2008
Father's Name : Mr. V.K Aurora
Father's Profession : Chief Engineer in P.H.E.D—Water Supply Department
Mother's Name : Mrs. Reva Aurora
Mother's Profession : Homemaker
Family Income : ₹7 lakhs (PA)

(The family income is 5 lakhs, but Gopalji throws in an extra two.)

Details of Siblings: Aman Aurora, 21 Years old, Brother, is doing Engg. From Bharti Vidyapeeth, Pune (Single)
Neeyati Aurora, 29 Years old, Sister, is a Doctor in Batra Medical College (Single)
(An unmarried sister of twenty-nine reflects badly on Namita, so her sister has been put at the very end of the biodata.)

The picture accompanying the biodata is of prime importance. Gopalji has a photographer on his payroll who takes appropriate biodata photographs, and is in charge of complexion photoshopping.

To find out more I speak with Sheena, the photographer. She tells me that she likes to take candid shots in natural home environments as opposed to studio shots because it 'shows more personality'. She shows me some of her work—a girl sitting on her bed hugging a petal-pink fluffy teddy bear, her long hair styled perfectly. Sheena points out that she is wearing a salwaar-kameez. Gopalji suggests that all the photographs be taken in Indian clothing or conservative western clothing, like a long skirt or jeans with a long-sleeved top. She shows me another one of a boy (in reality he is middle-aged) wearing a tight t-shirt and standing next to his car his hands folded self-consciously over his belly. Sheena says that she likes to portray her clients' hobbies or interests and passions through her photographs. The girl in the salwaar-kameez loves stuffed toys; the boy loves his cars. Another photograph appears with a television set in the background. This boy, she says, loves watching cartoons. I ask if people like reading, if she has shot any pictures with books. I imagine that if I got a biodata picture shot I would make sure I had a full bookshelf behind me. Sheena gives me a doubtful look. 'No, not really. Maybe magazines, but no,' she says shaking her head, 'not even that.'

Gopalji uses a few important points to guide the matchmaking process. He explains his method to me. The most important criteria for eligibility on both the boy's side and the girl's side is wealth. Caste is no longer the be all and end all of arranged marriages, explains Gopalji. It is perhaps not even a starting point. Wealth defines caste, and people want to marry into a family of equal prosperity. People prefer to stay within their communities, although communities have become fairly inclusive. So Aggarwals are happy to marry Gujaratis, Marathas, Jains, or Marwaris. Punjabis will marry Sindhis because they have a similar mentality.

I ask Gopalji what the average age of marriage at A to Z is. Gopalji says that over the past decade, the age is increasing for girls and boys. 'Today, the average age for marriage of girls is twenty-six, for boys, it is twenty-eight. Five years ago, the average age for girls was twenty-three, and for boys, it was twenty-six.' Gopalji says the timeline for marriage is completely random. 'Sometimes it happens instantaneously, the decision is taken at the first meeting, sometimes it takes a few years to get a girl married. That is why I ask families to start looking for their children, especially for their daughters, once they turn twenty-two. Girls begin to lose their innocent looks after twenty-five, and then it is very difficult for me to find anyone for them.'

Gopalji often mentions 'innocent looks'. If a girl is especially pretty, he won't say that she has a nice face, or even nice skin if she is fair. He will just say in admiration, 'What an innocent face'. I ask him what he means, and he isn't able to put it in words. 'Innocent just means innocent, like a small baby.' I wonder if this is part of the Indian obsession with virginity and purity.

According to Gopalji, for the girl's side, the second most important thing is the boy's career. Gopalji divides his clients into two broad categories—professionals and businessman. He usually matches people within these categories, because they possess the same 'family culture'. If the father owns a business the children either work in the family business, or set up their own. If the father is a professional, then the kids are usually professionals too. It is rare for these two categories to join in matrimonial alliance. It isn't that one is preferable over the other, but rather that everyone seems to want to marry their own kind—doctors want doctors, engineers want engineers, and businessmen want businessmen.

From the boy's perspective, the third criteria is looks. The girl should be good looking, especially if the boy is wealthy. Usually, girls are more willing to compromise on the looks of the boy. Family matters to the girl. It is important to see the mentality of the family. How is the mother-in-law? Will she let you go out of the house? If the girl likes to wear jeans and short skirts, will she be allowed to do that after marriage? If she is an independent-minded, working girl, will she be able to cope with a restrictive mother-in-law?

Gopalji's clients primarily consists of upper-middle class Punjabi and Marwari families. Different religious groups like Parsis, Muslims, Sikhs, and Christians have their own marriage brokers. Gopalji's most coveted clients are boys between the ages of twenty-four to twenty-eight—in the prime of their marital youth, because these are the most in demand. His least favourite clients are girls (though they are hardly girls anymore) above thirty-three—because he has the most trouble marrying them off. He has recently started charging a premium for registering female clients northwards of thirty.

When I ask Gopalji if he arranges matches between north and south Indians, he looks at me incredulously: north and south Indians never consider each other in an arranged setup. Though they may come from the same caste, their cultures and customs are too disparate. South Indians have their own marriage brokers. He has had over 20,000 clients in a decade as a marriage broker, but never has a south Indian person registered with him.

After Gopalji shortlists potential matches, he hands the baton over to the parents. 'Parents are very smart. They shortlist three or four boys. They don't pressurize the girl for one boy. They do the initial filtration, and the girl or the boy makes the final choice. This is good because parents observe many things, whereas the children are only interested in ego satisfaction. The family see the big picture, not the small things like the girls and boys do. Girls will say, 'Oh, his hair is less; we don't want to marry him.' Or the boy will say, 'Her skin is dark; I won't marry her.' The parents know their children best, and they can make better decisions for them.'

Gopalji's formula has been carefully developed and is time-tested. It is based on a few solid principles. The first is that the two families must meet before the girl and the boy do. For a first meeting it is standard for two entire families including grandparents, siblings and even close relatives to meet. 'If I ever have the kids meet first, I have gotten totally failed. It has been a total flop show. The parents have to meet first because they consider everything: money, education, values, and they can motivate the kids accordingly. Let me tell you an example. There were two families, Marwaris and Sindhis, and they like each other's biodatas. But I knew that this would never work because all Marwaris think Sindhis are snakes. I insisted that the families meet first so that they could see if they gelled. The parents met three times, and then the children. The kids had twenty-six meetings for twenty-six days, not skipping even a day. They observed each other carefully. They went to a bar; how much does the other person drink? What is the temperament after they drink? What kind of behaviour does he display when he is sad? How does she behave during her monthlies? Finally, they got married, and today they are happily married.'

Typically, Gopalji first meets both families individually, usually at their homes, so he can gauge their standard of living. He also likes to meet 'those in question' so that he can assess their personality types. If he feels that the two families, and those in question are compatible, then he organizes a joint meeting, always at the boy's side house. It is important for the girl's side to see the boy's home because this is where their daughter will live after marriage. After this initial meeting, the boy and girl are allowed to meet alone without supervision, though Gopalji carefully tracks their meeting and progress. If all goes well and everyone likes each other, then marriage discussions ensue. These negotiations are around how much the girl's family will spend on the wedding. Dowry, the act of giving or taking money or material assets from the bride during the time of marriage, is legally banned in India, yet it proliferates abundantly, albeit in a new form. Gopalji helps me understand.

Typically the first question that Gopalji will ask the family of the bride is how much they are willing to spend on the wedding. He then shares this number with other party, who then consider if the proposed wedding budget matches their 'status'. If not, then Gopalji will try to extract more money from the girl's side. The higher the 'wedding budget' and the more willing the girl's side is to spend on the wedding, the better the prospective grooms they can bag.

Money, Gopalji assures me, is *hardly ever* a problem. The purchasing power of the urban middle and upper-middle classes has increased tremendously (he relates it mostly to escalating land prices). Besides, a big wedding shows that a family has arrived.

STAR-CROSSED LOVERS

Gopalji's two least favourite people in the office are the two 'astro-boys', as he calls them, whose main job is to match birth charts with the help of efficient computer software. It isn't that he particularly dislikes them, it is more that he dislikes astrology in general, and he feels a great deal of pain in paying monthly salaries to his two astro-boys because so many parents insist on matching the birth charts of prospective grooms and brides.

When it comes to astrology, even the most educated people can be surprisingly superstitious. A friend of mine, a perfectly rational and intelligent student of science who studied at Stanford and then Harvard, refused to even *meet* a boy if their birth charts did not match. Then she fell in love with a man who was manglik, a man whose unfortunate alignment of stars made him somewhat of an astrological leper. She finally convinced her parents of the virtues of the man she hoped to be her husband, and they reluctantly blessed the star (un)crossed lovers. Could an alignment of the stars at the time of our birth dictate our future? Human beings have nearly touched the stars, how could we then let the intergalactic forces dictate our future?

The day that I turned twenty-five, an astrologer was unleashed on me too. To assuage their anxieties about my delayed marriage, my parents called an astrologer who plugged in my time and place of birth into his computer which threw up a quick astrological chart and told my parents that I would not get married for the next five years. My parents were infuriated by his analysis and they ordered the 'fraud' out of the house.

'The truth is that astrology is a long lost science and only 1 per cent of the astrologers know what they are talking about. Today, astrology is mostly used by fakes to make a quick buck and for parents to make excuses when they don't like a proposal,' declares Gopalji. It appears that astrology has other purposes too. 'If parents, especially the girl's side, really like a match then they will make fake birth charts so that they match.'

It is clear that astrology plays an inordinately important role in the marriage discussion, often making or breaking alliances. The practice of astrology is deep-set in the Hindu tradition, and it forecasts events in a person's life based on planetary influences. The underlying philosophy behind astrology is that your past life's karma dictates your present life. The importance of astrology can be revealed by glancing at newspaper matrimonial ads, many of which boast that the prospective bride/groom is 'non manglik' because being manglik or under the effect of the evil planet

Mars is an unfortunate circumstance in the matrimonial market.

To find out more about what all the fuss is about, I speak to K. N. Rao, a well-known astrologer, author and founder member of the world's largest school of astrology based in New Delhi. I meet Rao in his small apartment in the suburbs of Delhi. In a crowded office, the wizened Rao, with his snow-white beard and eyes clouded over with age, holds court. There are lots of people here; mostly middle-aged couples who have come to pose questions to Rao. I wait my turn while a worried couple inquires about their daughter's troubled marriage. Next up is an older couple who declare that their family is going through a bad financial period, and wish to know when it will end. All this while there is a cricket match on television, which Rao turns attentively to from time to time. Rao is well known for his accurate predictions of the Indian cricket team's performance.

Finally, it's my turn and we begin talking. When Rao was growing up (he is eighty-six now) kundlis (birth charts) were not matched with the same sort of fervour as they are today. Marriages were conducted within the caste, community, and most commonly between families who lived close by. Birth charts were typically matched only at the time of marriage to find a propitious muhurta or date and time of the marriage ceremony so that it could be performed under the most beneficial planetary energies.

Rao declares that it was only in post-colonial India that astrology began to play an important role in the matrimonial process. As families moved away from their ancestral villages in search of better prospects, it became harder to make informed matches, and that's when astrologers began playing an important role. Today, when so many marriages are being arranged through the newspaper and internet, often families know nothing about each other, so they turn to astrology—stoked by the fear of the unknown. Because of this fear, which has only risen with the climb in divorce rates, a whole industry has sprung up to match horoscopes and prescribe expensive pujas to solve future problems.

Rao strongly believes that most self-proclaimed pandits/astrologers are frauds and they use astrology to promote superstition and make money. For example, if two birth charts do not match, then often the man or woman is married first to a tree or pot, and then to his bride/groom. In recent times, this method made headlines when it was reported that actress Aishwarya Rai was first married to a tree before she married Abhishek Bachchan because of a peculiarity in her birth chart.[194] After this celebrity marriage made national headlines, many other young ladies were married to trees before their 'real' weddings.

During the last seventy years of his practice as an astrologer, Rao has come across people with well-matched horoscopes living in unhappy marriages, and ill-matched horoscopes living in peaceful marriages. An ideal match, he says, is based on social, financial and emotional reasons. An astrologer, based on the insights provided by horoscopes, can at best counsel a couple on ways of building a fulfilling marriage, but *cannot* predict the future, especially in these modern, 'egotistical' times. However, as in the olden days, astrology can also be used to calculate the most auspicious wedding time.

Scholar Rochona Majumdar who studies matrimony in her book, *Marriage and Modernity: Family Values in Colonial Bengal*, supports Rao's theory, and wonders whether the growing importance of astrology is because people are getting married with less information than they would have ideally liked about their partner. She writes, 'It is possible that in the absence of detailed genealogical information, knowledge that at least the stars were favourable to a prospective match comforted anxious parents. The urban astrologer in Calcutta owed his existence, in part at least, to this condition.'[195]

TROUBLE IN PARADISE

One slow, blisteringly hot and hopelessly slow summer day, with no electricity in the office, Gopalji's distress is palpable. His distress, unlike mine, is not related to the temperature. Gopalji has lost a key client, and he is furious. Facebook has emerged as a major problem in the marriage brokerage business; I have heard this from more than one broker. Matchmaking is all about access, and it is through Gopalji that parents get access to information. Now networks like Facebook give direct access, taking away some of the broker's advantage.

Gopalji explains, 'I introduced two parties. The girl's side was very wealthy, but the girl wasn't very good looking. She was dark-skinned and fat, and she was having some trouble finding a match. The boy was very handsome and a professional, but the status of his family was nowhere close to that of the girl's side. The girl's side rejected the boy's side. The girl's father gave me a cheque and told me to bring him matches and to work very hard on this case. During this time, the boy added the girl on Facebook and started liking her comments. They started doing things behind the scenes while I was hunting for matches for the girl. Then suddenly one day I find out from someone that the fat girl and the handsome boy are getting married. They didn't tell me, even though *I* was the one who introduced them. The girl's father told me that it was a 'love marriage!' And now those cheap bastards, the boy's side, won't pay me, and even the girl's side is not giving me the entire payment.'

When it rains, it pours; as if Gopal's mood weren't sour enough, one of his big-ticket clients, a girl's side party that owns a large chewing-tobacco company has cancelled a meeting, declaring that the girl has 'female problems', implying her period. Gopalji is apoplectic, so angry that the crown of his bald head has turned a peony pink. He had been thrilled when the parents of the two parties had agreed to take the matter forward. He had organized a meeting between the girl and the boy at a coffee shop in Delhi, and they were set to meet today—in exactly two hours. The 'female problem' excuse seems spurious to me. I wonder what had *really* happened. Has the young girl got cold feet?

Gopalji looks crestfallen, all the frustration has worn the poor man thin. Now he just seems afraid of losing business from the boy's side. He shrugs and looks at me glumly, 'Probably she got some better proposal. This marriage market is like the stock market, very volatile, you have to close deals quickly or they escape your hands.'

◆

Independent Contact for proposal for moderately fair, good looking, only son 5'11" Lking for smart, homely, height not less than 5'4" not desirous of working, qualified, lively, age between 24-26. Boy Divorcee, but only son of parents.

'The baraat was big and grand, with horses, elephants, and even camels. We made both the grandmothers sit on top of a rath (carriage) so they would not miss a thing. We didn't ask the girl's family for anything, no dowry, no wedding budget. When the girl left, they filled a Toyota Innova with her stuff and left. That is how *little* the girl brought when she came to us. The girl's side were from Haryana, so during the marriage we bought a car with Haryana license plates, so it *looked* like they brought something,' said Mr Gupta, speaking of his son's recent wedding and subsequent divorce.

I am at the home of the Guptas with Gopalji, posing as his associate. The Guptas are in the market for a new bride for their thirty-year-old-son who has separated from his wife and has recently filed for divorce. The divorce papers have not yet been signed, but the frantic search for a bride has already begun.

With Gopalji I go to many homes. I have never been to as many, and *such* a variety of Delhi homes in my life. In these homes I meet entire families: grandparents, sisters, sisters-in-law, brothers and brothers-in-law. I hold babies, I show biodatas, and I talk to 'those in question' about what they are looking for in a match. I eat many kinds of snacks—dhoklas at the Jain homes, kababs at Punjabi, imported biscuits at Sindhi. I have never tasted as many varieties of namkeens and biscuits.

The Guptas own a typical Marwari home. Marwaris are unusually abstemious, vegetarian, teetotal, and conduct their personal lives in a sober way. They are traditionally a business community and are best known for their ability to make money and keep it. Their homes, though, reflect their vision of the good life and are decorated in a particular style of opulence. The Guptas' house is of modest size. Although the home itself is not large, all the furniture is, and it overpowers the rooms. The central living room has massive velvet sofas with golden tassels, patterned marble floors, chandeliers in pink and gold. Everywhere there are 'showpieces'. Two large sculptures dominate the room: one of a mermaid with large breasts and golden hair, the other of a large, cerise-coloured Ganesha.

Mr Gupta is a snarky, stubby man with a thin, singsong voice. He looks perpetually constipated, barely opening his mouth while speaking. His jowls hang loose from his chin, and he strokes them regularly. He extols his son Vinay's virtues. 'He is a very good boy. He manages the entire business. I don't do a thing. He is also very well-mannered. He touches our feet every morning. When his grandparents come he presses their feet for one hour. He has been convent-educated and has always been a topper.'

He continues after a pause, wiping his hands on a yellow hand towel that he has laid on the arm rest of the sofa he is sitting on. 'We have no demand from the girl, but we want an unmarried girl. We are not so comfortable with divorced girls. Caste is also no bar as long as they are not different from us. Marathi and Gujarati are like us, we like them. We don't like Punjabis.'

Gopalji interjects, 'Mr Gupta, Punjabi girls are good looking. Your son is handsome, so you need a good looking girl.'

Mr Gupta considers, 'We can think about it. Basically, we need a girl who is friendly and has good values because she will not be in our control because we travel a lot.'

I have to satisfy my curiosity. 'Uncle, why have you advertised for a non-working girl? Is it a problem if she works? These days most lively and qualified girls do want a career, you know.'

'Beta, she can work of course. She can work with her husband. There is so much to be done in our business. She can handle cash if she wants to do finance, or she can do billboards if she wants to do marketing. But we don't want her working out of the house.'

'Why?' I press.

'Actually, we have had bad experience. That *other* girl,' he says referring to his soon to be ex-daughter-in-law. 'She was working with a company in Gurgaon as an architect. We *told* her not to work with someone else. We *told* her to work with us, to build houses for us. We are also in the real estate business. Initially she quit, but then her company called her back. She went to Gurgaon where her parents lived, and sometimes did not come back for two to three days, saying she was tired or there was a birthday or something. She also used to work late nights. We don't want to accuse anyone of anything, but then…she used to be alone at work, so far away, so…we didn't like it. Who knows what these girls do at the office so late?'

After a pause he says sternly, 'This time our main requirement is for a non-working girl *only*.'

He ponders for a second and then says, 'The problem is that she studied in Italy.' (She had attended a nine-month course, I find out.)

'Actually, from the beginning we said we didn't want an Italian. We didn't want an abroad girl.'

Talking about his son's broken marriage has stressed Mr Gupta out. His face turns greyish and he begins to sweat profusely. He mops his face with his yellow hand towel.

'Arre, Mr Gupta, no need to worry. I will find him someone,' says Gopalji patting him on the knee.

'*Of course* we are worried. He is divorced. This is the biggest failure of our lives,' Mr Gupta says in a small voice. 'Since the girl left, I have not worked at all. I just look at biodatas all day. We don't want our boy to be alone. It is not natural. We haven't told anyone that the girl has gone. After one year of marriage, people ask us when the good news is coming. We don't know what to say.'

He continues dolefully, 'We never even asked her to make tea. We gave her all the money to handle. We think to ourselves, why did the girl leave us and go?'

Vinay Gupta, the boy 'in question' is a pleasant looking man who smiles shyly and doesn't say anything in the fifteen minutes that he sits in on our meeting. Nothing except for the occasional officious, 'Yes papa', 'Ji papa'. His parents are in control of the process, and he doesn't seem to have anything to say for himself. Moreover, his parents seem more distressed about the breakup of his marriage than he does.

I ask him what he wants in a girl. He looks at me, then his father, and then replies, 'Whatever papaji wants.'

'What provisions have you kept for A to Z ?' asks Gopalji who has till now been listening patiently but is now beginning to look bored. 'There is a lot of work in this job.'

Mr Gupta is a real estate broker, and he believes that there is some similarity between his work and that of the marriage broker seated across from him. 'I understand, Gopalji. We have a property business and I deal with brokers all day. Disputed properties always take more time to sell. If it is a clean property we give brokers 2 per cent. If it is a dirty property we give them 4 per cent. We know that you will have to work hard to sell our property.'

At this point a young boy walks in. He is approaching us, but en route, Mr Gupta pulls him into his lap and smothers him.

'This is my daughter's son.'

'Hello beta,' says Gopalji

'He wanted to touch your feet, that was why he was coming to you. He stays very much in the culture,' says Mr Gupta proudly.

After drinking our tea, we get up to leave. Mr Gupta hands

Gopalji an envelope with a thick wad of cash, Mr Gupta smiles and says, alluding to the indolent Vinay, 'It is not a straightforward job. Clean, garden-facing properties that are in a good location get sold immediately. Properties that are in the alley, that are congested and illegal, are difficult to dispose of.'

As we are driving out of the neighbourhood, we stop at the local press-wallah. Here, by the side of the street a few men are busy ironing with industrial-size heavy irons. Gopalji takes out a ₹100 note, rolls down his window, and beckons to one of the press-wallahs.

'How are they?' he says pointing to the Guptas' house.

'Fine, sir.'

'Does the boy drink?

'Uh...' says the press-wallah looking uncomfortable.

'Tell me! I'll pay you more!'

'Sir, sometimes.'

'Ah! His biodata said teetotaller,' says Gopalji, with a knowing smile.

'How is his wife?' Gopalji asks.

'Sir, she has gone, not come back in a long time. We think, maybe divorce. She was very nice, sir. She was pretty and kind also.'

'Why did she leave?' asks Gopalji

'Sir, I think they were not having good time in bedroom.'

'How do you know?' asks Gopalji curiously.

'We found no stains on the clothes, sir. Also, bedroom lights always off very early. We can see from here, see,' he says pointing to the window. From where the press-wallah stands it is just possible to look into the young couple's bedroom. Even though Colonel Singh in the office will do a thorough background check, Gopal Suri likes to do a preliminary search. Gopalji thanks the press-wallah and we drive away. He says, 'See, Iraji, my job is not a simple one. Everyone is lying all the time, the parents, the boys, the girls. And then they expect me to find a good match for a lifelong marriage. Over the years I have learnt to tell the truth from the lies, and this is what makes me a good marriage broker.'

♦

At A to Z, a recent big-ticket client has caused a flurry. Manav is the handsome young son of industrialist whose biodata boasts a family income of a ridiculous ₹10,000 crore annually. Manav has recently completed his MBA in the US and is back in India, ripe for marriage. It is common knowledge that his family has employed twenty marriage brokers to find a match for the young scion. If Gopal Suri seals this deal, millions of rupees are to be made and he is determined to win this one.

Manav's family, though, has some specific requirements. They want a beautiful, humble girl who may not be 'monied' but who has class. She should not have studied abroad. His parents believe that an international education corrupts women. Manav's family has also specifically asked for a girl who wears full sleeves. This last request, I simply cannot understand.

One day I find Gopalji looking particularly happy. I comment on this. He beams, lowering his voice, looking around to make sure that none of the staff are around. 'I'm going to tell you this because you are close to me. I sent them my daughter's profile, and they liked it. They asked me whose biodata this was and who the father of this girl was. I told them that it was me, that *I* was the father of this daughter!'

He pulled up his daughter's carefully crafted biodata and showed me a picture of a smiling, plain-faced girl with Gopalji's weasel eyes.

I had not realized Gopalji harboured secret ambitions for his daughter to marry so well, but then again, I shouldn't be too surprised. Every parent in India wants nothing but the very best for their kids when it comes to marriage, so why shouldn't a marriage broker aim even higher?

COCKTAIL MATCHES

'The single most important criteria for eligibility in the Indian marriage market is wealth. Every family wants its match in terms of bank balance and rarely are they willing to compromise,' says Geeta Khanna, founder of Cocktail Matches, another New Delhi-based matchmaking service.

Geeta is a modern-day matchmaker or 'matrimonial consultant' as she introduces herself. She is in her late forties, fashionably dressed and sports a stylish coif. Her office is basically her home, and when I go to visit, she is in the midst of a gaggle of ladies feverishly discussing matrimony. This is a different set of people from the middle-class to upper-middle-class crowd that frequents A to Z matrimonial. These well-heeled ladies speaking in English, dressed in fashionable western outfits, are what Geeta likes to call 'the cocktail-going crowd', the upper crust of society, in other words.

The caste system is changing, Geeta tells me. Rather than 'Marwari, Rajput or Brahmin', it is now 'businessman from South Delhi, professional from Gurgaon, or doctor from a metro city'. The caste system, originally based on economics, was now reorganizing itself to suit modern needs and was based on a system of wealth. Geeta explains her modus operandi to me. 'I operate in a close-knit group of people, mostly setting up people from my social circle. It is much easier to check people out this way. Unlike most matrimonial services today, I run a very personalized, boutique matchmaking service. I handle all my clients myself, giving them the kind of attention that they deserve.'

Her style seemed to be distinctly different from A to Z, which was run as a business. Ironically, though, I discovered that despite the discrepancy in wealth and class, many of Geeta's and Gopalji's clients had similar concerns. Here, too, the marriage process seemed skewed in favour of men, and many of the parents that I meet at Geeta's worry that their daughters will never get married, and remain 'sitting at home'. I hear this phrase often at A to Z, 'ladki ghar pe bhaithi huee hai' (our girl is sitting at home), and even in this rich segment of society, I find the same paranoia.

Geeta tells me that in the marriage game the ball often lies in the boy's court. The girl's family often has to court the boy's side by displaying their wealth and ability to have a large wedding. Like Gopalji, a higher percentage of Geeta's clients are girls. For every three eligible bachelors, she has only one bachelorette. Geeta says that she often has to chase the boy's side to secure a good match. Geeta suggests that I meet one of her old clients, Anjali, to get an understanding of the factors at play to make a good match.

♦

Anjali's opulent Delhi home is typical of a sybaritic Delhi existence—plush velvet sofas, strange showpieces festooning the walls, and Nepali maids attired in frilly faux French designer uniforms.

Anjali comes from a middle-class family; her father is an engineer, and her mother a housewife. Geeta arranged her wedding to Gaurav who belongs to a wealthy Delhi family. The caveat was that Gaurav was divorced, after a short-lived marriage to his college sweetheart. Gaurav's divorced status was balanced by his wealth, and Anjali's middle-class status was made up for by her youth (she was twenty-two), her looks and her education.

Anjali speaks optimistically about the matrimonial process. 'In an arranged setup, it is really difficult to put your demands up front. Everything becomes much easier through a marriage broker. You can place all your requirements on the table, and you have a neutral party negotiating for you. This is really important because each family has their own set of expectations.'

Marriage brokers, though, like any other type of broker, can sometimes cause trouble. Making sure her mother-in-law is not around, Anjali whispers to me, 'You have to be really careful of these guys. My parents kept me away from them till the last stage, till it became absolutely crucial for them to see me. Sometimes these guys can be malicious if a family doesn't respond to their requests. They will spread rumours in the market. They say the boy has different 'preferences' implying homosexuality, or that a girl's 'character isn't right' (the standard line—iska character theek nahin hai). I'm not complaining. I am happily married so far, but I have heard some pretty terrible stories.'

Anjali continues, since her mother-in-law is nowhere in sight. 'I got lucky, because I wanted a rich boy, though we weren't rich. My parents were practical, and knew that we could only get a divorcee if we wanted wealth. So in my marriage process, this is what we focused on, and this is what we got.'

For some reason, Anjali seems to think that I have come here to get matrimonial advice from her. 'You should make a list of things that are most important to you and then give them to a marriage broker. You must also present the things that you just can't accept. For me, I did not want a dark guy. I didn't mind if he was short or fat. I told Geeta that I would not even look at a dark guy, no matter how rich.'

As Anjali harped on about marriage, I could have sworn she was talking about buying a car, or a dress, for that matter. It seemed to me that in many ways, marriage had been turned into a merger and acquisition where wealth rather than love was the bottom line.

◆

Mansi is my best friend, and though we are similar in so many ways, our nuptial journeys couldn't have been more different. Mansi is from a conservative Marwari business family living in Ahmedabad. She had just ended her relationship with a man in Mumbai because she wanted to get married (not because he was an amazing guy, but her parents were insisting that she tie the knot) and he did not. After that she decided to go down the easier-on-the-heart route of arranged marriage. So Mansi quit her marketing job in Delhi to move back home to Ahmedabad and hand over the job of finding her a partner to her parents.

As it happened, it was the venerable Gopalji who came to Mansi's rescue when she was going through the worst of her marriage anxiety. Her parents were desperate for her to get married and this stress had made her mother physically ill, her father emotionally. Gopal Suri added an inch to her height, knocked off a few kilos, and used Photoshop to lighten her skin tone by a few shades. A few weeks later, a candidate was chosen. Prem lived in Mumbai where he worked in his family's business. Mansi's father immediately flew to Mumbai to inspect Prem and the family. He approved. After going through a string of rejections, Mansi was ready to accept anyone who accepted her, as long as her father approved. On the face of it, Prem had everything that she was asking for in a man: he was kind, intelligent, and financially sound. He was not dashing like her ex-boyfriend, nor was he as cosmopolitan and well-travelled as she was. He didn't speak English in the polished way of the chattering classes, and he didn't dress in the fashionable way of her friends, but she was done with the humping and dumping game. Their common cultural background would hopefully fill in all the lacunae of love. And so they got engaged after one quick meeting.

I was happy for Mansi, but also a little disappointed. She would miss those moments of madness and crazy highs that come with love, but then she would also avoid the moments of angst, fighting and tumult. Maybe all of this would come after marriage, and hopefully so would the flutters of first love.

While Mansi found a husband through Gopalji, I hoped to find my husband through love.

I met Vinayak on the day of Holi—the festival of love. We were both silver-faced, our bodies splattered in pink, red and blue, and in the tradition of the festival, I had consumed so much bhang that the entire world seemed to spin round and round. After the drug-induced high wore off, my world continued to spin. At that time, Vinayak seemed perfect. Like me, he too had recently moved back to Delhi from the US and was finding his feet. We had common friends, and we spent endless hours together. He was bright, kind, and *real*. After a few months, when our relationship moved beyond flirtation into the realm of the serious, and as I found out more about him, my mind was lacerated with doubt. Could I marry him? He was from a conservative Marwari family and lived in a large joint family with an army of uncles, aunts and cousins. Vinayak was working for his father as was the tradition in his family, and was entirely dependent on him financially.

Vinayak's lifestyle in many ways seemed to be a cultural mismatch for someone like me who was brought up in a nuclear family. I was fiercely independent and I wasn't sure if I could marry a guy who depended to this extent on his family, and even lived with them. Vinayak and I were best friends, and worked well as boyfriend and girlfriend, but could we function as husband and wife? Would I be able to live with his parents for the rest of my life? Could I put up with Vinayak's financial dependence on his family? I wanted Vinayak to get a job and become independent from his parents, and he was confused about which path to take. We fought often, and sometimes I desperately wished that I could take the practical path of arranged marriage. If both people came from a similar cultural background, wouldn't marriage be easy? I decided to find out for myself.

◆

On paper, the boy was perfect. He worked in private equity, was Harvard-educated, tall and handsome, and we even had eleven friends in common on Facebook—friends in Boston, New York, Delhi and Mumbai, all the cities that we had both lived in.

I wanted to know how it felt to meet a total stranger with the idea of spending the rest of your life together, how the 'click' that Gopalji spoke about happened, what people meant when after twenty meetings, they knew that the twenty-first girl or boy was the 'one'. A hopeful inner voice of mine urged me to meet him. My main motive for meeting Nakul was to get more insight into the differences between love and arranged marriage for the book. But I was also secretly curious about him being a good match for me and wondered if the arranged marriage process could work for me, especially because I had been fighting more than usual with Vinayak. He wanted to get engaged but I wasn't sure if he was the right fit for me. If I did break up with Vinayak, I knew I could *not* bear going through the painful rigmarole of dating for a long while and an arranged marriage seemed like a relatively painless option at this point.

When I had looked at Nakul's biodata, he seemed to have some of things that I felt Vinayak was lacking. Research tells us that we are more compatible with people with similar life experiences, and Nakul reminded me so much of myself. We had a similar education—both of us had studied in Boston and done our MBAs—we had similar family backgrounds, and had spent our formative years in the US and India. Nakul seemed ideal. Though Gopalji usually discouraged it, I told him that I would meet only Nakul, not his parents or his other family members, because that would be too overwhelming.

When I revealed to my inner circle of friends that I was meeting someone with a view to an arranged marriage, they were not surprised, even though they all knew Vinayak. Many had been through this situation. They were dating men that they liked, but their parents pressured them to meet men that *they* did. Many would resist, but after a while ended up meeting these men, for no other reason than to placate their parents. One friend had a great relationship, but met a man through her parents, and immediately decided to marry him, because she thought he would make a good husband.

I had advice coming from all directions because everyone that I knew had at some point gone through the arranged marriage process. My friends regaled me with their matrimonial horror stories—a friend of mine had ruined her nuptial chances because she had gone back to the guy's hotel room after the first meeting. Another had blown it when she introduced a potential to her wayward friends, yet another because she smoked a cigarette. Mansi advised me, 'Let him make the effort, don't reveal too much.'

In an unusually bold step, Nakul flew down from Bombay to meet me. We had never even spoken on the phone, chatted, or emailed one another. We had only exchanged SMSs to confirm the time and venue of our meeting. This made me even more uncomfortable, first because of his apparent seriousness, and second because this earnestness further exemplified his good qualities. What if he actually turned out to be the one? Was I ready for this?

Nakul was everything that he promised to be. He was older than I had expected—thirty-six (his biodata had said thirty-four, I guess I had Gopalji to thank for this error) and he was sweet, kind, well-spoken, attentive, curious and funny. We had a lovely time over coffee, and agreed to meet again the following day. Though everything had gone well with Nakul, as the time approached to meet a second time, I did not want to see him again. All my nervous energy of the previous day had coalesced into dullness and other unfamiliar feelings that I could not quite understand. I was still nervous, but not in the fresh, light way of the day before. It didn't help that a vigilant Gopalji had taken a personal interest in this one and was keeping track of the meetings.

Somehow, something with Nakul seemed to be lacking in my mind. I couldn't put my finger on it, and I started harping on the smallest things: the elasticity of his socks, the unappealing computer bag that he carried, the unimpressive thickness of his hair. I felt a sinking feeling when I thought about Nakul, so I SMSed Vinayak telling him that I was thinking about him.

Gopalji was unnaturally clear-headed and had a vaunted prescience about these things; he was a matchmaker after all. He had told me to meet Nakul a minimum of three times. After that, he said, I would know. So I did just that.

The buccaneering Nakul flew down again to have dinner with me. As the waiters closed the restaurant, stacking the chairs and rolled the front entrance of the restaurant halfway down, Nakul and I talked about everything under the moon. The conversation was smooth, entertaining, and intelligent, but I felt nothing in my heart, my hands were cold, and a distasteful feeling oppressed me. I have no idea what unspoken covenant had been broken, or what unwritten law of nature had been transgressed, but when he dropped me to the car and said goodbye, I knew that I would never see him again. As he walked away, I only felt sharp relief. I immediately phoned Vinayak and told him that I loved him.

The truth was that it was difficult for me to accept this arranged marriage business, though I strongly wished that, like Mansi, I too could internalize my past calamities and find a way to sink into the 'comfort' of arranged marriage. It seemed to be so easy, so straightforward. With economics, social acceptability and background in place, marriage should be easy. I had seen so many of my friends and family, including my parents and sister, meet their spouse in an easy arranged marriage with none of the anxiety and heartburn of dating. It seemed perfect in theory, but the biggest hurdle towards an arranged marriage for me was my own mind.

According to Sudhir Kakar, 'Arranged marriages work best, and perhaps can only work, if the sexes are kept apart in youth and if marriages take place early, before young men and women have had an opportunity to compare a range of potential partners.'[196] Clearly this had not been the case for me. I had plenty, perhaps too much, interaction with the opposite sex so I wasn't mentally prepared to take on arranged marriage. Maybe if Nakul and I had met through friends, at a bar, or a nightclub, we could have had a perfectly natural, healthy relationship that may even have resulted in marriage. Just like if Vinayak and I had met through an arranged context, I would have rejected him after the first meeting, only based on his biodata, despite him being a lovely partner.

Sometimes I wondered if I had followed Gopalji's tailor-made format of our parents meeting first, could things have worked out differently for Nakul and me? But then again, I couldn't even imagine myself in that situation, despite having observed it so many times with Gopalji. Maybe I was being quixotic, but it seemed unnatural to think of marriage as a strategic transaction, or a calculated decision. It seemed stranger to make love to a man that I didn't really love. I wanted to actually *fall* in love with a loud bang and have scars and bruises to show for the fall. I wanted to date, to be best friends, to fight, to break up bitterly and to make up even more sweetly, and then one day, when the timing felt right, to get married. Though I had been brought up on a diet of arranged marriage, the later conditioning of my mind towards love and romance was much stronger than I had ever imagined. The meetings with Nakul had made me feel interminably uneasy and awfully awkward. It was like going on a single date, knowing that your choice would be for life, it was more pressure on the heart than I had ever imagined. Ultimately, an arranged marriage is about marrying a person who has the qualities you could fall in love with. Yet all my dating experiences had told me that love was a nebulous, intangible feeling. You couldn't put a value on it, and I certainly couldn't make it happen by matching myself to biodatas customized by Gopalji.

THE BIG FAT INDIAN WEDDING

On the eve of Gandhi Jayanti, a wedding that is a vulgar display of ostentation and wealth, to a degree I would have thought impossible even in a city renowned for its vulgar displays of wealth, is taking place on the outskirts of Delhi. The MC announces that today is an ideal day to get married since the following day, 2 October, is the birthday of the Father of our Nation. He isn't being the least sarcastic or ironic or maybe he sincerely believes that because the visage of the Mahatma adorns all Indian currency notes, including the ₹1,000 ones, he would have approved of the lakhs of rupees that are being spent on this wedding. In reality, Gandhiji had stated clearly and unequivocally that wedding ceremonies should be austere and focus on sacred rituals and simplicity.

The sangeet is taking place in the upmarket Chattarpur farms area; the theme is *Avatar*—based on the Hollywood blockbuster. A fifty-foot replica of the Tree of Souls stands in the centre of a ground the size of a football field—it is pretty impressive and I'm certain even James Cameron would find it commendable. Waiters are dressed as members of the Na'vi tribe, and state-of-the-art laser lighting and fog machines create an impression of being in an alternate universe. Cirque du Soleil dancers perform to popular Bollywood tunes before internationally acclaimed DJ Edward Maya takes over for the night. Like the over-applied rouge and glittering ornaments on the women, everything here appears tawdry, bordering on the burlesque.

Undulating patterns of strobe lights and shadows blend spectrally to create random forms. Against this storm of light and sound, young men and women from Delhi's swish set make small talk at the bar, decked out in jewels, dressed in slinky saris and sparkly lehengas. At one of the four bars, I watch a spectacular extravaganza—Na'vi tribe members ride human beings dressed as dragons and zip to and fro. Next, the 2,000 guests—parents, grandparents, children—watch a glittering Bollywood-esque dance performance that is staged by the bride's and groom's friends and family. As I watch, the sister of the bride gyrates with the liquid grace of a professional while a slew of male cousins prance around her. She is dancing to the song of the season, 'Chikni Chameli' which translates to 'Sexy Chameli', and alludes to a female prostitute named Chameli in another film. The lyrics go something like this:

> *Come, my evenings are lonely / I will share them with you… / With the fire of my body / I have come to light up cigarettes and joints / Sexy Chameli has come…*

Despite the somewhat risqué lyrics, the song is so popular even small children shimmy to it and mouth its lyrics. The show is impressive and it is apparent that the families and friends have spent weeks, perhaps even months, practicing their moves. The man behind the show is Rajender Masterji, a flamboyantly homosexual man with henna-orange hair, betel-stained teeth, wearing a body-hugging sequinned Lycra kurta and cat's-eye contact lenses. Masterji, as he is popularly known, is India's celebrity wedding dance choreographer. He began his career in Mumbai giving dance lessons to aspiring starlets, but today his main line of business is choreographing Bollywood dance sequences for mega-weddings. In the style of Bollywood movies, these dance sequences performed by friends and members of the family usually tell a story with intermittent mini skits narrating the couple's love story (even if the match is arranged).

It is only in the last few years (five to seven according to different choreographers that I have spoken with) that this Bollywood dance craze has become a standard at Indian weddings. According to Rajender Masterji, a series of hit Bollywood movies, like the blockbusters *Dil To Pagal Hai* (1997) and *Kuch Kuch Hota Hai* (1998) inspired people to stage their own dance performances. The popularity of these dance sequences has spawned an entire industry resulting in the proliferation of choreographers and dance studios that cater only to weddings.

In earlier, simpler times, the days preceding the actual wedding were reserved for auspicious rituals and ceremonies, but now with increasing disposable income and exposure to the West, these same rituals have taken on new forms. Until a decade ago, the sangeet was an innocuous affair, where women of the household got together to sing and dance to traditional folk ballads. Today, the sangeet is an ecstatic, protoplasmic affair straight out of the movies, where friends and family, men and women, children and adults, dance to hip-swinging sequences choreographed to Bollywood songs. Bollywood has invaded all aspects of the Indian wedding. Instead of the saris that her mother wore, today's bride wears a fancy lehenga inspired by a Bollywood star; wedding decor is inspired by Bollywood film sets, photographers make the bride and groom pose like Bollywood actors and videographers make wedding videos that are mini-Bollywood films, complete with song, dance, and drama. Bollywood celebrities too have capitalized on their popularity in the wedding arena and play a role in the most exorbitant weddings. For the small price of US$750,000 (₹4.6 crore), Shahrukh Khan, can reportedly be persuaded to make a celebrity appearance at any wedding. There is an industry 'A-list' for celebrity appearances, and even B- or C-grade stars have wedding attendance price tags.[197]

◆

Rohit, my companion for the evening, is most definitely drunk.

The cadence of his voice, the slur in his speech, his overly elaborate gestures are definite proof. We engage in some drunken chatter, and although I am a teetotaller, I have consumed a few Red Bulls, and am *feeling* drunk. Rohit has just returned from a four-day-long 'youngster's party' in Ibiza. He tells me about this latest trend: 'My friends don't know most of the people attending their weddings. Even if they want a small, private affair, their parents won't allow it, it is against social norms. You can't really get drunk, or have fun with all your aunties and uncles around, so nowadays everyone has a youngster's party attended only by "young" people, though they are all about thirty years old.'

Rohit now turns philosophical, 'Most big weddings are shit shows, there are thousands of people. To be honest, it's vulgar. It's sad. People want to remember these weddings by how opulent they are, and by going above and beyond the last big wedding. Isn't timelessness meant to be created by emotions? It seems far removed from what these functions are actually meant to be. A year later, you don't remember a thing, you just think about the next big party.'

Luckily for Rohit, the next big party is the next day at the mammoth wedding of a real estate baron's only daughter.

◆

At the entrance to the venue I am greeted by two life-size garlanded elephant sculptures. They are juxtaposed, unexpectedly, against an eerie, blue-eyed mime with his face spray-painted silver (thirty such mime artists have been flown in from France). The venue is so large that a fleet of golf carts is standing by to ferry people to the stage where the bride and groom stand to meet their guests. When I finally enter the actual venue—closer to an arena than a hall, I reel from the sensory overload. At one end, a women's choir sings devotional bhajans, in another corner, a group of saffron-clad young priests chant sacred mantras, on a balcony a small army of musicians play traditional Carnatic music.

There is also a fifty-foot-high wall with four rows of squares. Inside each square sits a musician playing an instrument. It is essentially a band on the wall. Next to these musicians is a bar where a bunch of kids have congregated. A few suited ruffians throw cocktail olives at a man sitting in one of the squares.

The newly-weds stand on a massive stage with octopus-like tentacles reaching up to the ceiling. Hundreds of visitors queue up to wish the couple, present them with gifts, and get photographed with them. There is a row of television screens on each side of the hall in the style of sporting events so that people far away from the stage can witness the activities. The sights and sounds are so overwhelming that all I can do is stare. I make my way to the front of this massive hall. I have to pause and rest in between, partly because this hall is so large, and partly because the sari that I have carelessly tied is threatening to fall off.

The wedding I am attending is typical of a big fat Indian wedding, and is no different from dozens of similar weddings that are taking place all across the country. Only the scale differs. I remember my own sister's recent wedding reception where a 'wedding set' had been constructed on a large barren ground, complete with a giant, wobbly wooden stage on which Anjani and Rahul stood for three hours while guests came and greeted them. The wedding set had various food stations—a Punjabi 'roadside dhaba' with a thatched roof, a cowboy bar with waiters wearing cowboy boots and hats, and a seafood station with a pile of sand as a makeshift beach. Our wedding planner made sure that we had an elaborate spread of food. I remember her words, 'The bride's family has to put up a show, and anyone you have interacted with in your lifetime has to be fed. An Indian wedding is like a mass charity event.' Except none of the guests that I saw during the course of that long evening struck me as being in the least bit malnourished.

The situation is similar at this big fat Delhi wedding too. I walk to the sprawling banquet featuring a variety of different cuisines—

French, Japanese, Thai, Mughlai; a seafood counter featuring lobster and Cambodian basa and a cheese counter with fifty varieties of cheese. The dessert counter has a chocolate fountain and twenty different kinds of comestibles. At the fruit counter people are hoarding fruit, pushing and shoving, and piling their plates high with peaches, strawberries, rambutans, mangosteens, and other varieties of imported fruit. A richly caparisoned lady ploughs through the crowd like a pocket battleship with her infant daughter—a plump child with salon curls and a frothy outfit—in tow. The infant daughter has three maids with her—one holds her bag, another her milk bottle, another the child herself. I look at the Northeastern maid carrying the small child and I wonder what she makes of all this. Her ₹6,000 a month salary is probably the cost per head at this wedding. She probably has a young child at home and ailing parents back in her village. And then she sees all of this. Enough to drive anyone wild, or at least crazy enough to hoard some fruit for herself.

Given the nationwide ostentatious, almost vulgar, spend on weddings there have already been efforts to regulate excess in weddings. Last year Kuruppasserry Varkey Thomas, the Minister of Consumer Affairs, suggested implementing a government cap on the number of wedding guests and the number of dishes that could be served, in response to the government's concerns.[198] To many it seems unethical that in a country where so many people are starving, such opulence should be allowed to go unchecked. There are also concerns about food that is wasted. In Assam, a Guest Control Order allows a maximum of a hundred guests at weddings. In Pakistan, where similar pomp and show is part of weddings, a government order has been passed which allows only two dishes to be served at all weddings. In 2004, the Jammu and Kashmir government passed an order restricting the numbers of people served at marriage receptions to 250 in the case of a vegetarian and 200 for non-vegetarian cuisine.[199] Unfortunately, the order was stayed by the High Court as people worried that these restrictions would hinder the growth of the wedding market and that the entire economy might stall as a result.

At a Haagen-Dazs ice-cream counter I encounter a saffron-robed priest carrying a small tattered leather briefcase eating a chocolate fudge bar. I ask him what time the wedding is. He replies with a breezy insouciance that the auspicious time for the wedding as per the birth charts of the to-be-wedded couple passed two hours ago. It doesn't matter now when the wedding rituals are performed. As rich and lavish as it is inside, just steps away from the entrance, the smell of open sewage pervades the air, along with the toxic fumes of a rotting corpse. There is a mini traffic jam and cars struggle to get out. Someone next to me says, 'Kutta mar gaya' (A dog died). Road kill lies in front of us, its skull flattened, further squished and ground by the wheels of a car. A row of luxury cars has been parked in front of the entrance including a Roll Royce, a Bentley and a Jaguar, blocking the way of the other guests. I see my friend Rohit walking fast towards an idling vehicle. I rush towards him, maybe he can give me a lift to my car. But there are people, cars, hounds and horses between us.

Rohit is sweating profusely, it is a hot night, and he is wearing heavy formal clothes. I catch his attention, and wave to him. He looks at me, befuddled by alcohol, sweat and the general confusion, and then comprehension slowly dawns. 'Hullo *dahling*. How are you?' he says. He gets into his car. 'How are you?' he asks again. Before I can answer, he quips, 'Good night, sweety!' and swiftly drives away.

Firecrackers erupt in the sky at midnight, industrial sized firecrackers that spell out the long names of the bride and groom. After a few minutes all that is left behind is a thick cloud of noxious fumes that obscure the moon and stars. Though the wedding is still going on inside, the venue is now being dismantled by a small army of workers. The façade of the entrance has been decorated entirely with red roses, perhaps a million roses were used tonight.

One worker is very carefully hand-picking roses with stalks out of a small mountain of red roses. I strike up a conversation with him. His daughter is getting married tomorrow. Fresh flowers are expensive, especially at this time of the year, and roses in particular are rare commodities. He is collecting the remains of the flowers from this wedding to use at his daughter's wedding. He tells me that he has been saving for his daughter's wedding for ten years. As dowry, he has given his prospective son-in-law's family a two-wheeler, a fridge and a gold chain. His daughter and son-in-law want to go on a honeymoon to Mumbai, and he will be paying for that too. He is worried about the expenses; even after all these years of saving, it is still not enough so he is trying to salvage things from this astronomical waste.

I also see an ambulance on-site, one of the musicians sitting in the square boxes has fallen down and broken a leg. Perhaps this was the man who was being pelted with olives. He tells me that he had been taken to the back and put in a room so that he wouldn't disrupt the wedding. It is only now that he is being treated. I ask him if I can help him in any way. He just shrugs and says that he is fine. He has only broken one leg and fractured a few ribs, it could have been worse. He doesn't seem to be angry at his fall or for being locked in a back room for an hour.

I am astonished by the equanimity with which the man seems to be taking his misfortune. We Indians believe in karma but what I've seen this evening should be enough to set off a whole series of uprisings. The maid whose own child lies awake at home while she mollycoddles a child dressed like a soufflé, the worker who picks dusty roses off the ground the night before his own daughter's wedding, the musician who is locked away in a dark room because he fails to entertain at a hedonistic wedding—do they all believe that they deserve the lives that they have, that it is their karma, that maybe their next lives or the one after that will be better if they suffer in silence in this one or are the hosts feeding them something that makes them play along?

It's ironic that in a country where 836 million people live on ₹20 per day, there are also those who spend US$11 billion (₹6, 68,538 crore) on a wedding per year.[200] It is rumoured that India's richest man, London-based billionaire Lakshmi Mittal spent over US$60 million (₹373 crore) when his daughter tied the knot in 2004. The five-day affair began with an engagement ceremony at the historic Palace of Versailles, followed by a sangeet party at the enchanting Jardin des Tuileries, where guests were entertained with a choreographed enactment of the love story between the bride and the groom, culminating in the wedding ceremony at the seventeenth-century château of Vaux-le-Vicomte. The show-stealer was a Bollywood extravaganza where Bollywood stars performed on stage ending with a surprise appearance by Kylie Minogue.[201] This wedding became the aspiration and the inspiration for a host of wealthy wannabes across the country leading to a series of knock-off weddings.

But not everyone can give their progeny a wedding like Lakshmi Mittal, and this drives many parents to make desperate, and sometimes financially detrimental, choices. Companies like GE Money India have introduced an 'auspicious' personal loan, exclusively for weddings, making borrowing money easy and quick.[202] Pension funds advertise investment schemes around a daughter's wedding.[203] Poor fathers will borrow from local shop owners at 22 per cent interest when banks deny them loans and mothers will sell their jewellery to finance their daughter's weddings. There are umpteen examples of families that have gone bankrupt after funding their daughter's lavish wedding and fulfilling ostentatious dowry demands. Yet there are no signs that the madness is going to go away.

◆

Marriage is undoubtedly the most veritable of Indian institutions, and pomp and show has been the mainstay of Indian weddings. For all Indian families, from the illiterate factory worker to the flamboyant real estate baron, the opulence of the wedding celebration is regarded as being directly proportionate to the financial and social status of the family. In a country with acute differences in lifestyles the one thing that binds the rich and the poor is the attitude towards marriage.

Contrary to what one expects, opulent weddings were not always part of Indian tradition. To see how Indian weddings have evolved and to understand how elaborate weddings have become an inherent part of our culture, I spent a day sifting through the wedding albums of my own family members—sepia-coloured photos of my parents' wedding thirty-three years ago, as well as fuzzy, black-and-white photos of my shy, nubile grandmother and stoic grandfather who met for the first time on their wedding day. I sat down with my mother and aunts and asked them what their weddings were like, and how they were celebrated. I knew that they grew up in decidedly simpler times but I was struck by the level of transformation between the past and the present, although only about twenty to thirty years had elapsed.

How had the simple, tasteful, meaningful Indian wedding that I studied in my families' photo albums and heard about from my mother, grandmother and aunts visibly morphed into the bloated, inappropriate, money-guzzling creature that passed for a wedding in these benighted times?

♦

As I'd already seen with Gopalji at A to Z, the wedding budget of the girl's family is the modern-day dowry that controls the possibilities of a girl marrying into a higher-status family. Traditionally, dowry or 'stridhan' was linked only to Hindu Brahmin weddings which defined different forms of ownership for women, including the times that women should receive gifts from their families particularly at the time of marriage.[204] Stridhan was regarded as a woman's wealth, a mark of a her social status and her safety net; her only resource when times were bad.

British colonial rule then codified Hindu marriage laws according to Brahminic customs, including dowry.[205] Further, in colonial times, because of the way in which the British rearranged property rights and the like, dowry became a means through which women became commodity, and an excuse to harass, abuse, blackmail and even murder women. However, when dowry became a threat to the well-being of women, the Government of India had to enact the Dowry Prohibition Act in 1961. (It was framed so that it had to be proved that dowry was given as an incentive, reason or reward for the marriage, which was almost impossible.) However, although dowry has been abolished by the law, it still prevails and has expanded to include all castes and religions. A 2012 survey by NDTV found that three out of every five Indians would pay dowry. The *form* of dowry though has changed, and is mainly seen in the form of elaborate weddings.

And dowry deaths continue to take place. Indian government statistics show that husbands and in-laws killed nearly 7,000 women in 2001 over inadequate dowry payments.[206] In 2010, 8,391 dowry death cases were reported across India, meaning a bride was burned every ninety minutes, according to statistics recently released by the National Crime Records Bureau.

As I researched further, I discovered that it had not always been that way. Dowry, as we know it today, has meant different things during different times, and it had strong links to British colonial laws. Author Veena Talwar Oldenburg in her book, *Dowry Murder: Reinvestigating a Cultural Whodunnit* provides a clear explanation. According to Oldenburg, '[d]owry has been changing so rapidly since the colonial period that it can be defined neither as the timeless stridhan, or women's wealth as described in the third-century *Dharmashastra*, nor as the lethal custom that allegedly provokes the murders of approximately six thousand women annually since 1985'.[207]

Oldenburg studied interviews conducted by the British in villages in Punjab in 1850 and found that none of them described dowry as gifts demanded by the groom's family. Instead those interviews describe dowry as a collection of voluntary gifts like clothes, jewellery, household goods and cash bestowed on the bride by the family and friends at the time of the wedding.[208] The British established individual property rights in land, in which only men were given the right to own land when previously land was a shared resource which provided sustenance, and in which men and women had equal rights. This radical change in property rights was detrimental to women's economic freedom. Cash and property began to play an increasing role in the composition of dowries as land became a marketable commodity in the colonial period and monetization became compulsory.[209]

Essentially, colonialism created only a tiny number of eligible males with proper employment or economic security but rising expectations. Mothers of daughters knew that a good dowry was now the hook to secure 'the catch'.[210]

Professor Veena Oldenburg explores other reasons why dowry became so entrenched in the wedding system.

She writes, 'The British reduction or outright abolition of the customary subsidies given to village heads by Hindu, Mughal, and Sikh rulers for the maintenance of the village *chaupal* (guest house), oil lamps, the upkeep of shrines and payment to the itinerant musicians made hospitality offered during weddings more costly for individual families. The inflation that accompanied the steady rise in the price of land stood on its head the old question of (movable) dowry for the daughters who married out of their villages as against (immovable) property for the sons who brought brides home. And as time went on, the increased circulation of cash and ever-broadening range of consumer goods, chiefly British imports, generated a clamour for these items to be included in dowries. A pair of shoes for the groom for walking, then a bicycle for greater mobility and now a motorcycle or even a car that costs lakhs of rupees could be on a groom's family's wish list.'

She concludes that 'the radical restructuring of land ownership and revenue collection, the accelerated monetization of the agrarian economy, urban growth, and the emergent middle-class values all worked to transform the dowry system itself.'[211]

Scholar Rochona Majumdar also traces these attitudes to reforms during the colonial period. The British reigned through two distinct legal codes, one of which was 'personal law', a category that differentiated between Hindus and Muslims and supposed that religious textual laws should govern domestic affairs. Marriage fell under 'personal law', and marriages became tied to property and inheritance. Majumdar describes reform efforts which aimed to repatriate marriage to the realm of the sacred. This included individual choices to curb the excess of wedding ceremonies, and marriage without dowry.[212]

◆

There is a bazaar-like frenzy at Emporio, a luxury shopping mall in New Delhi. Frantic brides-to-be with their eager mothers, trailed by harassed looking fathers and fiancées, are shopping up a storm. It is September, and the winter wedding season is just around the corner. Sparkling Swarovski-embossed trousseaux have to be tailored, gilded gifts have to be purchased, jewellery and gold has to be amassed. At a designer studio, a bride-to-be's father pays ₹1.25 crore in cash for the outfits that his daughter has just purchased. One of the glamorous outfits that the bride intends to wear for her engagement is a fuchsia-pink lehenga—heavily embroidered with gold lace and thread with a bikini-shaped navel-baring blouse made of nacreous crystals—which alone costs ₹15.25 lakh.

The shy, pretty bride-to-be, twirling the heart-shaped pink diamond engagement ring on her finger, speaks to me about her upcoming wedding, 'My wedding is the most important moment for me and also my family.' She has taken a full-time sabbatical from work to prepare for her wedding this winter. 'There is so much to do, I never imagined planning a wedding would be so difficult. I have five wedding planners, and over thirty people working full-time on my wedding. Organizing a wedding is practically like running a company. I have to import flowers and gifts from Thailand, Japan and Holland, I have to export invitations to people all over the world. I have to manage human resources, operations, PR and marketing. It is the best job experience I could have asked for,' she tells me with a laugh.

'Wedding retail is one of India's recession-free businesses,' says Diivyaa Gurwaara who organizes Bridal Asia, an annual wedding exhibition that brings together fashion and jewellery designers under one roof.[213] This bridal show sprawls over 40,000 square feet and has over 100,000 visitors. Bridal Asia is just one of such wedding exhibitions that are typically held at the beginning of the wedding season in cities across the country. Sales from such exhibitions are estimated to be over US$50 million (₹311 crore).[214] With the success of such ventures a street of permanent wedding malls with 400 stores dedicated to weddings has been built at a cost of US$16 million (₹99 crore) in Gurgaon, a suburb of Delhi.[215]

◆

I spot the Designer, one of the leading faces of Indian bridal fashion at an after-party at the finale of Delhi Fashion Week. I have to battle my way through a host of tall, sparsely dressed models giving each other lazy, sleepy smiles as they pull furiously on cigarettes. I finally get to the Designer and manage to tell him about the agenda of my book. We exchange BBM pins and agree to meet at his residence the following morning.

At 1 pm the next day, I enter the Designer's home, a bright panoply of colour, where I am made to wait for an hour-and-a-half. As per the servant-boy, the Designer has just woken up and has to perform his morning ablutions before he can meet me. I remind myself never to make an appointment with a fashion designer at a fashion show. The Designer finally arrives, dressed in a silk robe. His pallor is suggestive of a hangover. He seems dull and spiritless, so different from the man I met yesterday. I wonder if he even remembers me. Three double espressos and a two aloo paranthas later he is finally coherent, and now the conversation flows easily.

The Designer tells me that the wedding market has seen a transformation over the past decade, and today it's not just the brides who want trousseaux, their mothers and even grandmothers want to be dressed for what is (hopefully) a once in a lifetime event. The Indian buyer has become cosmopolitan and brand conscious and for weddings, branded clothes have become crucial. Every bride today aspires to wear designer lehengas. He waxes eloquent about a wedding lehenga for a 'very special A-list client' that he declares will be the most exclusive wedding outfit ever created in the history of contemporary Indian couture. It took the toil of a hundred of his most talented craft persons working over six months to craft it. 'It is hand embroidered by the finest hands in the trade on a gold, custom-woven fabric, with the finest precious and semi-precious gemstones like onyx from Madagascar, Peruvian opals, fresh water pearls and garnets, along with Swarovski crystals and antique metals.'

While I am speaking with the Designer, a stout, pudgy man with a moustache and thick glasses walks in. He introduces himself as 'Pagdiwala'. He points to a picture of Amitabh Bachchan and tells me that the day he tied Amitabhji's turban was the day that he felt God's blessings. 'I touched his head, his nose, his eyes. I tied a turban on his head! What more can a man ask for in life!'

He hands me his card in the shape of a small turban and says that he has diversified into a host of other businesses including bangles, horse and buggy, waiter uniforms, and event planning. When he finds out that I am a writer working on a book he tells me enthusiastically that he will plan my book launch. He unleashes a repository of eclectic ideas: the entrance will be a giant book, the tray will be a book, snacks will be little books, and he even offers to tie turbans at the book launch.

The Designer has also diversified, adding wedding decoration, flowers and wedding invitations to his business. The wedding card, the first announcement of the wedding is a crucial element of the Indian wedding. The Designer explains thumb rules to me. Traditional mithai is considered gauche and out of fashion. Swiss or French chocolate is considered much more elegant and fashionable. A simple card is not enough; invitations, like the weddings, have to be big. They have to make a statement, and they always have to come accompanied by gifts.

I have seen some bizarre wedding invitations reach my doorstep. I once received a wedding invitation in the shape of a small castle; another came armed with a box of Armani Dolce; once I even got a small trunk, each drawer of which held various goodies, including candles, dates and brownies. Most invitations come heavily armed with gifts, sweets, incense, silver trinkets amongst other highly disposable paraphernalia. I recall the reaction of an astonished invitee speaking of a fantastical wedding invitation which came accompanied by a golden Tirupati statuette. The invite to the wedding itself must have cost ₹25,000.

The speed of economic growth in India, responsible for the creation of overnight fortunes, is also creating a conspicuous, yet almost desperate type of consumption at weddings. Excess is in order in all departments of the Indian wedding industry, estimated to be a staggering US$ 25.5 billion (₹1,42,596 crore)—the economy of a small country, with an annual 20-25 per cent growth rate.[216] 'The average middle-class family spends more than ₹7.4 lakhs on a wedding, four times India's annual per capita GDP while expenses of a "good" wedding of a middle-class family is about ₹5 lakhs ($10,600), excluding jewellery', but the average budget is usually ₹1.5 million.[217] In Mumbai, a typical affluent family spends ₹60 to 70 lakh (not including jewellery and clothes) on a wedding. In Delhi, the figure is about twice as much.[218] To put all of this into perspective, an average American wedding costs approximately US$ 26,327 (₹16 lakh).[219] It is important to note that it is just not just Hindu weddings that are celebrated in this way, all weddings, even of faiths that have originated outside the subcontinent, such as Christianity or Islam, have Indian aspects to them, and differ quite dramatically from weddings in Islamic or Western countries. Most middle-class weddings across faiths will consist of a mehendi, a sangeet and a reception while the wedding ceremony itself will be different for each faith.

However, as more people choose partners of their own and have civil marriages, it is likely that a sizeable percentage of weddings in urban India, especially among working professionals will be smaller, more intimate affairs, celebrating the couple rather than their entire clans and communities.

But, for the moment, Indian weddings are celebrated as once-in-a-lifetime grandiose events. As one journalist correctly noted, 'An over-the-top wedding is an opportunity to bring together all these people under one supersize tent and to celebrate the core values that define Indian society. It is an occasion for joy, not just for the bride and groom but for all 25,000 of their closest relatives and friends.'[220]

THE BIGGER, FATTER MASS WEDDING

As I was to discover, Indian weddings could get much bigger than I could have possibly imagined.

Amravati is an unspectacular town. It boasts the tumult characteristic of any Indian town—stentorian car horns vying for supremacy, two- and three-wheelers swerving between cows and people, derelict buildings, shanty storefronts and colourful signage. It is the sixth most populated town in the state of Maharashtra and is conspicuous perhaps only for the Amravati Municipal Corporation, the first Municipal Corporation in India to privatize octroi, an archaic tax which, as of 2012, is levied only in Ethiopia and in the Indian state of Maharashtra.

Here in Amravati, I am attending a free-for-all marriage ceremony where an estimated 3,720 couples will be wed. I stand in the middle of a large field, my feet squelching in the slushy earth of the wedding grounds created at the centre of the city. Thousands of people are here to participate, to view and to wed in what is touted to be the largest communal wedding in the history of the planet. Ravi Rana, the politician-organizer of the event, has declared that he is aiming to find a place for the mass marriage in the Guinness Book of World Records.

There is wholesale confusion as the usual shambolic state of affairs that is to be encountered at any Indian wedding is multiplied 3,270 times. Families flutter around brides and grooms, the young brides-to-be in vermilion wedding saris, and the grooms festooned with king-size headgear, dressed in gold and cream. I stand inert—lost, confused and feeling part of the chaos. I am jolted back to reality when I am almost run over by an oncoming tractor that gives a long annoyed blast of its horn and flashes its headlights at me.

The highlight and reason for this event is the marriage of Ravi Rana, the chief organizer of this event, an MLA who decided to organize the mass marriage on the occasion of his own marriage to the pretty South Indian actress Navaneet Kaur. The co-sponsor of the ceremony is Baba Ramdev, the yoga guru who rose to national fame by propagating innovative breathing techniques. The expense for this event is estimated to be around ₹10 to 12 crore, which works out to approximately ₹33,000 per couple. This includes a free wedding ceremony, a wedding feast open to the wedding parties and their families, and also gifts for the couple. For Rana, this is an astute political decision. There is nothing that touches an Indian heart like marriage, and he intends to capitalize on this.

The scene today in this unspectacular city is nothing less than spectacular. The Science Core grounds are huge and erected on them are hundreds of brightly coloured pandals where wedding ceremonies will take place. I peep inside one tent and see a long line of mud kunds. On either side of the kunds, grooms sit facing their brides who have all powdered their faces into white masks with bright red lipstick. Rana and Navaneet, the celebrity couple sit far away from the crowds, on a massive stage on which a giant mandap has been constructed. A host of celebratory figures are meant to come to the event, including top politicians, industrialists and Bollywood actors; red velvet sofas have been laid out for them.

I am lost in the mass of people. The wedding ceremony is about to begin and families, brides and grooms are rushing to the pandals. I am feeling asphyxiated by all the shoving so I fix my gaze on a giant screen showing a smiling Rana and his bride, both dressed in gold. Rana's large nose sits like a beak above a toothy grin. Navaneet perfectly plays the part of the demure bride, looking down shyly, never bringing her eyes up to the camera. They are bowing down to touch the feet of various VIP guests. Baba Ramdev is dressed in saffron robes, his bare chest revealing a taut abdomen and a bony rib cage. He has a long droopy moustache, and a frightening smile. The camera zooms in. I look away. Suddenly there is a drone-like buzz in the air and several people rush towards the front of the ground. The thousand plus police who have been languorously milling around are suddenly attentive and they brandish their lathis, prodding at people for no apparent reason. It appears that the chief minister has arrived.

The smell and smoke of cheap, strong incense permeate the pandal where I stand. A skinny priest sits at the head of the long line of brides and grooms on a makeshift dais chanting Sanskrit mantras in a sonorous voice. His chants reverberate through the speakers in the tent while in the background squeaky piped shehnai music rises to a crescendo. Everywhere there are families dressed in wedding finery. Young girls with kohl-lined eyes flit about, dressed in bright sequinned lehengas and ornamental bindis; the boys are dressed in sherwanis, and kurta pajamas; some of them are in suits. When Vivek Oberoi, a fading Bollywood star arrives, several people dash off to the main stage to get a glimpse of him. One of the deserters includes the mother of a tearful bride-to-be. The bride looks at the ground, never raising her eyes to meet those of her prospective husband. The husband, a lanky young man wearing thick glasses, looks equally uncomfortable.

Hindu weddings take place in most of the pandals, but there is also a tent which features Muslim nikahs. The Muslim pandal is far less chaotic than the Hindu one. An imam with a fiery orange beard wearing a white-lace skull-cap is reciting verses from the Koran. Men and women are separated by a large white bed sheet that divides the pandal in two. The groom's faces are covered with a blanket of flowers attached to their headgear, and the brides are covered by burkhas or green and gold chunnis. Outside I see several wide-eyed Hindus looking on with trepidation at the solemn ceremony.

Other pandals are advertised: a Christian pandal, a Jain pandal, even a Buddhist pandal, but I am unable to locate any of them. I return to the Hindu pandal where I see several empty seats in the line-up of brides and grooms. A young bride, her face splattered with inflamed acne, set off by lips made up with shiny lipstick of the same colour, is on the verge of tears. I ask her where the groom is. Everyone is confused, a hirsute man, her older brother, looks furious, 'Woh saala bhag gayaa. (He ran away.) We'll find him, and then we'll show him,' he says cracking his long fingers. Then, much to my alarm, he pulls out a long knife from somewhere inside his pants. I urge him to put the weapon away and then ask him how the jilted bride met her groom. The brother tells me that they had only met the groom once through a marriage broker who had taken his cut and disappeared. They are trying to call him now, but his phone is switched off. The bride sits cowering in her seat and the family doesn't move. The ceremony isn't over. They will wait here till the end. There is still a chance that the groom may turn up.

The situation is better for the bride at the next kund. She seems enthralled by the occasion and sports a big smile, despite the fact that her nose has begun to bleed due to the large gold nose ring she is wearing. She is smiling so brightly that her mother comes and covers her face with her red pallu, whispering angrily in her ear. It isn't good behaviour for a bride to look so exuberant and happy. Hers, I find out, is a love marriage. The groom and she are neighbours in Amravati, he is a computer technician, and she a school teacher. Her name is Shilpy and she tells me that it was her dream to have the film star Shahrukh Khan attend her wedding. He was one of the guests advertised to grace the ceremony and that is why she is participating in the communal wedding. Shilpy asks her mother desperately if Shahrukh has arrived. There is no sign of him yet.

Amidst the chaos, I speak to a wrinkled farmer wearing a festive red turban. For him it's a package deal—three of his daughters are marrying three brothers. He tells me that he'd always wanted to give his daughters a grand wedding, but he wasn't able to afford it with the poor crop yields he's been having. His daughters are getting old and he feels that no one would have married them if he had waited. He has not been able to give a dowry to his sons-in-law though they have each demanded a two-wheeler. If this year's crop is good, he will buy them scooters, if not, a cycle will have to do.

The three grooms are seated next to each other in a line. The youngest brother is just a teenager and has a fine wispy moustache, and a shy smile plays on his lips as he steals glances at his young bride. All three sisters are dressed identically in red and gold saris, shiny gold baubles and blood-red bangles on their wrists. I ask one of the sisters, a grave-faced young girl who sits with a staid expression on her face, gazing into the holy fire: 'Are you happy to get married?'

'I don't know,' she mumbles from underneath her sari with a lack of visible emotion.

'Why? Aren't you excited?' I ask, hoping to get a more enthusiastic response.

'I don't know,' she replies.

'Do you like your husband?' I ask.

'I don't know,' she repeats with finality.

The plight of this poor farmer is the plight of many. The stupendous cost of today's weddings puts an intolerable strain on most middle-class families and makes weddings almost impossible for the poor. The only salvation they can hope for is the sort of mass wedding that's taking place here today or some other form of charity or state-based intervention that eases their burden.

Mass confusion takes place during the saptapadi (translated literally into seven steps) when each couple takes seven circles around the sacred fire solemnizing the marriage. Space is limited, and as couples attempt to walk around the havans, the brides and grooms bump into each other. Fighting and arguments break out. A band of dholak players arrives, beating jaunty rhythms, moving from couple to couple, demanding tips. In the background, the pandit bellows hoarsely into the mike, asking the disruptive dholak players to leave the tent and for people to stop fighting.

I try my luck at getting up on stage where Rana's special ceremonies are taking place. I push my way through the crowds of people, finally reaching the foot of the massive stage. Here I am denied entry. A bouncer asks me for my pass. I say that I am a journalist and he points sternly to a media tent where journalists are crowded around a screen watching the ceremony. I try to explain that I am writing a book but my explanations ricochet off his giant frame. After a while he only looks at me grimly and then ignores me completely. My only option now is to watch the ceremony on screen with the other journalists. At the media tent, free tea and snacks are offered and all the journalists are digging in. I ask a local Marathi journalist about his views on Rana's tactics.

'He is simply a devta,' he says staring in awe at Rana's golden persona on screen. 'He has made his people happy. This is what the kings used to do in the olden days. He is surely going to have a happy marriage, and be blessed with many sons.'

The journalist's words have a certain truth to them. From time immemorial, leaders have financed weddings to gather goodwill. Today scheming governments have realized the importance of marriage and are using weddings to their political advantage. Several states, including Karnataka, Andhra Pradesh and Maharashtra have set aside welfare funds for organizing mass marriage ceremonies according to caste, community and religion. Under state-run schemes, marriages are solemnized free of cost, and sometimes even dowry is offered in the form of gifts of household articles. On the face of it, it seems like a bright idea. Mass marriages can help the families of brides who incur the costs of hosting the wedding, it can curb unnecessary wedding spend, and can also ease the pressure of dowry.

Unfortunately, these schemes have evolved, like so many other things in India, into scams. Organizers get commissions from governments, middlemen make money by enlisting couples. They are also leading to bride kidnappings and fake marriages where married couples remarry just for gifts. State governments use marriage for their own strategic purposes. In Gujarat, on 27 February 2011, in memory of the Godhra train attack in 2002, a communal marriage was held to breed communal harmony— Muslim couples were wedded and the town's Hindu community was invited.[221] In Wadia, a locality that has been involved in prostitution (the village's men traditionally lived off the women's income from prostitution), women are married in mass ceremonies in an attempt to curb prostitution.[222] Madhya Pradesh has a marriage scheme called Mukhyamantri Kanyadan Yojana, literally meaning the Chief Minister Giving Away His Daughter Plan. An estimated 34,000 girls have been married off at a total cost of ₹42 crore under this scheme launched in 2006. The government of Madhya Pradesh has set aside a sum of ₹9,100 as wedding expenses for each girl, buying her a sari, anklets, a single bed, a mattress and a pressure cooker.[223] If the chief minister, or Mama (as he's called by the organizers), chooses to attend the wedding ceremony, the booty is expanded to include a gold mangalsutra, a steel cupboard and a gas stove. Wedding schemes in the state have been so successful that some say this is the secret behind the government's second term.

But these weddings also come with their fair share of controversy. Recently in Madhya Pradesh, hundreds of would-be-brides, mostly from poor tribal families, underwent virginity and pregnancy tests before they were allowed to participate in the mass marriage ceremony. According to reports, they were bullied into these examinations and were told that their refusal would mean that they wouldn't be allowed to participate and more importantly wouldn't be given their wedding gifts worth ₹6,500.[224] Of the 152 prospective brides tested, fourteen turned out to be pregnant and one was a minor.[225]

Back in Amravati, the wedding ceremony has come to an end. It is chaotic again, this time the chaos is coupled with emotion. Copious tears are shed, gifts are distributed, and there is much pushing and fighting to get to the food pandals where a wedding feast is on offer. I have been spending some time with Shilpy's family. When I go to congratulate her she takes my hand and pulls me into a smelly embrace. She points a hennaed finger at me and invites me to her home for a celebration. I take her address and promise to come.

The yoga guru Baba Ramdev begins to speak. The acoustics are poor, and it doesn't help that Baba is screaming into the mike. I struggle to understand what he is saying. I hear something along the lines of 'Get married, but be celibate. Remember Gandhiji. Save your semen'. It surely doesn't seem to be the most appropriate of wedding speeches. Celebratory firecrackers erupt in the sky, and smoke fills the area. Everyone looks on in glee. A cracker bursts fearfully close, and I think of what will happen if one of these crackers lands on any of the numerous canvas tents. There isn't a single fire escape in sight.

It is twilight now, and a hazy full moon rides low in the

sky. There are no clouds, no wind, and no stars visible because of the dust and the smoke of the fireworks display. Most of the guests have left and a slew of workers is taking down the pandals. The ground is littered with used plates, plastic cups, withered flowers and other debris. In the course of just a few hours, as the result of one political stunt, over 3,000 people have been made husband and wife.

I make my way to Shilpy's home which is in a crowded residential colony in Amravati city. Her squat, square house is painted entirely in baby pink and is lit up with strings of multicoloured flickering bulbs. The party is in full swing when I arrive. It is mostly 'youngsters'—the newly-weds, their siblings, cousins, and a few friends. Shilpy's mother and a few aunts are there to supervise the party.

A lanky boy, dressed in a shiny black suit, claiming to be Shilpy's brother, whispers in my ear, asking me if I want to 'take something'. I know from his tone that this 'taking' pertains to alcohol. I do not want to have a drink, but I am curious to see what the offerings are. I follow him into a small bedroom with peeling walls and a single wooden bed. A bar has been set up on a small wooden dressing table where a bottle of Old Monk rum, another of Smirnoff vodka, and a few dusty bottles of Kingfisher beer are on display.

Shilpy has changed from her wedding sari into a bright sequinned salwaar-kameez. She wears red and white plastic bangles that extend up to her elbows—the sign of a newly married bride. I ask her about her future plans, perhaps a honeymoon? She tells me excitedly that they will be going to Lonavala, a hill station outside Mumbai. I ask her if she enjoyed her mass marriage experience. She says that she is sad that Shahrukh didn't show up, but she didn't mind having Vivek Oberoi as a stand-in. She tells me dreamily that she will be able to tell her children and her grandchildren that a film star attended her wedding.

I am surprised to hear that even though Shilpy's is a love

match, a dowry is expected from her family, especially since they did not host the wedding. Shilpy will take with her gold jewellery, a dining room set, a bed, a sofa, and an air-cooler when she moves to the house that she will live in with her husband and in-laws, where she will continue her life as a teacher.

At around 11 p.m., I leave Shilpy's house, though there is no sign of the celebrations winding up. Bollywood music is blaring, and everyone is playing Antakshari. Many of the boys seem drunk to me, 'taking drinks' on the sly. I take an auto back to my hotel, a small derelict building that was advertised as a five-star hotel on the internet but, which I discover, is all of half a star.

I think back to the celebrations of the day. Marriage is an equalizer if there ever was one. In a country as diverse as India, the obsession with marriage is common to all—one of the few things crossing the lines of caste, wealth and social status. It is heartening to see so many people of different religions, castes, income levels, and from a range of professions including farmers, shopkeepers and school teachers, come together to celebrate what they believe is the biggest event of their lives. Nothing, not a medical camp nor an education programme, could have garnered Ravi Rana the goodwill that this event did.

As I navigate the alleys of a sleeping Amravati (except for, hopefully, 3,270 couples) I recall one particular incident from my eventful day. At the wedding kund where a painfully young boy was getting married to an equally juvenile girl, I had asked the boy why he was getting married. He had looked quizzically at his wife-to-be before turning to me with a wide-toothed grin and replying, 'Because Papa say so.' I then went and asked his Papa why marriage was so important. He gave me a questioning look. 'Because it is.' I persisted, trying to get a more convincing answer, but Papa wasn't especially forthcoming. Finally, fed up, he weightily said: 'Just because. This is the way that it was, this is the way it needs to be and this is the way it always will be.'

BREAK-UP

'*The Ideal Brahmin Marriage*' reads a large, garishly framed photograph of my elder sister's wedding that takes up prime wall space in my grandfather's living room in Ghaziabad, Uttar Pradesh. My grandfather has served a hat-trick term as the president of the All-World Brahmin Samaja whose primary focus is to set up marriages. Dadaji is known in many circles as a matchmaker par excellence and, for as long as I can remember, I have found endless streams of eager parents accompanied by their single sons and nubile daughters in his living room. Today, the scene in my octogenarian grandfather's living room is quite different. Dadaji, a lawyer by profession, is handling divorce with the same fervour and gusto as he once did marriage, and he is known in the same circles that lauded his matchmaking skills as a leading divorce counsellor.

On a recent visit, I found in my dadaji's living room none other than my cousin Chintoo. Growing up, we all thought that Chintoo had some form of disability because he never participated in our games, he just sat in a corner and stared at us. He would never speak to us, only make strange sounds from time to time and occasionally hit us for no reason. When Chintoo went to college, got a job and married a girl of his parents' choice, we were pleasantly surprised. Chintoo was normal after all. We were all shocked when, just a year after his marriage, Chintoo filed for divorce. It turned out that even after his nuptials, Chintoo had continued a romantic relationship with a long-time paramour whom his parents had not approved for marriage since she was not of the same caste. Following a digital trail, his new wife had caught Chintoo red-handed. To save face, Chintoo's parents told the family that the girl had the affair, not Chintoo, but the truth was eventually revealed to us by my grandfather who was Chintoo's chief counsel.

I ask grandfather if he finds divorce, especially in the case of someone like Chintoo, shocking since Dadaji himself is such a strong advocate of marriage.

'No,' is Dadaji's tempered response. 'It is part of Kalyug (the dark age predicted by the Hindu shastras). It is bound to happen, and it is my duty to deal with it,' he says steadfastly. So many things have changed in his lifetime and Dadaji applies the same tactic to face divorce as he does to the rest of his life. He deals with all things in life unemotionally, with the head and not the heart, with the precision and temperament of a surgeon—whether he understands them or not.

Perhaps the only thing that remains unchanged in that living room, preserved with the sanctity of a shrine, is that picture of my sister Ishani and her husband posing with my grandfather, whose beaming smile is as bright as the klieg lights under which they stand.

◆

Growing up, I hardly knew any Indian kids whose parents were divorced. Divorce was seen as a big misfortune which happened in the rarest of cases. I had the chance to see divorce close up when my masi (my mother's younger sister) got divorced after three years of marriage. Chhoti Masi had an arranged marriage to a man who lived in the US. Prima facie, he seemed well-to-do: he was an engineer at a large US corporate. However, when Chhoti Masi landed in the States after she was married, she was sent off to work loading trucks in a grocery store, to help with finances. When she quit her job, her in-laws and husband, who lived together in a one-bedroom flat, cruelly insulted her. Chhoti Masi gave the marriage everything she had, but eventually she returned to her parents' home in India. After her divorce she felt like a social pariah, so she sequestered herself away from family and friends and turned to spirituality to assuage her woes.

As a kid, my parents spoke about Chhoti Masi in hushed tones, lest her fate influence us girls. When I hit marriageable age, my parents often warned me, 'If you don't get married, you'll end up all alone like Babli.' When I got really annoyed, I would tell them: 'Well, if I get married to the *wrong* guy under pressure from you, then I may get divorced like Chhoti Masi too!' This statement always led to a quick termination of the marriage discussion.

Today, things have changed substantially, and thousands of Indian women like Chhoti Masi are making matrimonial choices that their mothers and grandmothers could hardly have dreamt of. This is a drastic change in attitude when, just a generation ago, divorce was considered a family shame. Today, divorce is no longer the anathema that it once was. The increase in divorce rates and the accompanying loss of taboo is apparent in newspaper matrimonials where divorce columns are getting longer by the day, and with the mushrooming of matrimonial sites like Secondshaadi.com. Divorce has even become a staple feature of the hugely popular family dramas that play on television and have millions glued to their screens. In the popular soap *Balika Vadhu* (Child Bride), the main character Anandi's divorce had viewers in tears, and her re-marriage to a handsome, suave government official had viewers celebrating and bursting firecrackers on the street.

For much of Indian history, divorce did not occur. Traditionally, Hindu weddings were not looked upon as merely a ceremony, but as a sacrosanct, religious act where multiple Hindu gods, the cosmos, the sun, the moon and the stars were all involved. Marriage is described in the shastras as a tradition where the body of the virgin bride merges into her husband's permanently and eternally and they become a single entity. It a holy sacrament and the gift of a girl to a suitable person is a sacred duty of the father for which the father gets great spiritual benefit. As recently as 1970, the Allahabad High Court declared the institution of matrimony under the Hindu law as a sacrament, not just a legal contract.

There were so few instances of divorce in Hindu marriage, that there is no word for it in the Hindi language. When divorce did happen in the Hindu tradition, it occurred in extraordinary circumstances—when a spouse was discovered to be insane or impotent, or if he/she had decided to renounce the world. Ancient texts like the *Naradasmriti* allow women to remarry in certain situations: if the man is impotent or decides to become an ascetic. In Muslim marriages, an option for divorce or talaaq did exist, but the Prophet cautioned that it was what Allah hated the most, and that it should happen only in the rarest of circumstances.

Today, the scene has changed considerably. In the 1970s and 1980s, the divorce rate in India was insignificant, ranging from 0.2 per cent to 0.14 per cent and barely touching 1 per cent of the total population.[226] An official national statistic on divorce is unavailable because divorce proceedings in India are dealt with at the state level, but the 2001 census (the last time a national divorce figure was available) estimated the national divorce rate to be as high as 7 per cent.[227] Though this number may pale in comparison to the 50 per cent divorce rates of the US, what is significant is the steep increase.

Examining divorce rates in Indian cities will give us a better idea of the enormous increase. In Delhi, touted to be the divorce capital of India, an estimated 9,000 divorce cases are filed every year.[228] This number is almost double of what was seen four years ago. In 2004, there were only two or three family courts; today there are seventeen. In Mumbai, the financial capital of the country, over the past decade, the number of divorces has increased by 86 per cent.[229] Since 1990, the annual number of divorce petitions filed in Mumbai has more than doubled, outpacing population growth.[230] In Bangalore, the IT capital of India, numbers indicate an increase of over 60 per cent.[231] A majority of those filing for divorce are young, in their twenties and thirties, and work in the city's corporate sector. In 2007, the Bangalore Mediation Centre was set up in the hope of disposing of the number of divorce cases; more than 1,783 cases were referred here in 2010-2011.[232]

States with high divorce rates include Kerala, India's most literate state, where the number of divorce cases has increased by 350 per cent in the past 10 years;[233] in Kolkata, 200 per cent in the past decade;[234] surprisingly, divorce has also gone up in Punjab and Haryana—both traditional agricultural states—by 150 per cent.[235]

In most marriages around the globe, the initial years are typically considered 'honeymoon' years, but for Indians they're usually the worst. Most divorces occur in the twenty-five to thirty-nine age group, and usually during the first five years of marriage.[236] Unlike in the West, where a common reason for divorce is the mid-life crisis, it is rare to see couples in their forties and fifties getting divorced. According to Dr Vijay Nagaswami, relationship counsellor and author of the New Indian Marriage Series, mid-life crises amongst Indians rarely end in divorce, but often in infidelity. Older couples in dysfunctional marriages remain together because of the taboo around divorce which they've grown up with, but younger couples have no such qualms and are quick to divorce.

The most apparent reason for the higher divorce rate is the financial independence of Indian women, which allows them to step out of unhappy marriages. Today, almost a third of India's 480 million jobs are held by women, and over the past decade, women's incomes have doubled in the cities. About 60 per cent of women in urban areas say they are responsible for everything that happens in their lives.[237] A higher focus on careers than on personal lives amongst women is a prominent game changer. In a study that surveyed over 1,000 women in the age groups of twenty to thirty in cities across the country, 93 per cent wanted to continue studying or working after marriage.[238]

Earlier when two families came together, the couple tried harder to adjust, because divorce was simply not a choice. But today because of their financial independence, and the consequent rise in confidence, the traditional view that women will accept and adjust to their husbands and their families no longer holds. Women are no longer ready to sacrifice their own happiness for the sake of the family. Individual happiness trumps all. Changes in the law too have helped divorce. Over the past decade, divorce laws have seen a lot of change, making it easier and faster to get a divorce.

According to Aarti Mundkur, a lawyer at the Alternative Law Forum, Bangalore, 'Women are able to split due to minor shifts in the law. Now, it's just a bit easier to live alone, rent a house, work in new sectors. If these (legal) conditions had existed earlier, we'd have seen the same divorce rates.'[239]

Before 1955, Hindus, Buddhists, Jains, and Sikhs had no option of divorce. Section 13 of the Hindu Marriage Act of 1955 legally introduced divorce in Hindu marriages if the divorce fell under the ambit of adultery, cruelty, renunciation of the world (a strange one), change of religion, or missing partner. These laws allowed divorce only if there was sufficient evidence of 'faults' even amongst couples who mutually wanted a divorce. These couples negotiated amongst themselves to determine uncontested claims of faults, and presented them to the courts. This fault-based system allowed for mutual consent divorce, but not unilateral divorce. In 1976, an amendment added mutual consent without a need to present 'faults'. In 2010, the Indian government responded to the vertiginous rise in marital breakups and the surging backlog in court cases by proposing an amendment that would make it easier and faster to get divorced. The new amendment proposes that couples show irretrievable breakdown of marriage or incompatibility and the six-month mandatory separation period be waived.

In her extensive study of divorce in India, psychologist Shaifali

Sandhya, author of *Love Will Follow: Why The Indian Marriage is Burning*, found another less apparent but important reason for marriages in India failing. Expectations of love and intimacy were not met for 70 per cent of couples. 'The biggest conflict is love,' says Sandhya. 'Marriage was historically about families, but couples now want to form their own unique territory. Women want love to be more active. That's a new thing.'[240] Sex too has become important to marriage, unlike the olden days where two people had sex only to procreate. According to a survey, 64 per cent of respondents said sex was 'very' or 'extremely important' to their marriage, and a third reported not being sexually satisfied in their existing marriages.[241] Sandhya also says that Indian couples are saddled with new, more 'Western' problems of work, sex and money, as well as the older problems of testy in-laws, overbearing relatives and children, creating a 'double whammy', and too much pressure to handle.

DOUBLE DIVORCEE

At the Sivananda Ashram in Kerala, Shiny stands out as the most ardent meditator. In the luminescent dawn, as the rest of us fidget in uncomfortable cross-legged positions on the cold, hard stone floors, Shiny's beatific face is the picture of peace. Strikingly handsome, with a lean, muscular 6'2" frame, he had caught my attention and one day over a cup of herbal tea, he and I got talking. I am at the ashram for a two-week yoga retreat, and he claims he is there indefinitely, on the run from his demonic wife of fifteen months in his hometown in Jalandhar, Punjab. He had packed his bags, written a letter to his father and his father-in-law announcing his wish to divorce his wife and boarded a train with no destination in mind. That journey eventually led him to the ashram, where he has now been for over two weeks with no intention of leaving anytime soon.

Over many hours of yoga and endless cups of tea, Shiny and I became fast friends. Little did I know then that this quiet man—with his studied look of calm—and I would become close friends, meeting year after year at the ashram to recharge our batteries and exchange stories. Three years later, as I research divorce, my first point of reference is Shiny. Of all the stories that I have encountered in my research, Shiny's is the most fascinating. First, because I have been a witness to it and second, because this is not Shiny's first, but second divorce.

The last time I saw Shiny was at the ashram in Kerala; he was ebullient, glowing with good health. Today, when I visit him and his family in Jalandhar, he looks tired and worn out. I ask him if the divorce has taken a toll on his health. His answer comes to me as somewhat of a shock—he has spent the last fortnight in prison. His bail application was rejected so he had to spend ten days in the lockup. His wife had filed a criminal case against him during the divorce proceedings. Despite his frazzled looks and jail-time, Shiny is in his usual good spirits. He laughs and tells me, 'It's like the ashram, really, the same bland food twice a day, the same early morning wake-up call and strict schedule. Everything felt the same to me, except that I was woken up by a bothersome policeman rather than ashram bells.'

As we drive through Jalandhar to reach Shiny's home, I observe that it looks just like any other Indian town—a once sleepy town now positively fizzing with new growth fuelled by new money, chaotic traffic, dusty parks, the ubiquitous MG Road and randomly placed statues of leaders, the only difference being that these ones wear turbans since we are in Punjab.

Shiny lives in a bustling residential colony on the outskirts of town which started out as a nine-house colony when his family first moved here. He proudly points out a glitzy mall that is being built around the corner that fuses Spanish architecture with Indian. A large signboard on the construction wall reads: *'The experience of a bazaar. The comfort of a mall'*. Shiny's family has grown with the neighbourhood. They started out as solidly middle class and over the past decade have ridden the Indian growth wave and are now upper-middle class. We drive by Shiny's factory where he works with his father. It is a small, rustic building with a big painted board that reads 'Dada Industries' where they manufacture bathroom fittings.

At Shiny's spacious home, I meet his mother. She is elderly, kind, and soft-spoken yet talkative. Shiny leaves me with her while he gets back to work. Auntyji and I settle in to talk while drinking cups of thick, syrupy chai. The television crackles in the background. Over the next few days I observe that it runs all day, mostly playing Hindi soap operas, Hindi news, and movies, and sometimes even National Geographic. Auntyji moved to Punjab from Uttar Pradesh as a young bride and quickly learnt to cook and speak Punjabi so she could cater to the needs of her husband. Even today, she wakes up at 6:45 a.m. to make hot tea for Shiny's father before he goes for his morning walk. After dinner when Shiny's father goes to bed, she always stays awake to clean and tidy up. She talks a lot about 'duty'. To her, and to many other Indian women of her generation, duty is marriage and marriage is duty. She talks about her husband as 'Uncleji' or 'Shiny's father', never referring to him by his name—a respectful form of address used by older Indian women for their husbands. When the timing seems right, I carefully broach the subject of Shiny's ongoing divorce. The old lady's face falls, and her wrinkles are suddenly marked. Shiny's second marriage, unlike his first one, was arranged. A woman of the same caste as Shiny's Brahmin family and from a comparable economic class was found through the matrimonial portal shaadi.com. Astrologers agreed that their birth charts were compatible, so all marked and matched, they quickly got married.

As a marriage broker later told me, 'A man in Punjab is like a bull; as long as he is virile, he can find a bride, no matter how many times he has been married before.' There was that, and Shilpa, Shiny's bride-to-be, was thirty-two, which, by Indian standards, was over the hill. According to Shiny, Shilpa was under pressure from her parents to get married, especially since her sisters and cousins were already settled. For Shilpa, Shiny fit the bill; he was handsome, his family was well-to-do, they were from the same caste and community, and their horoscopes matched. Shilpa and Shiny got married in a suitably ostentatious Punjabi way and quickly conceived a child. Six months after their daughter Pinky was born, all hell broke loose and Shiny fled from home to the ashram. Auntyji bemoans that Shilpa drove him up the wall and out of the house. As we talk about the divorce a sombre mood permeates the colourful living room we're sitting in. Auntyji repeats more than once how they were so loving towards her, how they opened their home and hearts to the 'girl' (as she calls Shilpa), but things still went awry.

'She did not adjust,' Auntyji says firmly, so Shiny was forced to do what he had to do. Auntyji believes that a woman should 'adjust' to her husband as she herself has done. But Shilpa, the product of a new generation and a new India, had different expectations from a man and marriage.

As the conversation steers on towards Shiny's life, Auntyji is uplifted, and her face lights up. Shiny has been a perfect son to her. She blushes as she tells me that Shiny was chosen to participate in a prestigious male beauty pageant, Mr India, in Mumbai. She says she was so proud to see her handsome son on television, and tells me how Shiny, a 'Punjab da puttar', had become the pride of Jalandhar and gone on to win the title. Shiny, being the deferential son that he was, turned down the modelling contract for the family business and less glamorous pastures of Punjab.

I ask if I can see photographs of Shiny's most recent wedding. Auntyji frowns and looks at me with a considered gaze, but she loves showing photographs so she eventually fishes out the photos, which are stacked away at the back of a cupboard. They have gathered a significant amount of dust, it is clear that they haven't been viewed for a while. Despite the festivities, there is an element of sobriety in all the photos, with Shiny and Shilpa flashing fake, bright smiles that get grimmer as the evening carries on. Auntyji points out all the relevant family members, though I can tell she is far less enthusiastic than she has been with the other photos. I take a chance and ask if we can see those photos of the first wedding too, but Auntyji apologizes and says grimly that Shiny has burnt all the photos from that wedding.

WITH PAPAJI AT DINNER

'Shiny has not given me thirty-five seconds of trouble in thirty-five years of life. He is a God-fearing and a good man,' proclaims Uncleji, Shiny's father, chomping methodically on his chicken.

'Yes, yes,' agrees his mother, nodding her head vigorously, and smiling at Shiny.

Then, as quickly as she smiled, her face falls. 'It is so sad that this happened to my son of all the people in the world,' she says and stares down into her plate. I have observed that she often falls into these moods in the midst of conversations.

Uncleji declares, 'Ira, when your father comes to Punjab, he is invited to stay here.'

'Thanks, Uncle, but what about my mom?' I ask.

'Father means the couple only. Both father and mother,' says Uncleji.

'Yes, beta. Your Uncleji, is right,' agrees Auntyji.

Over the past few days I have come to realize that Shiny's elderly father is a deeply conflicted individual. While he expresses deep reverence and respect for his wife, he has very clear-cut beliefs about a woman's role in the family and what her primary duty is—simply put, it is to serve her husband and her children.

Shiny is his father's son. Though he was deeply sensitive, caring and emotional, he had peculiar, rigid views that didn't seem to change despite his 'worldly' experiences. For example, sex. Shiny believes in what he calls the 'Indian Vedic culture of life'. According to his interpretation, the scriptures say that a physical relationship is important only to have children. Good sex, Shiny feels, does not guarantee a good relationship. To me, his interpretation seems unidimensional and also radical, more so for someone as emotional. But Shiny is set in his ways and views and was not willing to change, especially since love didn't work in his favour during his first marriage. Shiny had married from the heart the first time, but the second time around he changed his strategy, marrying strictly from the head. He had a checklist, and the woman who met his criteria would be the woman he would marry.

But in a modern day Indian marriage, it was not just the woman who needed to adapt in the marriage, but a man too. Shiny had told me that before his marriage, he had presented Shilpa with a list of duties and the things that his family expected of her; Shilpa had agreed to all of his conditions. After his first divorce he wanted to proceed 'by the book' (in this case the book was the ancient *Saptapadi*, the Hindu code for marriage) and that is why he wanted to make sure his second wife would be amenable, which she appeared to be.

The unfortunate truth was that a successful marriage couldn't be initiated by checking off a list, but Shiny refused to believe that.

◆

One evening Shiny takes me to Haveli, a large mock Punjabi village, complete with colourful dhabas, mud houses and turbaned waiters with impressive moustaches in colourful Punjabi garb. Shiny and I settle down cross-legged on a wooden coir-strung cot and order cups of rich almond milk and gobi paranthas. This place is, or at least was, special to Shiny because it is where his first wedding took place. He tells me that he hardly thinks about his first marriage anymore, and that this is one of the few times he has gone back over that period in his life. It was a love marriage, and the woman was five years older than him and he loved her deeply. Though she was not keen to get married because she didn't see herself as the 'marrying type', he had convinced her to marry him in 2005. The marriage lasted for two years before they mutually agreed to get divorced.

I ask Shiny why his marriage broke up. Shiny shrugs, giving me a resigned look.

'She was a nice, straightforward, truthful girl. She never wanted to get married, she always wanted to be single. I convinced her to get married.'

'Why did you try to convince her if you knew she never wanted to be married?' I ask.

'If you talk to any Indian girl, I'd say 70 per cent of them never want to get married. But 'no' means 'yes'. It's not a no no. If I had taken her at face value, we would've never gotten to be boyfriend-girlfriend. Some people say that love is blind. I was really blind and never saw the truth,' he says.

Shiny was blindly in love. His ex-wife, though, did not want to be married and did it out of a sense of duty. After all, every Indian girl is brought up thinking that marriage is the be-all and end-all of life.

Shiny looks away from me, his voice is cracking just a little bit.

'She asked for the divorce, and I agreed. I realized there was no point going back to broken relationships. They can never be made okay. It's like trying to put back broken pieces of glass. It's just going to cut your hands and it will never come back together in the same shape.'

While Shiny's first divorce was by mutual consent, his second divorce was contested. This is where the trouble lay. In India, except in cases of divorce by mutual consent, people are not entitled to a divorce because they have been separated. Everything has to be proven in court. A smart divorce strategy must be devised and a petition must be filed in court. The court then prescribes mandatory counselling sessions for the couple, which can go on for years, alongside court hearings. If couples get past this painful stage, then the battle for alimony begins because Indian law has no clear rules laid out and each case is dealt with individually.

It can be years before the marriage is finally nullified. According to estimates, there are 55,000 divorce cases pending in courts across the country.[242]

When Shiny filed for divorce, his wife resisted. Reacting to Shiny's divorce petition, Shilpa's father filed a police complaint accusing Shiny of domestic violence against his daughter and another charging Shiny and his entire family with dowry demands. This may seem like the hasty, hot-headed reaction of a madcap father, but the reality is that Shilpa's father's reaction is common. As Shiny explained to me, it is the 'typical way' for an urban, middle-class Indian family to react. Dowry laws were put into place to protect women and their families against dowry atrocities, but they were often misused. According to Shiny, poor women who really needed the law are not aware of it, and those who use the law are usually educated, urban women 'exploiting their ex-husbands'. Since a dowry complaint was filed, Shiny and his parents had to prove that they never asked for dowry, as opposed to the other way around. Knowing Shiny and his family, it was impossible that any of Shilpa's allegations were true.

The more I explored divorce cases, the more I realized how easy it was for women to be at the receiving end, and why they might be compelled to exploit the system. It is still common for Indian men, like Shiny, to live with their parents whose homes, property, and assets remain in their fathers' name. As maintenance or alimony is judged on the husband's income tax returns it makes it hard for a woman to demand a fair sum of money for maintenance. Many Indian men use this as a tactic to evade paying maintenance to their wives.

More often than not, says lawyer Shroff-Garg (author of *Breaking Up: Your Step-by-step Guide to Getting Divorced*), divorce cases end in a wrangle over money. 'There are never black-and-white cases. It's all grey. In the end, it's about buying your freedom. Either you pay money or take money. It's that simple.'[243] Maintenance remains a contentious subject in Indian divorces. In several Western countries, alimony is an obligation ordered by the court to the financially stronger spouse; in India it is not yet an absolute right of the seeker. The awarding of alimony, its amount, and its duration are determined based on the financial position and circumstances of the spouse. Women will let the legal proceedings drag on until they receive a satisfactory amount of money. Not giving a divorce is perhaps the only leverage they have.

Shiny's situation is not uncommon either. A study conducted by the NGOs Save Indian Family Foundation and My Nation, which looked at four aspects of domestic violence—economic, emotional, physical and sexual—in a sample survey of 1,650 urban men, found that 98 per cent of the respondents had suffered violence in these forms more than once.[244] Economic abuse was the most common, but so were nagging, grumbling, taunting, name-calling, refusing food, denying sexual intercourse, and throwing objects. The most serious of all was framing of false charges under the Indian Penal Code, just like Shilpa had done.

In a written testimony as a part of his divorce proceedings, Shiny shared his anguish and anxiety with the judge by presenting evidence of cruelty, the grounds on which he has filed for divorce. Shiny's frustration is evident in this twenty-page document, in which he shares incidents from his failed marriages. When he gets especially frustrated he writes in capital letters that are bold, and when he gets thoughtful, he puts in multiple ellipses.

Here is an excerpt from his affidavit:

> Before my marriage, I told Shilpa that I was a teetotaller. Shilpa told me that she is also almost one but occasionally she takes one or two drinks. I did not have a problem with that. After we got married, I realized that her 'occasion' is once every two or three months. Whenever we would go to a good eating-place she would need a drink. One day when we were at home she told me to get a drink (whisky) for her. I said to her, 'Go and get it yourself, it is in the

> cupboard.' My dad has a drink every evening, and all the arrangements are there. She refused to go, because she said she felt embarrassed to make a drink for herself. I felt so disgusted since I don't drink at all. I thought to myself, what will my father think, and what will the domestic help think about me. With a lot of courage and a straight face, I got a drink for her and thought the ordeal was over, but she sent me again to the whisky station saying, 'Ise theek karke laao, yeah mazedaar nahi hai' (Go fix this, there is no fun in this drink). I went all the way, did the horrible job, and prayed to God that no one was watching and darted back to my room. Sir, for a person who doesn't drink, and whose spouse has an impression in the house that she doesn't drink too, it's humiliating to do this service.

Shiny tells me that his lawyer deleted the above incident when the document was shown to the judge. Another incident was used instead.

> She used to kick boxes of food articles from our room like an angry footballer, in her fits of insane temperamental rages. Once, she kicked a box of mathis weighing appx 2.0 kgs from our room on the first floor. It landed in the ground floor—a heavy box like that could have hit anyone's head and could have easily injured that person, or maybe killed that person also.

◆

In the dirty, dusty alleys of New Delhi's Connaught Place, I circumvent cars, people and animals. I pass a McDonald's and a Costa Coffee, both of which reek of pesticide. At the law firm, sombre lawyers sit in crowded offices with stacks of papers everywhere, surrounded by enormous law books. Most lawyers' offices in India have this same aura—dim fluorescent lights;

thick, dusty piles of law books and lots of people crammed into one room. I have come to speak with Roopesh Sharma, Shiny's divorce lawyer, to get the final chapters of Shiny's story.

In order to give me the right perspective on divorce, Sharma first tells me the story of Manish Dalal's divorce.

As he entered the venue riding on a small white horse, dressed in his wedding finery, being trailed by his raucous baraat, Manish Dalal knew his life would never be the same again. Unfortunately, instead of walking seven times around the wedding fire to solemnize his marriage he walked and got burned in an entirely different way that fateful night.

Manish was stopped, horse, baraat and all, and told by his to-be-father-in-law that Nisha was refusing to marry him because Manish's family had demanded dowry and their family was unwilling to meet their demands. Overnight, the demure twenty-one-year-old Nisha Sharma became a national sensation, an anti-dowry heroine, praised for her brave rejection of her evil to-be husband. Famous politicians told the public that she was their daughter; handsome actors declared her their sister. Men queued up at her gate to ask for her hand in marriage. An interview on *The Oprah Winfrey Show* brought her international fame.

Manish, on the other hand, became the evil face of dowry. He was arrested on what was meant to be his wedding night and thrown into jail. Nisha and her family slapped dowry charges on him and his family claiming that they had asked for ₹12 lakh in cash and various household items, like a sofa, an AC and a fridge. The case went on for years; Manish and his parents went in and out of jail and the courts. Manish lost his job and was humiliated nationally and internationally. When all seemed to be lost for poor Manish, the case suddenly took a Bollywood-esque turn. Navneet Rai, a former classmate of Nisha's from engineering college, produced a marriage certificate and photos of what he claimed was their secret marriage ceremony. He claimed to be Nisha's jilted husband and declared that she had spurned Manish because she wanted to be with him. He demanded the restitution of his conjugal rights. By this time, though, Nisha was famous and being seen as a champion of women's rights. She was happily married to a third man and denounced the marriage certificate as fake.

Manish's legal team, bristling with confidence at this unforeseen stroke of luck, questioned how Manish could be charged with demanding dowry if Nisha had been married all along to someone else. Finally, after eleven long years, Manish and his family were acquitted. However, by this time, Nisha was the mother of a few children, nobody was interested in the case and poor Manish continued to be a pariah in the eyes of the few people who remembered him.

The Nisha Sharma case is similar to Shiny's, and Roopesh Sharma had represented Manish, so Shiny has hired Sharma to represent him.

I ask Sharma what will happen to my poor friend Shiny. Much to my relief Sharma doesn't seem to be too worried about his case. Over 60 per cent of contested divorces eventually go on to become divorces of mutual consent since it is difficult to prove mental or domestic cruelty. Cases go on in court for years, usually till one person decides to re-marry, and agrees to reach a settlement. The divorce then takes place by mutual consent. Shiny has already done his time in jail and it is unlikely that he will go behind bars again. The case will go on till Shilpa's family decides to end the trial and settle on a sum of money. In an ironic twist of fate it seems that divorce, like marriage, is simply a game of numbers.

◆

An adorable young girl dressed in a frothy pink and yellow frock runs past us, and Shiny's face suddenly lights up. He touches her hand as she runs past. I can tell he loves children. This toddler is just about the same age as his daughter, Pinky, whom he was forced to leave when she was only a few months old, because the trouble with his marriage had already begun.

In the labyrinthine legalities of divorces, economic tug-of-wars and, ultimately, broken families, what will happen to children? Many children will grow up in broken homes and there will surely be consequences.

'I don't want her growing up being taunted by children because her parents are divorced,' says Shiny, looking sadder than I had ever seen him. With a defeated expression, Shiny looks up at me, 'I wanted to get married desperately because it was my duty to my parents. I wanted to have a child desperately because it was my duty to my ancestors. I wanted to get a divorce because it was my duty to myself. How long can one keep doing their duty? When will *I* get to live?'

To this I had no answer. All weekend, I have heard of duty from Shiny and his parents. In this home, duty is of utmost importance. Shiny's mom lived to do her duty to her husband. Shiny's father worked and lived out of a sense of duty to his wife and son. Shiny's main goal in life now seemed to be performing his duty to his parents by taking care of them.

The concept of duty, or dharma, is ingrained in Hindu philosophy and is thought by many to be the most important pillar of life. My grandfather, to this day, leads his life based on dharma, doing what he *should* be doing, not what he *wants* to do. I don't think Dadaji has done anything in his life for the sake of just having a good time. My parents, too, lead their lives like this, though to a smaller extent than my grandfather. I do not follow my grandfather's or parents' way of life. I live a far more selfish life and I only care about dharma when it applies to me. I have a dharma to myself to fall in love with my husband. I have a dharma to myself to get divorced if I am deeply unhappy in my marriage. My dharma to myself is far more important than my dharma to anyone else—my parents or my progeny. Maybe I am selfish, or maybe it's just that my dharma has been diverted.

I feel dharma towards other things, like my work, my career, my creative spirit, my individuality. These are probably things Dadaji never felt.

Shiny is caught somewhere in-between. He has a duty to fall in love but then he also has a duty to his parents to have an arranged marriage; he has a duty to himself to get divorced, but then he also has a duty to keep his parents happy and safe and, at the same time, a duty to protect his daughter from ostracism. There is an entire generation of soldiers fighting this dharmic battle and people like me, Shiny and millions of others are caught in this crossfire.

GOLDEN TEMPLE

The sun rises on the Golden Temple, casting its iridescent rays on to the tranquil Pool of Nectar. There is not a single sound of human dissent despite the 20,000 odd people here, not a cry, not a squeal, not a laugh. Gentle hymns echo from the gilded sanctum sanctorum from which this holy shrine gets its popular name.

Shiny has brought me to this estuary of peace in Amritsar on the last day of my trip. Though this is a Sikh shrine, the Golden Temple is a place of worship for people across faiths. Shiny has offered to take me to more temples in the area that he regularly visits, but I refuse. One is enough for me. I enjoy temples, but the number of people that throng temples is increasing and they are exhausting to visit. In this fast-changing world, people like Shiny and Chhoti Masi are turning to religion and spirituality as an anchor more than ever before.

Shiny walks with a resigned gait and sloping shoulders, he prays ardently, prostrating himself at the entrance with his forehead on the cool marble floor. Shiny never wants to get married again, he wants to lead a spiritual life and be a good son to his parents, a good father to his daughter. In the early morning light Shiny's face is a perfect picture of peace, just the way I remember him from the Sivananda ashram. His trial is likely to go on for many years. The future is uncertain, but Shiny is optimistic. He holds to the one thing that he has now, an undefeatable faith in God.

◆

Back at home, I stay up reading the journal that Shiny kept before he separated from Shilpa. What strikes me most is that his estranged relationship is so much like mine. Vinayak and I have many of the same problems that Shiny and Shilpa had—money, family, his future, my future, our future, and our fights take on a similar tenor. As Shilpa told Shiny, I tell Vinayak that his best is not enough for me, that I deserve better. We both say really nasty things to each other, he gets angry and sinks into a hole. I feel for Shilpa because I can relate to her frustration. In these journals, Shilpa behaves like a monster, and at times, I do too.

What Vinayak and I share, that Shiny and Shilpa do not, is love. In an arranged marriage one is meant to marry from the head, not from the heart. Maybe Vinayak and I can work through it, because we are *both* willing to work and *want* it to work. Shiny uses his first marriage as an example of the lack of any guarantee of staying together in a love marriage, even with the best of intentions. That said, Shiny's first wife never had a desire to make the marriage work, just a sense that marriage was necessary. There was a mismatch of expectations, and this led them to exercise the freedom that they had and step out of an unhappy marriage.

As India falls in and out of love in droves, I wonder what is at the heart of the change. The old guard discourages love marriages, saying they lead to divorce. Statistically speaking they are correct, divorce *is* higher amongst couples who marry for love, but this is a chicken-and-egg argument. It can be argued that people who marry for love are those who broke free of societal norms in the first place and, in that same spirit of rebellion, are more likely to break free of unhappy, unsatisfactory marriages.

A 2005 study examining marriage satisfaction amongst Indian

couples in arranged marriages, and US couples in love marriages revealed that there was no difference in marriage satisfaction levels between the participants.[245] What was different between the two groups were their views on 'love wellness'. American couples thought that being in love was a strong indication of current and future marital success. Indian couples looked at things a little differently. They didn't expect love at the start of their marriage, they expected love to grow as they got to know each other.

According to the study, 'In arranged marriages, individuals marry according to family wishes, and the focus is on accepting and adjusting to their family's wishes. Thus love is viewed in a different manner by persons in India and is not seen as a necessary precursor to marriage. Instead, love is expected to grow as spouses learn more about each other as the years go by.'

The question then arises: Do arranged marriages fail because of a low level of intimacy and commitment? Some maybe, but not all. I have seen plenty of couples in arranged marriages deeply in love because they share the same values. Family involvement in arranged marriage is an added benefit because it breeds a deeper sense of commitment. Love over family is the modern Indian marriage mantra. One can argue that a higher marital dissolution rate is the price for our individual pursuits of happiness. Neither of these is going away anytime soon. So what happens to marriage then?

SHAH BANO

> In the heart of every Muslim woman in Bhopal survives a magical island. She traces it back to a vision, of four women who ruled and guided the destinies of the state for more than a hundred years. They ruled like men, rode horses and elephants, wore no veil, and were referred to as Nawabs. In today's Bhopal, a city that has moved like any other, their memories live on, striking echoes in the daily lives of people—Anees Jung, *Night of the New Moon*

The first divorce case any lawyer learns about is the Shah Bano case. When Shah Bano, a sixty-five-year-old Muslim woman asked for an increase of ₹80 to her ₹100 monthly maintenance from her ex-husband, little did she know that she would go down in Indian history and the judgment would spark off a communal war that would singe India for years to come.

The year was 1985 when the case that Shah Bano Begum from Indore had been contesting against her husband for seven years reached the Supreme Court of India. Her husband's lawyer argued that he had the right to be exempted from paying maintenance to his divorced wife as he was a Muslim and came under the jurisdiction of Shariah or Islamic law, not Indian civil law. Under Shariah, Muslim women had no right to alimony after the three-month iddat period[246] following the dissolution of the marriage. A Hindu judge ruled against her husband, stating that every Indian citizen came under the purview of Indian law. This caused an uproar among the conservative sections of the Muslim community, particularly members of the Muslim Personal Law Board, a body formed in 1973 to uphold Islamic values.

Shah Bano became a subject of parliamentary debate—should different communities have different personal laws? Then prime minister, Rajiv Gandhi, succumbed to pressure from Muslim fundamentalist groups demanding a separate Muslim law and in 1986, a retrograde law called the Muslim Women (Protection of Rights on Divorce) Act was passed. This act nullified the Shah Bano ruling in the Supreme Court, and stated that the Muslim personal law would be considered in all cases of Muslim women. Starting with this verdict, a series of incidents unfolded that antagonized the Hindu community and in their anger, Hindu right-wing groups demolished the Babri Masjid in Ayodhya. According to mythology this was the exact spot where the Hindu god Ram was born. This led to savage, bloody, communal riots across the country, in which thousands of people died.

Bhopal, the capital of Madhya Pradesh, is a sleepy town. It is also a beautiful town, situated on the banks of a glorious lake where the remains of Mughal rule are still visible in numerous structures. Many a tourist has stumbled upon Bhopal and been awestruck by its charm and cleanliness, wondering how it ever got left off the tourist map.

Unfortunately, Bhopal is world-famous for only one thing: the gas tragedy in 1984, under the shadow of which I was born: a disaster in which a chemical leak from the Union Carbide plant in town had a devastating effect—several thousand people were killed, and many thousands more were crippled for life. It is sad that this incident has tarnished the reputation of the city, for Bhopal is a unique town with a unique history. In Mughal times, the city of Bhopal was said to be the second most important Muslim city in India. In Bhopal, women ruled in dynastic succession throughout the nineteenth and twentieth centuries in spite of both British and Islamic strictures against female rule. Perhaps the most notable of the ruling Begums of Bhopal was the last Begum, Nawab Sultan Shahjahan Begum, a strong advocate for Muslim women's rights.

Since the time of Shah Bano, there has been much controversy and confusion around divorce and divorce laws amongst Muslim women. The situation has only worsened over the years, with the sharp rise in divorce rates amongst Muslims all over India, including Bhopal, and I have come to this town to understand why.

THE QAZI

I start my research at the Qaziat, the focal point of all matters of Islamic religious law in Bhopal, which is the office of the Qazi-e-Shahar—the judge ruling on all matters of Islamic law.

The Qaziat is contained in a sullen-looking building, the exterior of which has been painted a seasick green, and the interior of which has the distinct feel of a government office—a dank room with high ceilings and peeling walls that resemble feta cheese. Qazi Syed Mushtaq Ali Nadvi is an owl-eyed man with a long beard, dressed in a long, black, terylene jacket, a pair of badly cut white trousers, and a black skull cap.

Our ensuing conversation has more than a touch of irreverence to it. The first thing that he disdainfully tells me is that if I were a Muslim girl, he would not talk to me unless I covered my head. I am glad that I have a woollen scarf in my bag, which I wrap tightly around my head. The Qazi pounds facts about Muslim procedure like nikah (marriage) and talaaq (divorce) into my head, like nails into a piece of knotty wood.

The first talaaq is considered to be the first divorce. This is a revocable divorce and the husband and wife can get back together within the iddah period, measured by three menstrual cycles of the wife. Once the first iddah is complete, divorce is irrevocable, but the husband and wife can get another nikah if they choose. If the husband and wife have not sorted out their differences, then a second 'talaaq' is said, and another three-month iddah is completed. After the third iddah and final talaaq, husband and wife are declared 'ida', or separated.

During the separation period or iddah the woman receives iddat—a form of maintenance from her husband. After three months of the iddah, husband and wife are divorced and all maintenance is stopped. If a man proposes talaaq, he can divorce without his wife's consent, but he must pay her mehr (a sum decided before marriage) and also iddat. A woman, too, can ask for divorce through a khula, where she pays her husband dower, or property, but she cannot divorce without her husband's consent.

I understand that Muslim divorce laws are skewed in favour of men, and this explains the controversy. Indian Muslim laws also permit triple talaaq when a man simply utters 'talaaq, talaaq, talaaq', and the divorce is complete without separation. Certain Islamic countries, like Egypt, Iran, Jordan, Morocco, Yemen and Sudan, have banned unilateral triple talaaq through codified law.

It cannot be abolished in India unless the All Muslim Personal Law Board agrees to do so, but the all-male body is adamant about sticking to its old ways and at the moment there is little scope for change.

The Qazi is evasive on the subject of divorce. He does not divulge divorce numbers, though he is the man who knows it all because he signs off on all such decisions. I unsuccessfully probe him and eventually give up. When I ask him about the rise and reasons for it, he scowls at me. 'There has been a small rise, but that is inevitable.'

Why does he think there has been a *small* rise in divorce? I persist.

'It is because laws in Hindustan are very liberal. In Islamic law, no woman should live without a nikah. Today all sorts of bad things are happening because of this new free culture and new divorce laws,' he says.

I want to remind the Qazi that under Islamic law, divorce or talaaq has always existed. In many ways, the Quran is a forward-thinking text, and it forecasted that divorce would be an integral part of the marriage model in the future and gives clear-cut instructions on the execution of divorce.

Since the time of Shah Bano, the judgement has been overturned, and now all Muslim women have the choice to apply to Indian courts in the case of divorce. The Qazi, though, doesn't believe in courts and the Indian law. He believes that all Muslims should come to him to resolve all matters of marriage and divorce. It is a pity that this misogynistic Qazi is in charge of so many (married) lives.

I think back to the Begum of Bhopal who had built the Qaziat that we sat in. She was known best for mixing the traditional with the modern in just the right proportions. Clearly her ideals had long been forgotten.

I finally get the information that I want when I befriend one of the Qaziat bookkeepers, Ali, who informs me that over the past five years that he has been recording numbers, divorce has tripled, and many more women are now filing for divorce than men. He is keen to talk about divorce and launches into a personal tale.

Ali's twenty-five-year-old daughter has recently been divorced. She had an arranged marriage and went to live in Hyderabad with her husband. Before her marriage, she worked as a nurse in Bhopal, but in Hyderabad, her in-laws did not want her to work. The marriage lasted for a year before she moved back to Bhopal. Ali tells me that the reason his daughter divorced was simply because she wasn't happy and that she didn't love her husband. Ali ruminates, 'In our time, all this love-shove didn't exist. We just married the woman that our parents chose for us. Now girls have all these conditions. I don't understand my daughter, so how am I supposed to find her the right boy?'

Ali doesn't look particularly vexed about his daughter's future, perhaps because he sees so many cases of divorce that he has become desensitized. His daughter has resumed working as a nurse, and Ali is confident that she will re-marry one day. As I step out of the Qaziat, I see a group of men huddled in a circle, drinking cups of tea. They are dressed in loose kurta-pajamas and lace skullcaps. Their eyes are lined with kohl, they sport henna-ed beards, and their feet are encased in dusty plastic sandals. They are enveloped by that distinct air that bullies have, and passers-by, sensing it, stay a safe distance away from them. Ali whispers furtively in my ear that these men are agents.

'Agents?' I ask.

He explains to me that these agents offer husbands to newly divorced women. In return, they get a portion of the woman's mehr. Under Shariah law, a man is allowed four wives, so it is not difficult for these agents to find husbands for these recent divorcees. Ali tells me that most of these agents have married several times, and if they find a woman attractive, or if she comes with a handsome mehr from her ex-husband, they usually marry her themselves.

As I walk past these bullies, they quietly stare at me. Ali tells me later that the agents were inquiring about me, asking if I was on the market and how much my mehr was.

◆

Ghazala is a small dark woman. She is missing two front teeth, and her waist-long braid is grey, but she has a smooth, youthful face that makes her look years younger. Her husband Aftab is fair, elegantly handsome, with laughing eyes. They are an interesting pair, as opposite as opposites can be. He loves talking, whereas she has a calm, benign intensity and can listen for hours. He is jocular, always laughing, and she is serious, smiling rarely. Together they run an NGO in Bhopal, resolving conflicts in matters of matrimony. During my time in Bhopal, Ghazala, Aftab and I travel sandwiched together on his scooter: a thin Aftab, a plump Ghazala, and a tall me at the back, holding on for my life as we zip around visiting couples with interesting divorce case histories. One afternoon, the three of us visit Anjum and Amal, a couple who have recently been married, courtesy of Ghazala and Aftab's counselling.

When we arrive at their small home on a surprise visit, the couple is staring at the TV with blank-eyed expressions, huddled in thick winter coats and hats, given the cold weather and lack of heating. Everything in the house is neatly placed. The tidiness of the small hallway is juxtaposed against strident outbursts of fluorescent plastic blooms placed all over the house. A glass cabinet displays a collection of soft toys and plastic dolls. Amal works as a stenographer at the district court; Anjum runs a ladies' boutique from home. They have been married for six months; this is Anjum's second marriage and Amal's first.

Anjum talks about her first marriage with a nervous and haunted air. Things deteriorated when she discovered her husband having an affair with her sister-in-law (whose husband was in the Indian army and often away), whom he gave money to after sex. While married to her first husband, Anjum befriended Amal who was her sister-in-law's landlord. When Amal found Anjum's husband having sex with his tenant, he immediately reported this to Anjum.

'So you fell in love?' I ask Amal, and he smiles shyly.

'Very suddenly,' he said. 'After her divorce, I thought it was my duty to marry her.'

Amal tells me that according to Islam there should be no unmarried women in society, and it is the duty of a man to marry a woman. Amal takes this seriously, and when he saw Anjum in her awful situation, his heart went out to her. His parents, though, have not approved of his marriage to an older, divorced woman and have disowned him. He is hoping that their minds will change soon when they come to understand that he is following the Prophet's teaching.

Thirty-eight year old Anjum is the mother of two children, a twenty-year-old son, and a pretty eighteen-year-old daughter, both of whom live with her first husband. Anjum gets no maintenance from her husband. Despite his flagrant infidelity, the Qazi has not pushed him to give either the mehr or iddat and a battle in court will take years.

Anjum remembers the days after her talaaq, when she had no money and no home. She spent her three-month iddat period, during which she was prohibited from re-marrying, at her relatives' homes. Her children sneaked her money, food, and clothing. She says it was the worst time in her life.

Anjum's story is not uncommon in the Muslim world. Women divorce their husbands, yet they never get their mehr or iddat. The patriarchal Qaziat will do nothing about it, and battles in civil court take years. Divorce has always been a confusing and controversial subject in the Muslim world. Should it be dictated by the Qaziat or by civil laws in court? There are technically two sets of matrimonial laws for Indian Muslims—Islamic law, and civil law dictated by the constitution of India. Tradition encourages following the rules of the Qazi, but modern times mean the Indian courts increasingly hold sway.

According to Ghazala and Aftab, divorce rates among lower and middle-class Muslims in Bhopal have tripled in the past decade. The reasons they cite for increasing divorce are the ones that I have already come across—women's financial independence, less willingness to adjust, and changing expectations of marriage. There are a few things that are unique to Muslim marriage though. Divorce is relatively simple to get under Shariah, sometimes as easy as saying 'talaaq' three times. Muslim divorces are much easier to execute than Hindu divorces (or any other religion's for that matter), which entail many trips to court, expensive lawyer fees, etc. Divorce is less of a taboo in the Muslim community because it is mentioned in the Quran. The nikah is a contract between two people and the Quran has given every marriage the option of talaaq.

Ghazala and Aftab invite me to their home to have lunch. The tiny, crowded house is bustling with activity. An old lady, Ghazala's mother, is muttering to herself, lying on the couch under a thick quilt. Ghazala and Aftab's gregarious nineteen-year-old daughter, Baby, is cooking lunch. Rajini, a stout young lady with a sad, angry face is busy rolling candles. She was hired by Ghazala to work in the candle-making business after they met at a divorce counselling session. She was married at sixteen to a man in the village, but soon got a divorce because a city girl like her could not adjust to rural life. Though she is only twenty-three, she has lost faith in marriage.

Another woman, Kiran—a hired help, is flipping rotis on the stove. She smiles sweetly at me from the kitchen. I can tell that she wants to talk to me, but she is shy. Ghazala tells me that Kiran's husband has asked for a divorce twice and has even approached the courts, but Kiran refuses to give it to him. She has a young son, and she wants the father to be around when he is growing up.

Ghazala too has a story of divorce. Ghazala's eldest son, Baba, was divorced six months ago. He was married to Fatima, Ghazala's niece, in an arranged marriage. A few days after the wedding, Fatima collapsed. After a series of hospital visits and tests, the doctors diagnosed her with an incurable gastric condition and declared that she was unfit for married life, which basically meant that she was unfit to have children. Ghazala complains that her son only had intercourse with Fatima three times since she was too unwell most of the time. On those rare occasions, she lay in bed like a vegetable for days afterwards.

Ghazala insinuates that her relatives were aware of Fatima's condition. Arranged marriages can reveal unpleasant surprises, even when you marry within your extended family, which is standard practice in the Muslim community. After a year-and-a-half of marriage, during most of which Fatima was ill, Baba, encouraged by his parents, divorced Fatima.

As Ghazala narrates Baba's divorce story, I wonder if Baba would have divorced Fatima if there had been love in their marriage. In a contractual, arranged marriage such as his, being unaware of the spouse having an incurable condition is definite legal grounds for divorce. Poor Baba, I can only imagine his plight.

Baba, a sulky-faced young man, walks in while we are eating. He says hello and then disappears inside. Ghazala lowers her voice so that he can't hear us. She tells me that he is still reeling from his divorce and can't bear to hear the word 'divorce'. She laughs, saying that this is very hard to avoid, especially in the home of two divorce counsellors.

Making sure Baba is not around, Ghazala rummages in a cupboard and brings out some dusty photo albums. She tells me with pride that Baba's Mumbai wedding was lavish and celebrated with much dhoom-dhaam. Though her son is divorced, Ghazala is still proud of the wedding. I recall that Shiny's mother too felt this way when she showed me Shiny's wedding album. Sometimes in India, the wedding can be more important than the marriage. I remember a wedding planner once telling me that couples find it easier to call off the marriage than the wedding.

After lunch, Baby and I get chatting. Baby is a confident young woman studying Fine Arts at a local college. I ask her if many girls have boyfriends at her all-women's college.

Most girls have boyfriends, she says. The ones who appear to be the most conservative, dressed in abayas and burqas, are usually the most daring. Baby tells me that these girls go on dates stealthily, abandoning their burqas after college and cruising around town with their boyfriends. I am not surprised by what Baby tells me. On a trip to hill-top, a local tourist spot (aptly named because it sits on top of an isolated hill) and in the ubiquitous coffee shops scattered across town I notice many young couples romancing. I wonder how these young women navigate these two worlds—of strict tradition and of modern love. The changes that India is going through are hardest for women; will modern young Muslim women like Baby accept the antiquated practice of triple talaaq? And if not, how will they deal with it?

On my last day in Bhopal, I find myself back to where I started, at the Qaziat, where I attend an ijtimah—a congregation of Muslim women leaders.

In the large grounds, I see an endless sea of colourful burqas. Women are sitting on the floor, and women are giving fiery speeches in Urdu on the dais. Many children run around, while their mothers chat languorously, basking in the warm winter sun. Groups of women are sitting in circles and sharing their lunches. Others are sprawled on the mats, napping.

The one thing I notice is that all females—women, girls, and babies—are veiled. I too have wrapped a shawl around my head. I am shocked most by the miniature burqas that the little girls wear, some of them mere toddlers. Walking through the crowds I almost trip over a little girl, wobbly on her feet. She is wearing a baby pink burqa that matches her frock. This is the first time in

India that I have seen girls this young wear veils. When I tell my mother, who has lived on and off in Bhopal for the past thirty years, about the veils, she too is shocked. Bhopal has never had a tradition of the veil. In fact, the Begum had abolished purdah during her reign.

On stage, an old woman is speaking ardently, occasionally breaking into screechy screams. She speaks in Urdu, and the only words I understand in her inflammatory speech are 'United States of America'. Ghazala translates for me. The speaker is talking about how the United States of America is responsible for all terrorism, which in turn is responsible for giving Islam a bad name. Next, a flinty faced woman with eagle eyes comes on stage. She, too, speaks in Urdu, though she interjects her speech with some Hindi and English. I can tell by the way she speaks English that she is fairly well educated. In her thirty-minute speech she talks of how the US is home to 'think tanks' that control the media in all parts of the worlds. These think tanks, she says, are anti-Islam and are spreading anti-Islamic notions worldwide. Most other speakers continue in a similar vein. A man speaks bombastically on how Muslim men must discipline and tame the wife. Everyone seems to be listening calmly. I am surprised that some of these women haven't gotten up and thrown him off the stage because this is what I feel like doing. Ghazala too seems shocked by the things that we hear.

At the ijtimah, an event meant to spark positive discussion amongst Muslim women, fundamentalism is in full view. Speakers harp on about Islam protecting its traditions, which many speakers believe is under threat from America. I think back to a book I read by sociologist Anthony Giddens. He writes: 'Fundamentalism is a child of globalization, which it both responds to and utilizes. Fundamentalism isn't just the antithesis of globalizing modernity, but also poses questions to it, the most basic of which is, can we live in a world where nothing is sacred?'[247]

The women who I hear speaking on the dais, the Qazi and

the Muslim Law Board are fundamentalists who are trying to protect their tradition from a rapidly globalizing world. In a fast-changing society like India, religion is one the few things that remain constant. Fundamentalism is a call for people to stick to the old ways, to cling on to something from the past rather than make sense of the confusion that prevails.

On our way out, a grumpy old woman, with droopy features and a sagging face, stops to talk to us. Safina is Ghazala's friend and is on her way to meet the Qazi to resolve a worrisome problem. A fraudulent Qazi, a real menace to society, has set up shop in old Bhopal. This spurious Qazi has been signing off on talaaqs so that men can re-marry while he pockets the mehr that they should be paying their wives. He has also been performing nikahs without witnesses and the consent of family elders.

Ghazala suggests that the police be informed. Safina complains that the police did try to intervene, and the fake Qazi was briefly arrested, but there was an outcry, even by those that he had defrauded. People felt that a holy man should not be put behind bars. The fake Qazi was released and is now back to his old ways. Safina is hoping that the real Qazi will neutralize this fraud. I am not so optimistic. I see the Qazi approaching in the distance. Before he spots me, I quickly escape.

The word 'nibhana' has no exact equivalent in English. The closest translation that I can come up with is 'fulfil with a sense of duty', and the word is almost always used in the context of relationships, particularly marriage. It is a term that I hear a lot during the days that I am studying divorce. Elders say that the reason why there is so much divorce is because there is no concept of nibhana anymore. Young Indians do not want to stay the course of the marriage because they are impatient and are unwilling to change for anyone else. 'Wo nibha nahi sakte,' (They cannot fulfil their relationships), elders say with disappointed shakes of the head. Today's tempestuous generation is not willing to forsake its happiness, even temporarily, for the greater good of the family. Marriage, they say, takes time and patience. No marriage is perfect from the beginning.

Nibhana is a befitting word because so much is encapsulated in it. Marriage is, at the end of the day, a matter of staying the course, of adapting, of living not only for yourself but also for your family. But individuality too is increasingly important, especially in young India. Marriage in India is going through a change like it has never seen before. Divorce can be argued to be a good thing. It signals the liberation of women who are willing and able to say no and step out of awful situations. It can also be argued as a damaging consequence, especially if there are children involved.

The tenfold increase in divorce rate is severely detrimental to the development of children and for the first time in this country, a large number of kids will be raised in single parent homes. On the flip side, maybe a lot more women and men will be in equal relationships. As nibhana loses its place in shifting Indian society, a new Hindi word for divorce might just usurp its place in our vernacular.

MODERN LOVE

LIVING IN

Beaming like a newly-wed bride, Garima eagerly shows me around her studio apartment in Model Town. The small apartment is decorated with black-and-white pictures of her partner Suketu and herself. Carefully tended money plants bloom in wine bottles. Suketu plays with a small kitten on the zebra-print futon, a stereo warbles out Hindi tunes in the background. Suketu is now lying on his back, and a tiny second kitten, the size of a rat and the colour of curdled milk, crawls on to his forehead. The original kitten, quite a bit bigger than the milky runt, is now on his stomach. Garima lets out a shriek of joy, runs into her bedroom and brings out a heavyweight camera and starts taking photos. Suketu poses languorously, professionally.

It seems to be nuptial heaven in this small apartment, except Garima and Suketu never want to get married. They have been living together for the past six months after having dated for a year. Garima, my newly hired research assistant, had invited me over to her apartment across town to play chess and to meet her two adopted kittens, Pugli (silly) and Pidi (tiny). I wasn't particularly interested in either activity, but I was curious to check out Garima's digs, and meet Suketu, the boyfriend whom she lived with and spoke so much about.

Suketu is dourly enigmatic and less friendly than I had imagined. He is reticent, and when he does speak, he has a strange spasmodic way of speaking—fast, in convulsive sentences, the words bumping into each other. He is very evidently conscious of his good looks—the chiselled jaw, the large prominent forehead, the sideburns trimmed sharp as knives, and shoulder-length hair which he wears in a tight, greasy ponytail held by a feminine velvet scrunchy. He perches tentatively on a sofa, holding a joint aslant, which he passes on to Garima, who then passes it along to me.

I ask Garima about her thoughts on marriage, and she grimaces, 'I don't believe in marriage. Marriage slows you down. I believe in living life in small instalments.'

Suketu adds to this, 'We believe in living life light. Marriage makes things so heavy. This is much simpler. Who wants to bear the brunt of eventual marriage, eventual in-laws, eventual children and eventual grief?'

'For the year that we were dating, we were practically living together in Suketu's hostel room. Getting an apartment together was the natural next step. We give each other a lot of space because we know that people have a high propensity of taking over each other's lives. We don't want that,' says Garima taking deep drags of the joint, the end of which is so close to her fingertips that I am afraid she will burn herself.

Garima and Suketu question the entire concept of marriage. Garima's mother threw away her career as a schoolteacher for her father and she sees her parent's joyless marriage, arranged when her mom was sixteen, as a habit more than a choice and something she will never opt for. Why should she? She needs no man to support her, so why would she ruin her life with marriage?

Soon the apartment is sheathed in a nimbus of smoke. Suketu begins talking, fuelled by the joint, 'It was difficult finding an apartment, and most realtors immediately refused when they found out we were not married. They don't want singles, because they think they are trouble, but when they found out we were a couple, but not married, they thought we were criminals or worse. They may have overlooked criminal records but wouldn't rent to us. Fortunately for us, the woman who owns this apartment got divorced here. You know how people are so stupidly superstitious, no one was renting the place and that's how we got it,' he says with a grin.

I had heard these complaints before. It was difficult for unmarried couples to rent apartments. Often realtors told potential tenants to get married and then to return.

'What about friends and family, do they know?' I asked.

'We try not to tell too many people because we know how cheap mentalities are. Eventually people find out, you know how nosy they are. Our friends thought it was a bold step, but also a good idea, especially because we save so much money,' says Suketu.

'Now our place is party central and all our friends are following suit,' adds Garima.

Garima tells me that she was the focus of neighbourhood opprobrium for a while. She heard people whispering not so discreetly about the slut who lived in the divorcee's apartment, who smoked cigarettes on the balcony. She, being a woman, bore the brunt of the abuse. Suketu was regarded as a bystander, even a victim.

'It's been six months now, and we have been accepted by the community. It's typical Indian schizophrenia. While something is hot they go crazy over it, and they'll forget about it just as quickly, especially when you send them birthday cake or Diwali sweets,' says Garima.

As for parents, they both shrug, and Suketu says, 'We have our own lives now. They live far away and can't really dictate our lives. I don't talk to my parents about my personal life. And they don't really ask.'

Today, unmarried couples living together is not the norm. Instances like Garima and Suketu's are still rare, but they are common enough for laws to be changed. In early 2010, a landmark verdict by the Supreme Court legalized live-in relationships in India. The apex court stated that if two sound-minded adults of the opposite sex wanted to live together without getting married, it was not a crime. This verdict was reached in response to twenty-two charges of criminal offence filed in 2005 against South Indian actress Khushboo after her statement to magazines supporting live-in relationships and premarital sex in India. The argument of the counsel was that her endorsing premarital sex would adversely affect the minds of young people, which would lead to the decay of the country's moral values. The response of the three-judge bench was that two people living together was not an offensive act. They justified their stance saying that according to Hindu mythology, even Lord Krishna and Radha lived together.

The Supreme Court went on to state that a live-in relationship qualified as a 'relationship in the nature of marriage', if four requirements are met. First, the couple must hold themselves out to society as being akin to spouses. Second, they must be of legal age to marry. Third, they must be qualified to enter into a legal marriage, and fourth they must have voluntarily cohabited for a significant period of time. Such a relationship would come under the jurisdiction of the Protection of Women from Domestic Violence Act, and the Hindu Marriage Act of 1976 would allow for children from such a relationship to be legitimate, establishing succession and property rights.

Most Indian parents believe that live-in relationships are anathema. Even after two people get engaged, meetings between them are monitored because the widely held belief is that intimacy creates contempt. You risk learning about the deficiencies of your partner, and you may opt out, whereas after marriage you won't have any choice but to adjust. Perhaps the most significant issue is that of the woman's chastity. Most Indian parents feel a perverse sense of duty towards their daughter's chastity and fear greatly that it may be lost. Live-in relationships bring their worst fear to life.

Today in urban India, many young Indians are questioning the views of their parents. They watch television shows like *Friends*, and they wonder how they can spend the rest of their lives with someone without a thorough understanding of their habits, their peccadillos, and their peculiarities, which only comes with intimate knowledge of one another. Kareena Kapoor, a Bollywood star, and an icon to millions of young people recently spoke out in public in support of live-in relationships. She said, 'we shouldn't try to be traditional when we are living in a modern world... We only claim to understand the modern values in our society, but unfortunately, in our minds, we are still stuck in a time frame of years ago.'[248]

The age-old formula of marry first and then love will follow is being questioned as people become keenly interested in romance, love, self-discovery and exploration. People are becoming increasingly experimental, and marriage is competing with new relationship paradigms—dating, live-in relationships, and even more brazen options such as open marriages. And if somewhere love follows, elsewhere it fades. Ninety-four percent of Indian couples say they're 'happy' in their relationships, but the majority of the same sample group say they would not marry the same person or marry at all if given a choice again.[249] 'Unless we're ready to discard our new notion of marriage as a personal domain rather than a cultural or familial one, we'd better get used to its vulnerabilities, which are entwined with these higher standards of love and empathy.'[250]

New relationship paradigms are emerging because of a change in middle-class morality and decreasing stigma. A greater number of working women are able to withstand social pressures due to their relative economic independence. As more and more young people move away from home to study and work there are greater opportunities for experimenting with relationships other than marriage. There is also a slow change in the idea of marriage providing a 'happily-ever-after'. Another significant aspect that has affected relationships is the loosening of the belief that the most significant form of sexual relationship is the one that relates to reproduction.[251]

I met Garima while conducting interviews for a research assistant to help me with my book. Garima, twenty-six at the time, was finishing up her PhD, and was a lecturer.

Though Garima was not the most qualified of the candidates I had interviewed, I felt like she was the most intelligent and understood the kinds of things that the job demanded—identifying interviewees, recording, and then transcribing the hundreds of interviews I would be conducting around the country. We got along well, and I could imagine spending an extended amount of time with her. Also, since she was the same age as me, I thought that she would provide an interesting perspective.

Although Garima isn't beautiful in the classical way, she is attractive, with her small, curvaceous body, her gamine haircut, her baccate nose and pixie-like face. She is a bright girl, and I can see how she may have had her way with men. When I had interviewed her, she had laughed and told me that she was a connoisseur of sex. I was sold, and I hired her on the spot.

Over the months that Garima worked for me, I got to know her well, and many things about her lifestyle stunned me. She slept only three to four hours a night, she drank and got stoned regularly (I guessed ten times a week) and she missed thirty working days (of a part-time job) on account of either funerals or weddings.

One day, two hours after her reporting time, Garima sauntered into my office. Her hair was in disarray, her face was coated with a layer of oil and dullness, and her breath stank of garlic. She was fretting because she hadn't got her period yet and she was afraid she was pregnant. She was furious with Suketu for letting this happen. She told me that Suketu was a worthless guy, she was the one paying all of his bills, that all he did was lie on their couch and feed the kittens. If she was pregnant, who would pay for the abortion?

She had asked Suketu to contribute to the household expenses, so he had finally taken up a job at a Cafe Coffee Day. He felt that this was below his dignity and that he was much too intellectual for this kind of work. She said that he preferred taking worthless courses billed to his parents and surviving at her expense. Now, to make it all worse, he had made her pregnant, because he disliked wearing a condom, because that too hurt his male pride. Garima was obviously in no mood to work.

Suketu had just finished a master's in psychology at Delhi University and was now doing a graphic designing course. He was unsure about what he wanted to do in terms of a career, but he wanted to build up his resume by taking short courses, standard approach used by students taking advantage of the booming and inexpensive private education industry in India.

I found it ironic that Suketu's parents paid for his classes, but he didn't feel the need to tell them about his living arrangements. Not that he was very different in his attitude from many of his peers—many kids feel it is their parents' duty to look after them as long as they are alive, and their parents seem to go along with it. As long as this equation continued, nothing would change.

Technically, Garima had had sex when she was twelve years old, with another girl, who stuck a finger inside her. Mamta was her best friend and they did everything together; they studied together, played cricket together and even bathed together. One day Mamta suggested that they play a new role-play game, not their usual favourites, doctor-doctor, or teacher-teacher, but mummy-papa. According to Mamta's rules, based on keenly observing her parents, both of them had to take off their frocks, slips, and panties and lie naked together underneath the sheets. Mamta had kissed her on her mouth, touched her everywhere, stuck her pinkie finger inside her 'pee-pee', and Garima hadn't stopped her. It had felt strange, and she had felt nervous, like she felt before her exams, and somehow she hadn't minded the pain.

Even though Garima's first sexual experience happened early in life (though she didn't realize it till much later), her first sex education came at the age of fifteen. She had been waiting in an auto rickshaw outside the bank while her mother ran in to deposit some cheques. There must have been a long queue because Garima was waiting for quite a while. The auto driver turned around and asked her if she knew how she was born. The auto driver was young, sixteen or seventeen, she remembers, and painfully thin, with a tiny head. He didn't look particularly dangerous, so Garima didn't think twice about chatting with him.

'Yes,' she had said, 'I was born from my mother's stomach.'

'But how?' he had persisted. 'Do you know how?'

'Yes, my mamma became pregnant, and then I was born.'

'But how did she become pregnant?'

'Like all mothers do,' she had replied coolly.

At fifteen, she didn't know much about sex, her parents never talked about, she never spoke about it with friends, nothing was shown on TV, and the age of the internet hadn't yet arrived. The auto driver had put his hand on the bulge in his pants. 'This goes inside your pee-pee. Touch it,' he had said, and she had. This is when her mom hopped back in to the auto, and they had quickly buzzed away.

What Garima experienced is not uncommon. Studies show that over 50 per cent of children in India are sexually abused, a rate that is higher than in any other country.[252] In a repressive sexual culture with sex education almost non-existent, sexual abuse in India is becoming a serious enough problem that the government passed the Protection of Children from Sexual Offences Act in 2012.

Another evening, while playing chess at Garima and Suketu's, I find myself caught in the midst of a heated discussion, the subject of which makes me feel impossibly old and behind the curve in terms of sexual knowledge. The discussion is based around how all of us are inherently bisexual, but that society's contracts have screwed us up. I knew Garima had had several lesbian experiences, the most recent one with her first cousin. I hadn't inquired about Suketu's sexual tendencies, but based on the conversation,

I gathered that he'd had at least a few homosexual experiences, as had many of their friends. I could not contribute in any productive fashion to this conversation since I had never had any of these experiences that they said were so common. I felt immobilized in amber and wondered if my attitude was retrograde. Suketu, Garima and I are all the same age, but it seems that the disconnect between us in terms of sexual experience is vast. I wonder how I'd got left behind, especially since I was the one who was the most widely travelled and exposed to the world.

As I am mulling over this, a couple enter the apartment—a frail, pleasant girl, who drops off some groceries on the kitchen counter and smiles politely at me; she is with an equally pleasant boy. They go into Garima's bedroom, shutting the door. A few minutes later the door opens to let Pugli in, and then a few minutes later, a bare arm sticks out to let in Pidi. A few minutes later, I hear what are the unmistakable sounds of tender intimacy, which make me increasingly uncomfortable. Suketu and Garima, though, do not flinch, and continue to discuss bisexuality. Sounds of violent lovemaking ricochet off my eardrums. The sounds are so overwhelming that I can't help but visualize what is happening inside the bedroom. They don't even seem to be trying to do it quietly, but except for me, no one here is self-conscious, not the frail couple nor their hosts. Suketu looks at me and smiles, 'If you think this is loud, you should hear the couple next door. They break the bed.'

I hear frantic shrieks, clearly the end is near, and then gasps, and then shortly afterwards, the cats are let out. Twenty minutes later, the frail couple emerge, they uncork beers and are unreserved about their satiation and delight, kissing each other tenderly in the kitchen. I can't look them in the face after what I have heard, so I decide to leave.

The sticky evening has melted into a deliciously cool, cloudless night. Everywhere there are people, crowds and crowds of people, miniature cars crammed with people, rickshaws, a family of four, sometimes even five or six on a motorbike meant for two, two children squeezed in between an overweight mother, and a father sitting on the tip of the nose-shaped seat. One tiny bump and he would so easily slide off.

In this overcrowded country, places for physical intimacy are limited; parks are crucial sites, and so are cars, if you are lucky enough to own one. Few young people live on their own. Economist Abhijit Banerjee in a recent article alludes to the inequality of access to sex that he feels is leading to greater sexual violence. He writes, 'If you are poor in urban India or even middle class and 25, you have be very lucky to have a room of your own in the family home, let alone a separate apartment that you can call your own. I remember walking home from our mutual adda one evening some 30 years ago in Kolkata with an acquaintance who lived somewhere in the neighbourhood, feeling slightly puzzled when he stopped on the way to have one more cup of tea before he went home. It was late, past dinnertime so I asked naively, "Tea this late?" He hesitated for a moment and then explained—he goes home after everyone else has eaten because there is no place to sit or sleep till they have all had dinner and gone to bed and the dining area is vacated. He was substantially older than me, perhaps 25 and had some kind of job, but clearly there was no way he could afford to get married—where would they sit together, where would they sleep?'[253]

It was understandable then that Garima and Suketu's friends would come over to have sex, there were just three people listening. In the hostel where they lived, there are probably one hundred. After spending all those years in America, I believe in space, lots of it. I need my space, from my boyfriend, from my parents, sometimes even from myself, but the concept of personal space simply does not exist here. Most people have never had their own room growing up, they have never had their own hostel rooms, they have never lived alone, and they probably never will. So they learn to share everything, particularly, especially—space. Even the most intimate of activities, like having sex is done in shared spaces, with everyone around shutting their eyes and ignoring it, pretending nothing is happening. It is normal to have sex like this, they saw their parents doing it when they were growing up, muffling their moans with their pillows, and now they were doing it themselves.

After six months of Garima's employment, which consisted of hanging out in my small home office after arriving straight from long, hedonistic nights (the telltale signs showing), napping on my couch curled up in a little ball, and taking showers in my bathroom, I took the difficult decision of firing her. The ex-corporate in me demanded some modicum of propriety. Unfortunately, she was quite unhappy, but I had little choice. Most, if not all, of our attempts at 'work' had been futile. She had been hired to help me research my book, and had quite gratefully become a subject when I had asked her to, but she failed to strike a balance between subject and researcher.

A few months later, I received a surprise phone call from Suketu asking me if I wanted to go for a motorcycle ride. He was persistent, and I was curious about why he wanted to meet me. The first thing Suketu told me when we met was that he had broken up with Garima. He had moved into a hostel, and she into a smaller, cheaper apartment. She was still teaching and had almost completed her PhD.

That windy, silver-mooned night, Suketu opened up to me. He told me of his love for Garima, and how he had imagined living the rest of his life with her, wandering, learning, exploring. When they broke up, he felt he had to radically change his lifestyle to cope with the grief. He quit his job at the coffee shop, applied for a PhD, and visited his parents in his Kolkata. Shockingly, he admitted that he was even thinking of an arranged marriage.

'She cheated on me, and I didn't like that, that too with that ex of hers. I want to be with someone, but don't trust my choice, so maybe an arranged marriage is better,' he said with a resigned sigh.

'That ex in Bangalore?' I asked. Garima had spoken profusely of her divorced ex-boyfriend.

'Ya, that dweeb. She went to Bangalore for some work and stayed with him. I didn't like that, but it was okay because she didn't have a place to stay. When she came back, she wouldn't have sex with me for, like, two weeks, and I knew something was wrong. I read her journal, and well, you know. It was the beginning of the end,' said Suketu.

Garima was an avid journal-keeper. I remembered this from the time she was working for me. When she was supposed to be researching, I often caught her scribbling away in her candy-coloured notebook.

After an ice cream at India Gate, Suketu dropped me home. I gave him a hug and asked him to stay in touch. I wasn't sure why Suketu had called me. Maybe he thought that Garima still worked for me and I could give him some information about her. He had seemed disappointed when I told him that she no longer did. I was sad about Garima and Suketu's break-up. They were happy together, at least most of the time. I also knew that they loved each other. Perhaps in the world of arranged marriages, they would have been long married, but that isn't what they wanted. They wanted to be weightless, to travel through life without the excess baggage of permanent relationships.

I found both Garima and Suketu to be in lock-step with their counterparts in cities like Los Angeles or London where there is a well-established culture of dating and alternative relationships. There, people travel on a road well-travelled by previous generations. In India, most of the previous generations have had arranged marriages and a large part of society, like the narrow-minded realtors, or Garima and Suketu's parents, are not accepting of new sorts of romantic arrangements. This makes it more difficult for a young couple to stay together. The necessary support to nurture a relationship is missing, especially a relationship as difficult as marriage. That is why Suketu was now considering an arranged marriage. He had told me that he couldn't handle the pain of another heartbreak. He had gotten used to living with a woman, he enjoyed it, so maybe marriage, even an arranged marriage, wasn't so bad after all.

From a live-in relationship to an arranged marriage was an extreme reaction. Suketu with his wild hair, listening to jazz music, strumming his guitar, smoking a joint, was this just a modern facade? Did he truly feel like having an arranged marriage? Who really knew. All one could really say was that India was changing at a break-neck pace, and it was quite a ride for someone like Suketu. It was a constant yo-yo between the past and the present, between East and West, between the glittery new ideals on TV and the dusty, outdated ones of earlier generations. I guess it was to be expected that he would be a little, if not, highly, confused.

That night as I lay in bed listening to the rain pounding on my window, I couldn't get Suketu and Garima out of my mind. On a whim, I decided to call Garima, though we hadn't spoken since I'd fired her. She told me that she'd moved to Bangalore temporarily to live with her new boyfriend. She was taking a sabbatical from her PhD and had quit her teaching job. Her new boyfriend made a lot of money, and she didn't have much to worry about. She said she really liked it there, and that she was working on a book, also on love, sex, and marriage. She claimed to have found a publisher. I figured she was doing this because she was angry with me for letting her go.

'What about your career?' I asked. 'Don't you want that?'

Garima had seemed so focused on her career, putting it above everything else in life. It seemed very unlike the Garima that I had known to throw it all away for a man. She had seemed determined that these were the mistakes that her mother had made, and that she must not, in any circumstance, make.

'Well... You know,' she replied. 'The old life is waiting for me. I can go back to all of that whenever I want. This new life though, this is something new and exciting, a new city, a new man, a new project. It's inspiring. Plus, it's not like I'm marrying him. He isn't even properly divorced yet.'

I wondered if Garima and Suketu's liberation came from a true desire for freedom or was it that they were just rebelling against the strict society they were brought up in. After so many years of repression, had they gone off on an extreme tangent?

OPEN MARRIAGE

When Suganda met Shammi she was a virgin. Not only was she a virgin, she had never kissed a man, or even held a male hand, save her younger brother's, which her parents began reprimanding her for when he turned fifteen.

Suganda's parents had found Shammi's profile in the matrimonial section of *The Times of India*, and a week after the Sunday ad came out, Suganda was sitting face-to-face with a shy, fresh-faced man of twenty-one. She had turned eighteen just a week ago, and her parents were anxious to get her married. Suganda knew that the things that mattered to her in a man didn't matter to her parents. When she had presented her father with her criteria he had laughed at her, and had told her gently that she had a lot to learn in life. What mattered to her most was that the man be handsome and tall (she stood at 5'6" herself, well above the average height for an Indian woman). It was also important that he rode a motorcycle, and that he enjoyed Bollywood movies with the same fervour that she did (she hadn't missed a first day first show of any Salman Khan film for the past five years). To her parents, what mattered most was their reputation in the Jat community that they were part of, and their wealth, which they assessed based on the acreage of their land holdings and the size of their house. Suganda was the older, prettier of two sisters, fair as fresh milk, and her parents had high hopes for her. Shammi, their latest find, seemed to fit the bill. His family had significant land holdings in Haryana, even though they did not have an active family business. Shammi was a recent graduate of the Haryana University and held a BA in Finance. He was hoping to set up a shop selling imported perfumes, CDs, and electronics in Delhi. Shammi was the first and last boy that Suganda had 'seen' for marriage. She only saw him once before their wedding day, in the living room of Shammi's parents' home in Rohtak, Haryana. Much to her delight, he was quite handsome, even though he was of wheatish complexion. He had a head of glossy hair settled with heavily scented pomade, nicely shaped eyebrows, a well-shaped nose (this came as a relief to her because Jats were infamous for their hook-noses), and though he wasn't particularly tall, he more than made up for it by the width of his chest. She couldn't get as good a look as she would have liked to because she couldn't stare at him openly in front of his parents. She was expected to be the demure, shy bride, with her eyes cast down—this only helped her get a detailed view of Shammi's footwear. The only time she got to see Shammi's face was when she was sent to sit with him in the corner of the same living room, so that they could 'get to know each other'. This lasted all of ten minutes after which they were summoned back.

Suganda was not the first girl that Shammi had seen for marriage. He had been looking at girls for the past six months now. His family had seen about a dozen girls and had shortlisted six for his approval. He had rejected all six. Only four of them were appropriately fair-skinned for him (and he could tell the difference between make-up fair, powder-fair and real fair) and not all of them were well endowed enough for his liking. There was one woman who had been well endowed, but she had been well endowed all over and he didn't like fat women. He took his own body seriously, doing his chest and bicep exercises daily. His keen sense of observation informed him that all Indian ladies gained weight after marriage, and if this was her situation at her most nubile time, he only dreaded what would come later. Suganda, though, was adequately fair, slim, and he gleefully observed that she had a generous bosom.

They were married two months later, and Shammi used the dowry money that he got from Suganda's parents to put down a deposit on an apartment in North Delhi, and much to Suganda's delight, he bought a Hero Honda motorcycle.

Eleven years from the day of their marriage, much has changed in the lives of Shammi and Suganda. Shammi never got around to opening his store, though Suganda tells me that he tried many things, imp-ex (import-export), real estate, furniture and upholstery, but nothing ever really worked out. As the years went by, Shammi realized he was passionate about music and had taken various DJ-ing courses. He loved English music, especially pop, and he was now the in-house DJ at a newly opened Gurgaon nightclub.

Though Shammi's career didn't turn out the way he had planned, something financially fortuitous did happen to him. The price of the agricultural land that his family owned in Gurgaon increased exponentially every year, as thousands of acres of agricultural land was sold to real estate developers in the hopes of solving the housing crunch that Delhi faced.

Shammi's family was one of the hundreds of farmer families who benefited from the escalation of prices of agricultural land; they sold their land which was added to a land bank and promptly converted into a gargantuan 500-apartment building township, of which his family were promised five three-bedroom apartments upon completion. Of these five apartments, three were given to Shammi. Today, the substantial rental income that Shammi and Suganda receive from these apartments sustains their lifestyle, paying for all their expenses, allowing them to save enough to feel responsible.

In these eleven years, the world around them had changed. Gurgaon, a sleepy village where once turbaned farmers tilled the land, where water buffaloes wallowed in the shallows of the Damdama Lake, where cows and goats roamed free in the sepia-toned landscape, has expanded into a metropolis of colossal highways, fluorescent SEZs, and gated apartment buildings. The Haryana that they grew up in seems so lost that at times they feel like it may never even have existed. Suganda drives a golden Honda car. She had never imagined that she would be in the driver's seat, and that too in her own vehicle. The knick-knacks that Shammi strove to smuggle into India, and so much more are available in the hulking malls neighbouring their apartment complex. Their children go to school in a neat, yellow school bus; Shammi and Suganda both remember the bullock cart that took them to school. Life today has a glitter that it never had before.

Fortunes, finances, and land deals aside, perhaps the most critical change that has taken place in the lives of Shammi and Suganda, besides the birth of their now six-year-old twin boys, Ram and Shyam, is the change in their selves. Suganda can't imagine what she had been back then, an inexperienced young girl who made painful love to a man she had only known for a few hours. Shammi can't believe that he was once a foppish young man who oiled his chest and whose life-long dream was to start a shop selling women's perfumes.

At first glance, Suganda and Shammi seem like an ordinary young couple, somewhat gilded by the prodigious change of urbanization, but they have a secret that lifts them out of the ordinary—almost a decade after their arranged marriage, they have agreed to live in an open marriage.

In India, where marriage is sacrosanct, an open marriage is an outrageous arrangement, but I have observed from the prolific online advertisements, chat groups and hearsay, that it is happening more and more across all strata of society.

Shammi and Suganda had no option but to get married. For both of them it was a mandatory step into adulthood, and they only began exploring their sexuality *after* their marriage. Shammi and Suganda married at a young age, burdened by the social definition of marriage, and of what they were expected to be, but the world around them had changed so much that they found it difficult to be living with the antique conventions of their youth. Like Shammi and Suganda, there are millions of people out there who were married young to partners of their parents' choice, and as they came of age so did the world around them though marriage remained important for the sake for their families.

In India, marriage has important legal and social dimensions, and the married couple continues to be the legally recognized unit for aspects such as property ownership, succession etc. There is also a strong social stigma against children not born into marriage. Though there has been a loosening of norms around relationships other than marriage, there is at the same time a continuing emphasis on marriage.

I meet Suganda at her apartment. She is in the midst of launching her own fashion label and I am overwhelmed by the chaos. The twins are clinging furiously to each other, screaming at the tops of their lungs, and the teenage maid who couldn't have been a day over thirteen is on the verge of tears. Suganda is the picture of rage as she yells at the tailor who has ruined an outfit. Most aggravating, though, is her Blackberry that goes off on regular intervals, playing the popular Black Eyed Peas song 'I Gotta Feeling'. And then, just as quickly as it had started, the storm passes (though it returns at regular intervals). The kids are absorbed in the jetsam of my handbag, the tailor has walked out of the apartment, abandoning the blouses, and the battery of the Blackberry has finally (and thankfully) run out of juice. Suganda is now ready to talk.

When Suganda was married, she was fresh out of college with a degree in Mass Communications from Panipat University. She never actually went to college though, she simply showed up for her exams and paid off the admissions officer. She had a flair for design and had been much too busy helping her cousins prepare their wedding trousseaux. On the year-round carousel of weddings, she had no time to attend classes. Today, Suganda has turned her passion for clothes into a busy business. She designs and tailors salwaar-kameez and saris for a clothing store located in one of the neighbouring malls dedicated to weddings. She has now decided to launch her own 'designer label' and has named it 'Suggi' after her name Suganda. She has converted one of the three bedrooms in her apartment into a manufacturing unit, where two tailors sit at sewing machines, stitching the florid fabric into designs that I observe she pulls off the internet and from fashion magazines.

Suganda speaks to me candidly about her open marriage. Both she and her husband have affairs but remain committed to each other. They are both open-minded individuals in creative fields and an open relationship allows them to explore connections with other people that they never had a chance to experience when young.

It all started three years ago when Suganda found incriminating text messages on Shammi's phone. At the same time she had found herself insanely attracted to one of their tenants, a 6'2" young American whose hair was as golden as the mustard that grew on her parents' farm, and whose eyes were as blue as the cloudless summer sky. When she found the SMSs on her husband's phone, she didn't feel anger or sadness as she thought she would. Instead she felt interminable relief that she was not the only one who was having wayward thoughts.

She wasn't sure how Shammi would respond to her adultery; after all, he was an Indian man. But she also knew that he was more open-minded than their fathers. Perhaps Shammi would be able to accept it, especially if she accepted his misdemeanours.

'One day I confronted him about the messages and he told me that he liked a girl in his nightclub, but only sexually. I told him that I had romantic feelings towards John. I was scared at first, you never know with men. But he just simply shook his head and told me that he understood. I am not sure exactly when we came to our open understanding. It's not like we ever sat down and talked about it. He saw me hanging out with John, I saw him with the women from the club. And basically we just sort of got with it,' says Suganda.

I meet Shammi at the nightclub. It is 6 p.m. in the evening, and he too has just arrived. The air has a sickly-sweet odour of stale alcohol, and the floors are so sticky that each step of mine sounds like a thunderous rip. I immediately like Shammi. He is a soft-spoken man with kind, smiling eyes. He has a hard body that speaks of many hours spent at the gym. He is wearing a faded black tank top with a pair of fatigues and sports an untrimmed beard. A large eagle tattoo is embossed on a sinewy bicep. He speaks mostly in English and Punjabi and chain smokes a pack of Indonesian clove cigarettes Gudang Garams.

'Suganda and I were young when we got hitched, yaar,' he began. 'We did it for our parents, not for ourselves. We really love each other, but life is all about experiences, and we don't want to deny that to each other. Life is short, and we both want to live it.'

'Would you ever consider ending the marriage?' I ask.

'No chance!' he retorts. 'I love Suggi. She is my best friend. We have grown up together, and I can't imagine being married to anyone else. Also, I would never break up my family, I love them all too much for that. My affairs are different—they are for masti, for mazaa, not for love.'

I ask him if their friends know about their arrangement. He shrugs, the smile disappearing from his face.

'Some do. Many found out, you know how gossip travels. Most people are shocked. I don't care though, our relationship is honest and happy. That is a lot more than most of our friends can say about their marriages. Most people just live through their unhappy marriages lying to each other. The husbands cheat on their wives with cheap women. The wives have no freedom and have affairs with the servants and drivers,' he says grimacing in disgust.

'The truth is that ours is a case of modern love,' he says

smiling his infectious smile.

What Shammi tells me is not far from the truth. A survey conducted in 2011 amongst people living in urban India shed some light on extramarital relationships. A whopping 23 per cent men confessed to having an affair as against 8 per cent women. Of these a surprising 37 per cent female respondents said that their spouse knew about their affairs.[254] These figures were bolstered by a similar survey by *Outlook* magazine in which 25.4 per cent people confessed that they have had sex with someone outside of their marriage. (Of these 48.4 per cent of respondents have slept with their friends/batchmates, 14.3 per cent with their colleagues, 11.7 per cent with their neighbours, 9.1 per cent with their spouse's friends and 5.5 per cent with relatives.)[255]

I recall my conversation with psychotherapist Dr Vijay Nagaswami, who told me that extramarital affairs were more rampant today than ever before. Extramarital affairs are not a new phenomenon in this country. There are several references, even in the *Mahabharata*—in the story of Svetaketu, the son of the great sage Uddalaka, whose mother is taken away by a guest for sexual intercourse. We also find Krishna willing to give his wife and sons to his friends and Karna declaring that he will give his wives and children to the man who can show him where Arjuna can be found. In the *Niruttara Tantra* as also in other Tantras, it is said that a worshipper will not gain virtues or merit unless he sexually unites with a married woman.[256]

As society got more rigid, strict monogamy became the norm, especially for women. Today, it appears extramarital affairs happen not with religious sanction, but with moral sanction, sometimes even with the permission of the spouse. In Shammi and Suganda's relationship there seemed to be a sort of equality, there weren't glaring double standards that one usually saw in Indian marriages.

To me it seemed that Shammi and Suganda had skipped the normal trajectory of Western-style romance that involves dating, premarital sex and break-ups. They have followed the traditional track of arranged marriage and suddenly veered off-road to enter into a brazen, undefined open marriage. Neither of them seemed to be resentful, but were rather like overgrown teenagers enjoying the youth that they never had the chance to live, their adulthood a zone of adolescent desperation.

For Shammi, finding girls was never difficult, especially of late. Monstrous call-centres have been mushrooming around Gurgaon, and there has been an influx of young girls from around the country who have moved here, free for the first time from the prying eyes of parents and college matrons. These girls frequent the nightclub on the weekends (it doubles up as a hookah bar during the week). Most of these young girls find DJ Shammi irresistible, and he is spoilt for choice.

It is not so easy for Suganda. She recognizes the pitfalls of being older. She has lost her figure after the birth of the twins, and her breasts too have lost their firmness, no matter how many chest exercises she does. She realizes that she will never find 'true love' with the men she meets through online dating sites and chat rooms.

John, the American with the eyes of a celestial blue, was the second man that Suganda had ever had sex with. The count has gone up since then, but she refused to reveal how many. Her experience with John was so revelatory that it bordered on the mystical. It's not like she didn't like sex with Shammi, it's just that it had become so old, such a routine, and it was profoundly non-erotic. John, on the other hand, was foreign, mysterious and strange in the sexiest of ways. John performed hours of cunnilingus on her, a first-of-a-kind experience, something her husband had always thought of as vile and obscene. She found her first experience of cunnilingus to be extremely pleasurable, and she felt stimulated like never before. Suganda tells me that sex is different with every person, not better or worse, just different. What she loves most, even more than the sex, is what comes with the affair: the discovery, the suspense of the chase, and the thrill of the illicit romance.

Shammi and her husband haven't had sex for a while, almost two years now.

'Isn't that a crucial part of a marriage?' I ask.

'Our relationship isn't about that anymore. It's about family,' she says thoughtfully.

She adds, a little defensively now, 'You'll know once you get married what it feels like to be with the same person, night in and night out. We share a bed, a bathroom, we are not conscious when I am having my monthlies or when he has gas. Sex is just an act between us, it doesn't mean much anymore. With other people it is definitely more exciting.'

I am curious about the dynamics of an open marriage. There doesn't seem to be any tension between husband and wife, not in the weeks that I have known them. Instead there seems to be a mutual tolerance, and a comfortable companionship. But I could also see that nuances were lost. They didn't joke around, not the way Garima and Suketu had. The inflections were missing, the small things that built up into big things, the kiss on the cheek, the holding of hands, the arm around the shoulder, all seemed to be gone.

One day, as I am playing with the twins, a shrieking Suganda runs into the room, telling me that Shammi has been in an accident, and we must go to the hospital immediately. I freeze with fear. I have grown to like the hulking Shammi, so gentle with the twins, sweet to his wife, and who has welcomed me into his life without any suspicions.

Suganda, her two tailors and I pile into her car, and zip to Medanta Hospital. There are people everywhere. In India, guest policies are never followed, and when any member of the family is admitted, protocol prescribes that the entire family camp out till the patient is discharged. A few strange looking hipsters lurk outside Shammi's room. I guess that they are from the club. Apparently, Shammi was driving to the club, when a stray dog came in the way. He swerved his bike to avoid the dog, lost his balance, and fell into a ditch. Suganda is weeping uncontrollably. 'A dog! A bloody dog!' whimpers Suganda through her tears. 'You know how Shammi loves dogs. That bloody dog! That fucking mongrel. He got away. He is probably enjoying life right now, and poor Shammi...' Her face suffuses with grief.

At that moment the doctor appears, and since a hyperventilating Suganda is in no state to talk, I step forward. The doctor declares that Shammi is alive and well. He has broken three ribs and his right leg is in a cast. He has also suffered a head injury, but it is nothing to worry about. The doctor's prognosis is that Shammi is fine save the broken bones, and will be discharged within a few days.

A few hours later, two sets of worried-looking parents come in from Haryana: Shammi's from Rohtak and Suganda's from Panipat. Suganda immediately covers her head with her chunni and touches her in-laws' feet in the traditional way. She speaks in hushed, quiet tones, so different from her usual manner of speaking and fawns over her in-laws, pressing her mother-in-law's forehead and her father-in-law's feet. The modern Suganda of the open marriage and of internet adultery is suddenly transformed into the shy bahu, who refers to Shammi respectfully in the third person as 'jee,' or 'woh'. I find Suganda's behaviour odd, to say the least. It is as if she has a dual personality, one side of which rebels against societal norms and pressures by indulging in illicit love affairs, while the other side plays the obsequious, traditional bahu that she has been brought up to be.

A few days later I visit a recuperating Shammi at home. He is sitting on the sofa in the living room, his broken leg propped up on a pile of pillows. He is surrounded on all sides by piles of colourful saris and is flipping through a copy of *Femina*. Suganda is fussing about him, wearing an infelicitous combination of a lacy red nightie and rubber slippers. Ram and Shyam are installed in each crook of their father's arms slurping on Maggi noodles and watching cartoons.

Shammi and I fall into easy conversation. He talks a lot about the past. His life has been confusing and disordered, and I gather that he is trying to recover some semblance of normalcy.

He tells me in a ruminative vein, 'You know, during my recent near-death experience, I realized something. Actually, I realized many things.'

He reaches out to Suganda and squeezes her hand. He hugs one of the twins tightly to his chest. He is rethinking his DJ career. Maybe he could get into real estate or the stock market or maybe even help Suganda with her flourishing business.

'After the accident, when I came so close to dying, so close to losing them, I realized how few things matter in life, and that my family is really all that I have.'

THE SWING

What aroused Vishal most were sexual acts he craved but were not available to him in real life with his wife, such as fellatio, which his wife did not enjoy giving and anal sex, which she found dirty and painful. Vishal didn't feel right paying for sex, he wanted to be with 'normal, everyday' people: the kind girl in the next cubicle, his neighbour's buxom wife, and especially his elder brother's sweet-scented, fresh-faced wife. Vishal admitted that he had once picked up a pillow-lipped, saggy-breasted prostitute wearing a sparkly red salwaar-kameez, her talon-like nails varnished black at GB Road but quickly deposited her back with a ₹100 tip when he imagined all the potential diseases she could be carrying.

Vishal thought back with nostalgia to the six months he had spent in Texas—sent by his IT company for a project—where he spent the icy nights carousing in the streets, exploring adventurous orgies advertised online, and titillating swing clubs, where he was pleased that women found him dashing and exotic.

As he lay next to his sleeping wife, whom he loved dearly, and desperately wanted to have intercourse with, his member swelling underneath the drawstrings of his pajamas, he had a brilliant revelation. Why couldn't he himself start a swingers' club? He had extensive experience, and he remained an active participant in online sex chat groups. Seeing the strong online interest, and given his foreign connections, which he steadfastly maintained, he could easily put a group together.

He looked at his wife, sleeping as peacefully as a child next to him, and stroked her silky hair. Neelam, though she didn't like to have sex often, liked to watch pornography. They had been married six years ago in an arranged-cum-love marriage. His parents had seen her advertisement in a newspaper, and as soon as he had glimpsed the slender woman with the gentle eyes, he knew that he would marry her.

On my quest to understand modern love, I had explored a live-in relationship which rejected marriage and an open marriage where each partner explored their sexuality individually while maintaining their marriage. The third and most radical idea to me was that of swingers' clubs where couples explored their sexual selves not just with each other but with other people as well. I had come across swingers' clubs in the upper echelons of society, but it was not unexpected that a Western-educated and influenced elite would be involved in these sorts of lascivious activities. What was surprising was how these ideas had spread to other levels of society. The internet revealed that all of India's metro cities had multiple swingers' clubs.

I find Vishal Chaudhry on the internet. He is a short, worried-looking, rotund engineer, who works in the back-office of an American IT firm in Delhi. He and I are interviewing a fresh batch of candidates for his swingers' club one steamy, humid morning, and trying to keep our cool by sipping on iced coffee. Vishal has a laptop displaying an Excel sheet on which he intends to rank couples under heads such as 'confidence', 'looks', and 'the X-factor'. He has already sent in questionnaires to interested couples, which he has studied carefully. This process is tried and tested, and over the two years that Vishal has run this club, he claims to have interviewed over a hundred couples. Vishal keeps in touch with an American friend of his from his days in Texas—Cherry, who runs a swingers' club there. She gives him tips and advice on how to break into the Indian market though she has never been to India. Vishal has agreed to let me witness this meeting only on one condition—that I tell people that I too am a participant in his nocturnal rendezvous. Basically, I am being used as a prop to attract people to Vishal's club, which he has named 'The Swing', after his Texan favourite. I have negotiated with Vishal and told him that I will agree to his conditions only if he agrees to mine—I want to attend the next swingers' party as an observer. One of Vishal's most stringent rules is that only couples are allowed to be a part of the club. Singles are strictly not allowed, except for him. He allows couples to participate only after screening them, to make sure that both members want to participate of their own volition because he has had a few unpleasant experiences when husbands forced their wives into swinging. 'It's a highly unpleasant experience, especially for me,' he says with a look of disdain. 'Even one nervous wreck can ruin the mood of the party. That's all it takes. One time this lady started crying, and that was the end of the party. After that, I've been very strict.'

Today Vishal will interview three couples who have applied online to be a part of the next club night. At 3:15, our first couple walks into Cafe Coffee Day. Vishal is polite and curt, never over-friendly. He says that he has to maintain an air of professionalism because people are scared. The top fear in people's minds is that they will be filmed. A few years ago, a scandal broke when explicit footage of two students of Delhi's Modern School having sex on the school campus, shot by a mobile phone, was circulated extensively on the internet. A fracas followed, involving the national media, parliament, and the right-wing Hindu party, the Shiv Sena, demanding that the government ban mobile phones in schools. According to Vishal, the greatest fear for prospective club members is that Vishal may be filming their activities, or that he runs some sort of seedy sex racket.

'That is why it is necessary for them to see nice people like you and I, so that they understand that the club has high standards,' says Vishal, adopting a sort of professorial air.

The young couple that sit in front of us couldn't be more different from each other. The boy, twenty-three, is craggy-featured with a thin, wispy moustache that looks like a calligrapher's mistake. The girl is a lot more attractive in comparison, with small, pleasant features, and long hair that is black, smooth, and so shiny that it practically reflects the light. They have been dating for eight years, and are engaged to be married. Both work for large corporations in Delhi. They read about Vishal's club in an online chat room and want to further explore their sexuality.

Vishal seems to be delighted, and he whispers to me that they are his 'ideal couple'. He has dealt with many rascals and posers in his club, and now he can really tell those who are genuinely interested from those with perverted interests. Vishal's voice rises with excitement as he speaks to the couple.

No one actually has intercourse during these parties, Vishal explains. Sometimes people use the club as a pick-up joint. To avoid this problem, only couples in serious relationships are allowed into his club, and they are given a space to sexually experiment with each other and also with other couples through a variety of techniques that he has learnt in the US. The club is free at the moment, but he encourages donations.

There seemed to be a lot of rules for something that was meant to be all about freedom.

The young couple listen excitedly and only ask if there would be any recordings, to which Vishal declares that everything is extremely private and no cell phones are allowed in his club meetings.

After the couple leave, and while we wait for our next interviewees, I ask Vishal why, if couples didn't swap partners, or have intercourse, there is any reason to have the club.

Vishal explains that young couples wishing to overcome boredom could be stimulated while preserving the 'sanctity' of their relationship. Middle-aged couples could once again, or perhaps for the first time (since many of them are in arranged marriages) experience the élan of youthful courtship. These same people could then divert this awakened sexual energy into their own relationships. When men saw their wives arousing other men, they would become aroused by her themselves, while women, particularly those who had been married at a young age, could experience with a new man the feeling of being desired. For many couples, according to Vishal, his club could reinvigorate a dead marriage.

The second couple, a middle-aged pair, walk in. They had written in saying they were thirty, but they seem to be closer to forty-five. The woman has a pockmarked face and thinning hair, she wears a loose kaftan and tight jeans. The older man has short hair, a gentle smile, and close-set eyes with a slightly somnolent expression. They are both shy, and despite their age, seem to be far more nervous than the previous couple. They don't seem to really understand why they are here. To stimulate conversation, the unflappable Vishal asks them about their hobbies. Neither says anything at first, and after a while the man stutters, 'Watching TV'. Vishal cringes.

During interviews Vishal says he always asks about hobbies. If a candidate says 'watching TV or movies', or 'surfing the net', he does not approve. He considers that to be boring, lacking a sense of curiosity or adventure. He is pleased when he hears that the couple reads books or travels. These are his favourites, and the people he aspires to convert into swingers. Travelling, especially, seems to be a quality that translated well into club membership.

After they leave, I ask him if he thinks they would qualify.

'If I don't have enough couples, maybe. They are too old, and they scare the younger ones off. Which girl would want to pleasure her boyfriend in front of a man who looks like her father?'

Next to arrive is a couple who speak to Vishal mostly in Hindi. They seem to be the least affluent of the lot. Dilip works at a McDonald's as a senior staff member. His wife, Isha is a tiny, gnome-like woman, who smiles at me a lot. She has clearly dressed up for the interview, and appears to be floating in a sparkly, yellow sari. She hardly speaks or understands English, but when Vishal asks her if she would like to participate in the swinging club, she just giggles and nods her head. Her husband nudges her and smiles, 'Yeh to tera idea tha' (This was your idea). She had found Vishal's website while surfing the internet at the internet cafe that her brother owns, and had been curious to test it out. Her husband of two years had immediately liked the idea, and they had applied. These two seemed so unlike anyone I would have thought would want to participate in such an activity. They are the lower end of middle class, not as 'westernized', which though non-pc sometimes seemed a fairly accurate way of gauging class in India. I wonder if they know what they are in for or what a swingers' club is intended to do. As Vishal explains stuff to them, they listen with blank expressions. Dilip assures Vishal that both he and Priya are interested.

After they leave, Vishal sighs deeply. Initially he had seemed suspicious of Dilip, thinking that he may have forced Isha into this, but Isha seemed to be as enthusiastic, if not more than Dilip and Vishal has made it clear that enthusiasm is what matters the most.

Now that the interviews are over, I ask Vishal who has made the cut.

'Couple Number 1 is ideal. As for the oldies, it seems unlikely, but I won't rule them out. Older couples are more likely to give contributions, and I need that. Right now all the expenses are coming out of my pocket. I eventually hope to make some money with this club, charging for membership once people realize what a unique concept this is,' says Vishal.

◆

For the party in the evening, Vishal has brought along a bag containing many types of erotic paraphernalia, most of which has been sent to him courtesy the Texan, Cherry. These include a rabbit shaped vibrator, dill-pickle-shaped-dildos, neon-coloured cock rings, cheap lacy garter belts and packs of fruit-flavoured condoms. He is also carrying a box full of novels with salacious titles, backdated copies of pornographic magazines displaying photos of nude men and women, erect male genitals and baby-pink vaginas with fashionable, cropped hair-cuts. Vishal scatters these items around the small apartment rented for the night from a real estate broker friend. The rather unprepossessing apartment is in an obscure colony in Noida, a suburb of Delhi. Vishal never holds these parties at home. There are stains mottling the omelette coloured walls. The only source of ventilation is two small windows. I help Vishal set up the various props that he has brought to decorate the apartment—an old wooden chair with a hole in the seat that he calls a 'lick chair', a 5"x5" cardboard board with circles cut in various spots that he calls the grope wall, and a bundle of cushions in what he calls the 'play area'. Vishal has brought along a few bottles of alcohol, to 'relax the mood of the party'. To mark my contribution, I have brought along some namkeen—salted peanuts, and potato chips—not knowing what else to contribute. I am nervous about the proceedings of the evening, but equally I am curious to see how the motley crew that Vishal has assembled will get on with each other.

THE PARTY

The description of America's first public swingers' club—Plato's in New York, which opened in 1977—by Jon Hart, who interviewed owner and promoter Larry Levenson, gives us an idea of what the first Western swingers' clubs looked like:

> At Plato's, clothing was strictly optional, Levenson told me that first day in the cab. There was a buffet, a game

room, a dance floor, an enormous Jacuzzi, and a mammoth swimming pool. In the back, there were private rooms for intimate acts. And right off the dance floor, sectioned off with plants, was Plato's piece de resistance: the mat room, where exhibitionistic couples engaged in group activity... Once inside, couples participated in an unspoken tango. "If you wanted to make it with somebody, you reached over and caressed their leg. If your hand was not removed and the leg did not move away, you knew you were in... Once you take your clothes off, everyone's the same. Nudity is the great equalizer," said Levenson. "Bus drivers were partying with doctors and Wall Street people. No one cared about materialistic things or how much money you made. It was all about having a good time and making each other feel good."[257]

Though I didn't expect anything as outrageous as this description, I wondered how India's swingers' clubs would compare.

Seated on a lick chair, poor Isha is terrified as her husband clumsily tries to undo her sari. She stands in just her petticoat and blouse, her arms clutched over her chest. Vishal is the perfect picture of authority, dressed smartly in a white kurta pajama. There is a visible confidence in his demeanour, a new swagger in his step. He walks over to the couple and says something to Dilip, who is practically jumping with nervous energy. With some hesitation, Isha sits down and slowly lifts her petticoat. Vishal then instructs Dilip to slide underneath the chair, but Isha continues to look highly uncomfortable.

There are three other couples in the small living room— Couple Number 1 from the coffee shop; Couple Number 2—a young, trendy couple in their early twenties whom I haven't met before, and Couple Number 3—the older couple from the interview whom Vishal had decided to include after all. Couple Number 2 is hanging around in the 'play area' sipping on Bacardi

Breezers waiting for Vishal to set up a porn film on the laptop.

Couple Number 3 stands in the corner staring intently at the other couples in the room. I am technically Vishal's partner for the night, since his wife does not participate in these activities, though according to our terms and conditions, I would not actually take part, but just hang around. I busy myself serving drinks and the snacks I had brought.

Vishal is demonstrating the grope wall to Isha and Dilip. He encourages Dilip to take off his pants and stand behind the wall, while Isha closes her eyes and reaches out through the holes to touch Dilip. Vishal is urging the older couple to join Isha and Dilip, but they just look on with disdain. Suddenly, I notice them looking in *my* direction. At one point 'Tom', as the man introduced himself, unfurls a glowing smile at me, inviting me to join him at the lick chair. I quickly excuse myself and go into the kitchen. The older couple have two beers each and then leave the party prematurely.

The rest of the evening goes off rather uneventfully. Both young couples snuggle with their partners in the play area watching porn. Isha and Dilip are like capering young children in a toyshop, and they are back at the lick chair, Isha much happier now with her canary-yellow sari abandoned on the dusty, stained, tiled floors.

Vishal ends the party abruptly at 10 p.m. He turns on the lights leaving poor Isha cowering in the corner behind her husband, suddenly shy. He aggressively asks for donations, the young couples hand out a few hundred rupees, Isha and Dilip, a hundred. The dour older couple have left ₹500.

The party has been somewhat anti-climactic for me. I had expected prodigious amounts of booze, posturing, flirtation and maybe even sex. Although Vishal's club is a far cry from Plato's, he is not disheartened and explains to me that it is a step-by-step process. First couples experiment with each other, only when they are comfortable doing so in a public setting can they experiment with other couples. People are shy, and a bit wary, and he has to make them comfortable.

'This is India, after all. It isn't Texas, no matter how hard I try. These guys will get to the Texan standard, but at the moment they have absolutely no idea about anything. They don't know anything about sex, they have never seen a sex toy or quality porn,' says Vishal with authority.

On my way home, I give Isha and Dilip a lift. They are thrilled by their experience, shocked that they have landed upon something so genuine. They wax eloquent about 'Vishal Guru'. They hope they are invited next time, and before getting out of the car, Isha in her untidily draped sari and freshly applied plum-red lipstick, asks me, joining her hands in obeisance, if I could put in a word with Vishal to make sure they are called back.

Though the Delhi version of 'The Swing' was less brazen than the Texan version, it seemed to be at some level successful. Vishal's efforts at mimicry had given way to something organic and self-indulgent, an American concept but uniquely Indian in its execution. At some level, the couples were being educated about sexual experimentation. It would be a while before they got to the level of Plato's, but Vishal's club revealed that people across the board—students, and middle-aged couples alike were open to experimentation.

A week after the swingers' party, I visit Vishal. He suggests that we go out for coffee. Over all the days that I have been visiting, he has not suggested this, so it comes as a bit of a surprise to me, but I agree. In the small coffee joint named Blah Blah, a dim aqueous light fills the room. The air is hot and wheels of smoke whirl around the room. The crowd is young—high school and college students. Vishal and I are definitely out of place—the portly, balding Vishal more so than I. Vishal leads me upstairs to what he says is the 'private area', which is basically little bamboo huts, where young couples snuggle, most of them staring into laptops and expertly sucking at hookahs. I glimpse on all the screens the ubiquitous blue and white colours of Facebook. It is a muggy day, and I am breaking into a sweat. Vishal is sweating profusely, and he takes out a small towel from his pocket to rub his face dry. I suggest we move to the downstairs area, but a waiter brings a small, noisy cooler blasting out welcome spurts of cool air. Vishal is not his normal, self-assured, loquacious self. He seems shifty and nervous, shaking his legs, and cracking his fingers.

We sit down and Vishal edges closer to me. I begin to back off when Vishal squeaks, 'Please don't move away.' I get a whiff of something and I realize that Vishal is drunk. I chastise myself for not noticing the smell earlier on the motorbike, but that said, I had been wearing a gigantic, suffocating helmet.

I quickly scoot away.

'I love you,' says Vishal in a small voice. He adds. 'I think you love me too.'

'Um, no, Vishal, I don't love you,' I say.

He looks crestfallen. 'Then why are you spending so much time with me?'

'I told you, Vishal. I'm a writer, I write books. I'm writing a book on all of the stuff that you are doing with your club,' I say sternly.

'I guess,' he mutters softly.

He edges closer, till I feel his leg brushing against mine. I quickly move away.

'Actually,' he says, 'I don't like my wife much. She troubles me a lot. She is complaining about my club business. I thought maybe you and I…because you understand me.'

I am shocked that Vishal has misunderstood my friendliness for romance. I figured that, of all people, Vishal, with his swingers' club, would be open-minded, especially since I had made my intentions so clear. Then again, I suppose poor Vishal is a confused man living in a perplexing, changing society. Though Vishal wants to re-enact his brief stint in Texas here in India, and hankers to live with the same openness, that seems impossible for the moment. Indian society is changing, but there is some way to go before people can do as they please, and until then there will be a whole lot of turbulence with people like Vishal bearing the brunt of it.

Vishal stands up, wavering unsteadily. I tell him that maybe he should sit down.

My first instinct is to be scared, but then, I'm not sure what I should be scared of—this strange, funny man, half a foot shorter than me, who I am sure if push came to shove, I could take down? I decide that I should be calm and understanding. I couldn't hit Vishal. No, I simply couldn't do anything to poor Vishal, except feel sorry for him.

'Vishal,' I say as firmly as I can. 'I think you have the wrong impression. Maybe we shouldn't be meeting anymore.'

Vishal blanches and looks as if he is about to be sick, or worse, start to cry. Before anything disastrous happens, I quickly thank him for all his help, and rush out of the coffee shop. Before I go I turn around to take a look at Vishal, just to make sure he hasn't fallen. He is sitting calmly, staring with a particular curiosity at the young couple in the booth next door.

TANGO

Tonight's gig is at Tango, Shillong's most popular pub, located in the basement of a derelict building in Police Bazaar, the commercial centre of Shillong. In this small, curious pop-up nightclub in the distant northeastern town of Shillong, the crowd is more cosmopolitan than at any of the parties that I have been to in Delhi or Mumbai. At this moment I could be in an underground New York City nightclub. Boys kiss girls, girls kiss boys, people sing and jive, moving their bodies with abandon. Everywhere there are couples—on the sofa, in the dark shadowy corners, and no one seems to heed them. In a top Delhi nightclub, where the cover charge is ₹5,000 per person, I have never seen, nor can I imagine this kind of pumping energy, this flagrant openness. I listen to the unfamiliar music, watching Tips perform her best on home turf, the audience cheering her on, singing and dancing, sassy, confident, and full of new hope. I haven't listened to much Blues, and in the beginning, the music is jarring to my ears, the beat unfamiliar, the cadence unnatural. Besides, the acoustics of this club are not particularly good. For one, the shape of this decrepit, musty room is strange: I count seven or maybe eight corners. Second, we are underground, in a sort of basement, and the ceiling is low. Third, there isn't much space. The small room is crammed with two bars and crowds of sofas and chairs. There isn't even a stage, and the lead singers of the band, Tips and Rudy, are performing in one corner.

I don't usually attend concerts and do not understand the draw of live music. I grew up in the age of DJs—invisible forces, unknown faces hidden in corners of nightclubs, whose only identity is the music they blare out. Then, suddenly, apropos of nothing at all, I begin to understand the music. The change is unexpected. I start enjoying the regularity of the drums, the sound of Rudy's guitar, and most of all, Tips's crooning, which had previously given me a headache. I begin to understand the power of performance. Holding a red guitar, singing into a microphone decorated with butterflies, and wearing a slinky red dress with her hair pulled back tight, Tips is simply ravishing.

Tips's complete unconcern about elegance or show only underlines the impact of her extraordinary face, of her whole persona. Before she begins to sing, she seems to withdraw for an instant, half closing her brown eyes, turning her head away from the microphone as if she were saying a prayer. Right after a peppy track, Tips breaks into a Khasi folk song—the Peace Prayer—and suddenly the room becomes quiet, people stop dancing and stand still, their heads bowed down, the way one does during the national anthem. A lot of people here can relate to this folk song, which was an anthem during the decades of insurgency in the Northeast. And then just as suddenly, the drums break out and they start jamming, this time a Buddy Guy cover, and the room is once again alive.

SHILLONG

Shillong is the capital of Meghalaya, a small hill state in the northeastern part of India. During colonial times, it became the cultural capital of the Northeast after the British established it as the capital of Greater Assam in 1864, which gave birth to a bustling town. In recent times, it has made a name for itself as the rock capital of India because of the number of local music bands here.

Shillong is the abode of three matrilineal tribes: the Khasis, Jaintias and Garos, of which the majority are Khasis. There is no written history of the tribes and much of it is still oral (the Khasi language had no script till the Christian Missionaries introduced it) so there is still some confusion about antecedents, dates and origins. It is thought that the original Khasis migrated to present-day India from Cambodia. Since Khasi men were primarily hunters with a high rate of mortality, a matrilineal system was adopted. Within the Khasi matrilineal system the khadduh or the youngest daughter is the custodian of the family wealth, rites and religion. The youngest daughter plays the role of the eldest son in patriarchal communities.

Shillong was a Khasi hamlet before the British came and paved the way for missionaries, the first of whom, the Welsh Calvinist Methodists, set up their missions in the hills in 1841. About 70 per cent of Khasis today have converted to Christianity.[258] With the spread of Christianity, the khadduh no longer plays a religious role but continues to inherit the family wealth. The children born to Khasi parents take the last name of the mother, though the father is allowed to retain his own last name. Today most Khasis, even those who practice Christianity, follow Khasi Customary Laws, which are practiced though Siems—village headmen—and District Courts.

As I explore Khasi culture some more, I realize that the 'modern love' erupting in pockets across the country is not just a Western construct. The truth is that India too offered these experiences when our society was a more open, creative, accepting one. A few of these traditions remain today. The Khasis are not the only matrilineal tribe in the country, there are a number of other tribes—the Todas of Tamil Nadu, Nairs of Kerala and Bunts of Karnataka—who showcase the diversity of relationship paradigms that India once offered, but which have slowly deteriorated over time.

Even today some adivasis, or tribal communities, encourage some liberal practices. Several adivasi communities have communal dormitories to encourage healthy adolescent sexual liaisons. One of the most well organized forms of communal dormitories is among the Murias of Bastar in Chhattisgarh.

In his book *The Muria and Their Ghotul* Verrier Elwin describes the typical 'ghotul' or dormitory: 'The typical ghotul will stand in the middle of the village inside a spacious compound surrounded by wooden stakes. There will be a large central house with a deep verandah, perhaps more than one open hut, and a number of small ones. There may be a wooden vagina carved on the central pillar of the house, or a drawing of a boy with an enormous penis and a girl in his arms.'[259]

For the child, the ghotul as described by Elwin is 'a school of sexual manners, a society of his own and in time an introduction to fulfilment of sexual life. In other words, it fills what is a remarkable gap in Western society—a community of adolescents and near-adolescents who are free to behave as they wish, enjoy sexual freedom without a sense of guilt and who invent their own disciplines'.[260]

The average ghotul has twenty members, everyone abides by the strict rules and has equal sexual privileges. No boy or girl is allowed to sleep with the same partner for more than three days. If they do, they are punished and banned from the ghotul. When a girl is married she can never come back, though there may be a final ceremony during which she massages every boy for the last time. A boy continues coming to the ghotul for three to four months after his marriage, after which he throws a feast for everyone to mark the end of his ghotul days.[261]

Quite remarkably, pregnancy is an infrequent problem in the ghotul. It was calculated that in 220 ghotuls there was only a low 4 per cent chance of pregnancy.[262] In the Muria tribe, men and women are not segregated, there is no discrimination on the basis of gender, and there is almost no sexual harassment or violence. The Murias show us that ancient practices are stunningly modern and are finding a place for themselves in modern times.

KONG PAT

My first meeting in Shillong is with Patricia Mukhim, or Kong Pat as she is known in these parts. She is the editor-in-chief of Shillong's largest English daily—*The Shillong Times*—and one of the most highly respected and well-known women of Shillong. Apart from being an award-winning journalist (she has won the Padma Shri), Kong Pat is an activist working on a variety of local issues, including marriage laws. She is also the khadduh, or youngest daughter, and has inherited the house that we sit in today.

Kong (or 'aunt', a term of respect) Pat is immaculately dressed in a Jainsem, the traditional Khasi dress, and sports a stylish haircut. We sit in her office, a small, low-roofed room filled with books. I squeeze myself on to a tiny wooden chair, and feel like a burly, dishevelled giant in front of this tiny, elegant woman. I begin my conversation with Kong Pat by asking her about marriage in the Khasi culture. 'It's simple. We fall in love, and we start living together, *this* is our Khasi culture,' says Kong Pat proudly. She continues, 'We are a sexual and sensual people and till the Christians came we didn't think formal marriage was so important. If people cohabit, they are considered man and wife. Many still live together without being married.'

The traditional Khasi attitude towards marriage is a liberal one, showcasing an open mindset where live-in relationships are widely accepted, and a formal marriage doesn't prove anything. Young people choose their own spouses, and then simply move in together if they want to declare their relationship to the world. In most cases, the man moves into the woman's home with her family.

Kong Pat tells me that her nuptial life has followed a typical Khasi trajectory. She has had four children from three different men. Her first marriage (in the Khasi sense, because they weren't formally married) was at the age of sixteen, the second at twenty, and the third at twenty-eight. She has had children with all of them, though she only formally married her last partner, a Tamil pilot in the air force. She tells me that they divorced because they were culturally too far apart. She is now single and enjoys it.

Despite the liberal attitude towards marriage, there are certain downsides, Kong Pat explains. Amongst the Khasis, there is an increasing number of abandoned women and single mother households. Even though a large percentage of the population is Christian, including Kong Pat herself, Khasi traditions are followed and there are no provisions for maintenance in Khasi law if the man deserts the mother of his child. In the olden days, the kur (clan) was responsible for all of its members, but in modern-day society, the kur doesn't perform these functions. Kong Pat has been deserted by two men, the fathers of her first two children, and now is on the board of an organization which is pushing for laws making formal registration of marriage mandatory so that women can get maintenance for their children from deserter husbands

Kong Pat tells me that live-in relationships are common amongst the Khasis today. She believes that it is a positive thing, and she encourages all her children to do this before they get married. She talks to me about a discussion she had with her daughter-in-law regarding infidelity in marriage. Her daughter-in-law says that she would never be able to accept her husband being with another woman. 'It is natural that at certain point in time a man looks at other women for stimulation, be it intellectual or emotional. Suppose a man has a girlfriend, but supports you, maintains you, what is the problem then? This has been Khasi society in the past. Many men have had three-four wives. In our times, we were more open-minded, not because we had to be, but because we wanted to be,' she says firmly.

What about the other way around? Would it be okay for a woman to take another partner?

'Why not!' says Kong Pat. 'I am the best example of this. It is all about understanding and openness between two partners, which did exist in the Khasi culture of the past before we had Christian guilt and Hindu obsession with purity enter our culture.'

I ask Kong Pat about the influence of Christianity on Khasi life. She considers, then explains, 'Christianity here is skin-deep. It may affect the religious practices that we follow, but many Khasis become Christians at the end of their lives, maybe just to make sure they get a spot to get buried. Not all is bad, there have been many positive influences such as education and healthcare but the missionaries tried to impose a certain way of life that wasn't the original Khasi way of life. Our tribal culture is intrinsically open and non-judgmental. Christianity is all about judgment and sin. The only thing that Khasi culture says is that the man should not have an affair while his wife is pregnant, because she then may have trouble in delivering the child.'

On sex, Kong Pat simply says that Khasis have always been able to sexually express themselves, whether it is through their mating rites, dances or songs. Khasis regard sexual repression as the worst form of repression, and instances of rape, sexual harassment, and eve teasing, commonplace elsewhere in the country, especially in the 'rogue' states of Bihar and Uttar Pradesh, are unheard of here. Women are highly respected, and problems of female foeticide and infanticide are unimaginable amongst the Khasis who celebrate the birth of a daughter. Kong Pat has recently lost her youngest daughter, the khadduh, to a heart condition. As she speaks about her daughter, whose picture in a frilly, white wedding gown hangs on the wall with a rosary strung around it, she maintains a steady expression despite the sadness creeping into her voice. 'Sometimes we can't associate with Indians, maybe that is why we feel like we aren't really one of them. We don't understand how people in the rest of this country can kill their daughters. Here, our daughters are more precious to us than even our sons.'

It seems like the liberal ways of the Khasis are leading to a certain number of problems in these modern times. Some months ago, there was a brouhaha in Delhi over the suicide of a Northeastern student—Dana Sangma. It received extensive media coverage because Dana was the niece of Meghalaya Chief Minister Mukul Sangma. Dana's suicide was one in a series of recent suicides amongst Northeastern college students allegedly due to discrimination and harassment. The police are finally taking action, putting together a plan to protect female students from the Northeast.

I ask Kong Pat about this suicide and she speaks to me passionately, since she, like many Northeastern women who leave their homeland, has been subject to discrimination. Kong Pat explains to me that the economies of Northeastern states like Meghalaya are struggling and job opportunities are nearly non-existent, so young people look for jobs in the mainland where they are coveted since they speak English well and are well-turned-out. When they arrive on the Indian mainland, Northeastern women act like they do back home, freely and openly interacting with men, conducting sexual affairs, and this often leads to teasing and harassment. There is a strong prejudice against women from the Northeast in many parts of the mainland leading to a lot of strife, and in some extreme situations like Dana, even suicide.

In Shillong too, the free mixing of the sexes in Khasi society has led to problems recently. Teenage pregnancy has soared, and maternal mortality and abortion rates are higher than they have ever been. Kong Pat fears that the Khasis are becoming increasingly licentious and that Khasi youth are abusing the 'freeness' of the traditional culture by having too many sexual partners.

I ponder over my conversation with Kong Pat as I walk to my next meeting. In Shillong I have been walking everywhere, trading in the flats that I normally walk in for a pair of unfashionable but comfortable sneakers, which I need to navigate the precarious traffic and to trudge up the exhausting winding roads. I realize that there is a certain amount of truth to what Kong Pat said about society here being open. I notice that young people mingle freely, men and women hold hands in public, and this seems to be the norm. As I walk, I am surrounded by many young people, men and women in equal numbers, dressed in the latest fashions, skinny jeans, tight, brightly coloured t-shirts, and high heels. In my linen pants and kurta, I feel like a troll in front of these fashionistas. I am also fascinated by how these young people traverse the steep streets with alarming dexterity in their trendy, inexpensive and more likely than not, ergonomically incorrect shoes.

I think back to my extensive travels, from Kashmir, the northern-most state of India, to Kanyakumari, the southern-most tip, and I realize that I have never felt as safe, or as comfortable walking around as I do here in Shillong. There are no men bumping into me, groping my behind, or brushing past me and 'accidentally' touching me. There are no prying stares, looks that are often more threatening than touches, even though I look distinctly different from anyone on the streets, standing a foot above most here. They don't need to segregate men and women for fear of violence or harassment, because that culture of fear and segregation which is entrenched in so many Indian cities, simply does not exist.

On a recent trip to Lucknow, the capital of Uttar Pradesh, I was shocked because I didn't see women anywhere. I calculated that the ratio of men to women on the streets was something like thirty-five men for one woman. I had stopped to buy a bottle of water and asked the man behind the counter where the women were. He looked at me as if I were dim-witted and replied, 'At home, where they should be. Where else would they be?'

◆

Mervin's features are strikingly different from most Northeasterners. He is Kong Pat's son with her third husband, the Tamil pilot, and he looks more South Indian than Northeastern. The feature that sets most people from this region apart is their almond-shaped eyes, but Mervin's are round as saucers. Kong Pat has sent me across to meet her thirty-year-old son to find out more about how young Khasis deal with their relationships. I meet him on the campus of the Indian Institute of Management, Shillong, a newly set up branch of the premier Indian business school, where Mervin is the head of Public Relations.

The term has not yet started, and the campus is deserted. It has just rained, and the lush campus is a dazzling emerald green. Mervin is a warm young man, and he talks to me about his relationship. His wife is a khadduh, the youngest daughter, so after he started dating her four years ago, he moved into her family home. They had a daughter two years later, and only formally married six months ago. I ask him if moving in with his in-laws into a joint family, where his wife's siblings lived under the same roof, was problematic for him. Mervin tells me that it was, but he had little choice in this matter, as this is an age-old tradition. He adds that marrying the youngest daughter is a major responsibility since she is expected to take care of her parents and the well-being of her home and family, unlike the rest of India where the woman moves into the man's home to take care of *his* family.

I ask Mervin what young people from his community and peer group think about love, marriage and sex. Mervin estimates that close to 50 per cent of the people he knows are living together with their partners and children, though they are not formally married. In his own case too, he was married only after the birth of his first child. He explains that the single biggest problem in the area is sex education. Like the rest of the country, there is no sex education here, but unlike the rest of the country, there is no stigma attached to sex. This has led to major problems of unplanned pregnancy. The church is trying to launch sex education programmes, but they are sporadic and ill-planned.

Mervin suggests that we visit Father Cella, who runs the Don Bosco Youth Centre, the largest youth centre in the area, to find out more. Mervin and I navigate the narrow winding streets and the traffic of Shillong, and fetch up at the youth centre, which sits in the heart of town and is a hub of Shillong's social and spiritual activity.

Father Cella came to India from Malta in 1956 as a member of the Catholic Church with a mission to convert tribal Khasis following their indigenous Seng Khasi religion to Catholicism. He started the youth centre twenty years ago. Here he offers everything from Sunday church service to Alcoholics Anonymous meetings, to music classes. To counter the burgeoning problem of teenage pregnancy, Father Cella has recently started sex education classes. He immediately hands me a pile of flimsy safe sex brochures, which he keeps handy to give to all young people.

'We are taking the worst of the West,' says Father Cella.' I am not sure where we are heading, but at the moment the situation is looking grimmer than in my fifty-six years in this country,' adds the eighty-five-year-old pastor. 'The last time this sort of change happened was when the British came and conversion happened, but that change was gentle compared to this one.'

Father Cella explains to me with a defeated look in his old eyes that there has been a steady deterioration of Khasi culture over the past decade, especially in the past five years. Alcohol and premarital sex are the two biggest problems, leading to teenage pregnancies and depression. According to Meren Lonkumer et al., the internet and mobile phones have worsened the situation by providing easy access to pornography and sex-related material.

The lethal brew of unhindered and unrestrained access to alcohol and women (since mixing between the two sexes is not taboo) is such a heady concoction that teenage or premarital sex is a natural progression, often with disastrous consequences.[263]

Father Cella tells me that according to the Khasi tradition, the clan would take responsibility for orphans, the destitute and old people. Today, babies are being abandoned and orphanages have sprung up, there are old age homes because people have migrated, leaving their elderly parents behind. These are problems that were never meant to exist in the Khasi culture, but they have become endemic today.

The repercussions of modernity have been dire for the Khasis, and Mervin tells me that to understand the thrust of the problems I must speak with a member of the SRT or Syngkhong Rympei Thymmai (Association for New Hearths), an organization formed in 1990 whose main objective is to change the Khasi system from a matrilineal to a patrilineal one, something that a few tribes in India, like the Nairs of Kerala have done to cope with the challenges of modern times.

◆

On a blistering hot day, I set out to meet with a senior member of the SRT who has chosen to remain anonymous.

'Do you wonder why the men here drink here so much—why alcoholism is such a problem?' says the squat, rubicund man with a fiery attitude. I say yes, this was something that I had indeed wondered about. Alcoholism is a major problem in Shillong, and much of the Northeast, where levels of alcohol consumption are some of the highest in the country.

He flutters his hands like two birds in flight, spits out the betel that he has been chewing and inserts another leaf into his mouth. 'The men feel useless. We don't have any dignity in this culture,' he says.

'That's why our society has become so screwed up. Our great

Khasi race, and the women (sic) have been through its heyday. Earlier Khasi men were hunters, they were often killed in the jungles, so it made sense to leave everything to a woman. We aren't hunters no more, so we want our rights back!'

The main complaint of the SRT is that there is no centre of real authority in the modern Khasi family and that the father is not respected since he is not related by flesh and blood to his wife's clan. The SRT argues that the role of the father is crucial because he gives not only his personality and dignity to his children, but also his flesh and blood through procreation. The issue of property succession too has become an important one since, according to Khasi law, only a woman is allowed to inherit property. If a family does not have a daughter, they either adopt a girl, or pass on the property to the youngest daughter of the mother's sister.

He launches into a fiery diatribe. 'The Indian government shouldn't be imposing any laws on us Khasis. What do they know? We are not the same as the Indians. We are totally different, our origin is different, we think differently. They call us chinky, those Indians. We are more like the Chinese, or maybe the Koreans. The Korean culture is really popular amongst the youth here.'

I ask him, because I cannot resist the question, if he has met any Chinese or Korean people.

He croaks out a 'No' and then adds, 'But I don't really care. We are like them.'

Before I leave, hurrying, because this man seems to be in a violent mood, he says to me with an angry look on his face.

'Times have changed. Meghalaya has changed, and we Khasis must change with the times.'

SOULMATE

Growing up, Tipriti didn't know she was beautiful. As a recalcitrant student in Shillong and later at boarding school at Kalimpong, Darjeeling, she thought she was ugly, so ugly that she pretended to be a boy. She dressed in loose jeans and muscle shirts. Her hair was cropped to the skull, and she sported a skinny rat-tail. At nineteen, when she met Rudy Wallang at his recording studio to record a hymn for a pastor, her life took an unexpected turn. From a gospel singer at church, she became a back-up singer in Rudy's band Mojo, and in less than a year she was the lead vocalist for Soulmate, the Blues band she formed with her own soulmate, mentor, lover, best friend, and father-figure, Rudy Wallang.

Tipriti 'Tips' Kharbangar is a well-known face of the Indian music scene. She is the face of Blues band Soulmate, the poster child of Shillong. Tips's beauty stuns me. Her long hair is dark golden-brown, the colour of a bay mare's glossy coat, a relic of her Scottish ancestry. Her skin is fairer than the Khasi ivory, and her strawberry shaped mouth is stained a deep red from the betel that she chews. Her most magnificent features though are her eyes. They are large, a deep chocolate brown, and lined with thick, dark kohl. The look in her eyes is wild. I can't figure out what it is—unbridled hope, fear, or grief. I am intrigued by this young Khasi woman, a role model for all the other young Khasi women around, and want to understand her perspective on relationships. As I spend time with Tips, in her home, in the cafes she frequents, during Soulmate practice sessions, and with her friends and family, I realize that it isn't easy or joyful being a woman in Khasi society. On the surface it may seem like a lovely, free place where young people, especially women, can do as they like in their relationships, but underneath the shiny veneer lurks a different story.

'I've got the blues real bad,' Tips tells me with an acerbic laugh. She adds, 'I had a traumatic childhood, that's where I get my blues from, and they are deeper than anyone else's I know.'

As her parents' only daughter, Tips is the khadduh. She tells me that being a khadduh doesn't mean that you are brought up like a princess. Instead, she was brought up like a boy and was expected to take care of her family, which she does today. She has built the small hilltop house with her earnings from music, where she lives with her family.

'We didn't have a normal childhood. While other kids were playing, my brother and I were bleeding in a corner,' she says talking about the abuse from her alcoholic father.

'I was a tomboy because it was easier going through what I did being a boy. Being a girl, I couldn't handle it. In school, all the boys were scared of me. I felt that I was ugly, that no one liked me. When I met Rudy, I was still a boy. It's only after I met him, after he told me that I was beautiful that I became interested in myself, in doing up my face before gigs, in looking like a girl. Now I can say that I'm a woman,' says Tips with a fierce expression in her eyes.

However 'modern' Shillong appeared to be, relationships in Khasi society weren't simple. The first thing that Tips tells me about Rudy is that he is a wonderful father, and that she is envious of the way he treats his children, the eldest of whom is just a few years younger than her. Her own childhood is scarred by memories of her drunken father, and she is fascinated by Rudy's love for his children. She doesn't blame her father for what he did. It wasn't his fault that he didn't know how to be a father, or how to treat her because he had never had a father. Her father never met the Scottish army man who gave his mother three children and then left in 1947 when the British left India, never to come back again

The community in Shillong is more ethnically diverse than people imagine. There are all sorts of genes floating around, and it is not uncommon to see brilliant blue eyes, blonde hair, or very fair skin. The British made Shillong their home for over a century; many Khasis have at least one foreign grandparent, usually men who were here with the army and then returned with their ilk once the British left India. During those times, sticking to their beliefs, Khasi women never doubted the legitimacy of their liaisons with British men and looked upon these men as their husbands. Most people I meet in Shillong speak of their foreign ancestry proudly, decorating their living room with photos of their foreign grandparents, yet hardly any of them have ever met them. When I ask if their grandmothers had legally married these men, most of them don't really know, saying that in Khasi custom marriage on paper doesn't hold much value. Yet the fact remains that a large number of Khasi children were deserted by their fathers and this has led to many complications in today's Khasi society.

I ask Tips about her mother.

'My mom is a strong woman. I look up to her,' she says speaking of the timid woman with the tired smile and the betel stained teeth who sings Carole King songs, though she doesn't speak much English.

'Everything that I have done in my life is just to make her happy,' she says.

'Is she happy?' I ask

Tips has a doubtful look on her face. 'Maybe.'

Tips tells me about the struggle she went through with her family, and the pain her mother felt when she and Rudy began dating. For all their open-mindedness, what the Khasis seemed to have in common with the rest of their countrymen is a sense of hypocrisy. In Khasi society, an older man being with a younger woman is not uncommon, yet people gossiped when Tips and Rudy got together, calling Tips a 'slut' and chastising Rudy for being with a younger woman even though several of them have similar age differences in their relationships.

'I guess that's one of the downsides of being a clan. People love gossiping about each other and it permanently damaged my mother who cares so much about society and reputation,' said Tips dolefully.

She shrugs off her sadness and says she thinks Rudy was a godsend. In Rudy, she saw the father that she never had, and she was immediately attracted to him, despite the twenty-one-year age difference and the fact that he was married with four children. It was Rudy who introduced her to the Blues, through which she found a way of letting go.

◆

When Rudy speaks of his ex-wife, he lowers his voice, out of respect to the deceased. His face suffuses with grief, and he tells me that he tried his best to hold the marriage together, and he was always a good father to his children.

Rudy was not deeply in love with Aarti when he married her. He had only known her for two months, and had married her because she was pregnant. Even though Aarti and he didn't have much in common in terms of family or interests, it seemed to him the right thing to do. Aarti quickly converted from her Seng Khasi religion to Catholicism, so that Rudy and she could marry in church. Aarti never liked Shillong; she preferred the buzz of a big city like Bangalore, where she had lived before they were married. She regretted the marriage, but had little choice but to marry the father of her unborn child. With Rudy away on tour with his band Mojo, Aarti resorted to alcohol, a problem that spiralled out of control, and to which she eventually lost her life. They were married for ten years and had four children together, after which they divorced. Aarti died years ago of alcohol poisoning, about the time that Tips and Rudy met.

'Reincarnation is as important for the living as it is for the dead. I think of this line when I think of Tips. When everything in my life was so dark, like an angel, she walked into my studio, and I fell in love,' says Rudy.

'I guess we all have our blues. I have my blues, she has her blues, we even have our blues together, and that is what makes us sing,' he adds with a sad smile.

The next time I meet Tips, we are outside the hospital. It looks like she may have drunk too much. There are dark circles under her eyes, and her eyes are tinted crimson. She stares at me with a sort of benign intensity, face clammy, hands folded across the chest, head bowed as if paying homage to something. Tips is at the hospital to meet her elder brother, who has been in and out of hospitals and rehab centres for the past five years. He has been an alcoholic for almost half his life and is now dying of cirrhosis of the liver. She doesn't blame her brother for being an alcoholic, it helped him deal with the pain of their childhood. She too could have easily become an alcoholic but was saved because of her music and Rudy.

Tips has had a difficult childhood and has deep scars to show, but she is not the only one. Much of Shillong is mired in confusion, and as this idyllic place opens up to the world, there is a violent clash of cultures, within and outside. The shift from their indigenous beliefs to Christianity may have been skin-deep for people of this region, but it seems to me that the current shift—to a modern, consumerist culture—is the more deep and soul-shifting one. As the world changes, revolving on its axis, there are things that we take away from it, things that we hold on to, and things that we let go of. While we wait for this age to set, I can only wonder what the repercussions for a generation, for a nation, and for the world beyond will be.

EPILOGUE

A TALE OF TWO REVOLUTIONS

My assumption, when I first set out to write this book, was that India was going through a sexual revolution. The change was all around me, on billboards, on television screens, in chains of coffee shops and on college campuses. Instead, what I discovered was that there was not one, but *two* revolutions coursing through India's social landscape—the sex revolution, and the love revolution.

I had hypothesized that sex, love, and marriage were all part of *one* revolution; after all these three often do come together. I had expected to see trends, to cull statistics to reach neat conclusions—and to wrap everything up with a pretty red bow. This was not so easy. Every time I was close to cementing a theory, something, or someone would come along and dislodge it. It seemed that for every truth, there was an equal and opposite untruth. Through the course of my research, even my fundamental premise for writing the book—that India was going through a sexual revolution—was tested.

I referred to experts—academics, social workers, lawmakers, government officials and several others—to make sense of what was happening. From Shiny to Dr Kothari, from my grandfather's living room to dorm rooms in Bangalore, as I traversed India, I realized that there was much more at play.

Though the participants and forces behind both revolutions

were the same, they were happening separately, in spite of each other, but *also* as a result of each other. It was a bit like that well-known chicken-and-egg question—which came first: the love revolution or the sex revolution? In India, it seems, it is all happening contemporaneously.

As I expected, young people are having premarital sex, same sex relations have been decriminalized and re-criminalized, more people are defiantly declaring their sexual preferences, and women are demanding their sexual rights. Essentially, sex is coming out of the bedroom and on to the streets. And the love revolution has led to the break-up of the arranged marriage as more people decide to marry for love rather than community or caste. Priya and Kartikey, and the numerous other couples I interviewed are examples of the love revolution. They fell in love, and married against the wishes of their families and communities, but they did not believe in premarital sex and consummated their love only after marriage.

Then there are people who are part of the sex revolution. People like Shammi and Suganda who had a traditional arranged marriage, but took the renegade route of having sexual affairs while remaining tied to their tradition. Or others like Prayag and his girlfriends, who were having sex before marriage, but who may not be able to handle the emotional baggage that comes with the physical aspect. So while all these people may not be (at the moment) part of one revolution, they could be part of another. It is inevitable though that at some point in the future these two revolutions will meet.

Another important point that I discovered for both revolutions is that they were happening at different speeds in different ways across the country. So we may have an upper-middle-class Delhi gal who dresses as she wants, has sex with whom she wants and marries whomever she wants. Then we may have another young woman, who lives right next door to her, who may not have *any* of these choices. She has been sequestered at home her entire life, and will be expected to marry someone of her parents' choice. All this while, she may be having a secret affair online, but no one will ever know. Here, we have one young woman who is in the advanced stage of both revolutions, and then another, who is part of the first stages.

The love revolution will lead to the breakdown of the traditional arranged marriage. This is significant, because it also means the breakdown of the joint family, of caste and community identity, and as divorce rates skyrocket, perhaps also of marriage itself. The switch from arranged to love marriage will be a slow, gradual one, but it is happening nonetheless, particularly in urban India. The India of ten years ago was substantially different from the India of today, and the India a decade from now will continue on the path that we have paved.

The sex revolution does not just concern the physical act of sex. It is about changing laws, about loosening censors, and about more sexual liberty. It is about seeing women choosing to wear what they want and about accepting gays in our communities. It is about the burgeoning prostitution industry and pornography. It is about escaping hypocrisy and realizing we are making change happen. Above all, it is about exposing an entire generation to a heavily sexualized culture which is seeping into their lives.

The multifaceted fallout of sexual liberation, a lot of which are already manifesting in ugly ways, will be unwanted teenage pregnancies, sexually transmitted diseases and infections, the continuation of female foeticide, disturbing sexual violence and harassment that we have already been witness to, all of which will tear India apart. Until the state provides adequate infrastructure to support the sexual revolution, we will continue to see and read hackneyed stories of violence against women. And, while laws may change and be strengthened, mindsets will have to follow suit. It is our moral imperative as Indians to support this change.

WHAT KIND OF REVOLUTION IS IT?

To understand more about what the consequences of India's revolution will be, it is crucial for us to understand what kind of revolution we are in the midst of. Is it like the love and sexual revolutions of the West, or is it something different?

I argue that India is going through a different kind of revolution, one that can be compared to China's in many ways. In the West, the love and sex revolution took the linear route—first came the love revolution, in which family and community involvement in the marital choices of young people diminished, and then came the sex revolution, whose hallmarks included multiple sex partners, the celebration of nudity, full sexual expression no matter what one's sexuality or sexual orientation was, the rejection of all forms of censorship[264] and reliable contraceptives.

In his classic work *The History of Sexuality,* philosopher and social theorist Michel Foucault differentiates between two types of erotic cultures. An Eastern culture is endowed with an *ars erotica* (the erotic art), where sexuality is seen as way of life, and is part of the soul, whereas Western societies like America, England and France see sex as *scientia sexualis* (a scientific act) and treat it as a mere biological act. According to Foucault's theory, historically, India and China have had similar views on sex. Also, like in India, in China, 'the pendulum swung unevenly, from unprecedented sexual liberalism under the Tang Dynasty to repressive orthodoxy under the Qing Dynasty, with lots of back and forth in between. Puritanism reached its peak in the Mao era, when prostitution was all but eradicated along with almost all public references to sex.'[265] China's sexual revolution began in the early 1980s with Deng Xiaoping's policy of 'reform and opening up'.

Today, the Chinese revolution, like the Indian one, is an urban phenomenon, and has left the countryside relatively untouched. As Richard Burger writes in his book *Behind the Red Door,* in China, most twenty-somethings have moved from villages to find work in urban areas. Tens of millions of young migrant workers who move to towns and cities often frequent internet cafes where they use social media to find dates and make friends. This, amongst many other reasons of a burgeoning sexualized culture, sounds eerily similar to India's revolution.

Since we have historically and culturally had similar experiences with sex, and our current revolutions have similar characteristics, it makes sense to see what China's biggest problems are to forecast our own. What I see as *both* China's and India's biggest problem is the looming gender imbalance. For all the dramatic changes in China's sexual landscape since the 1970s perhaps nothing will have a more dramatic effect than this. This imbalance has led to a jump in crime and violence in both countries already. Some Chinese sex experts predict that this trend will be accompanied by a significant rise in HIV/AIDS and other sexually transmitted diseases. A high male to female ratio also increases the chances of a woman becoming pregnant before marriage. Some say that these bare branches (like those discussed in the 'Dark Side' chapter) will turn to homosexuality because of a lack of other options.[266]

The gender imbalance also affects the love revolution. After years of research, Dr Robert Epstein, a Harvard University psychologist and professor, has concluded that a higher number of males than females leads to society becoming more conservative. In this case, arranged marriage will prevail, and all the positives of the love revolution will go out of the window.

Society benefits from the revolution of the kind that India is going through. There is greater gender equality, more freedom for women, an increasing culture of respect and tolerance in marriage, and the waning of homophobia. Yet no revolution comes without its fair share of casualties, and it is important to address the revolution's excesses, the worrisome side effects and the constant tug of war between past and future.

THE ROAD AHEAD

Most likely, the struggle will continue. As India's past pushes against its present, there is an eternal war between social conservative prudes and a new generation of Western-influenced young people. In the present moment, thanks to globalization and technology, I see the libertine making his way to the top, but that could easily turn, like it has before. As economist Joan Robinson famously said, 'Whatever you can rightly say about India, the opposite is also true'.

All we can do in a constantly changing India is to brace and prepare ourselves. Sex education in our country remains woefully inadequate, our government has to rid itself of its squeamish views and tell it the way it is. We desperately need more support systems—legal, mental, social, etc. or else young people like Aasimah will keep falling through the gaps.

India has the chance to overcome her past prejudices and recognize sexual and marital freedom as a fundamental human right. We may never again be a society devoted to sexual practices as we once were, but we are on our way—however slowly and treacherously—to greater sexual openness, tolerance and freedom.

On a personal note, this book was transformational in more ways than one, and through the stories that I captured, I learnt much about myself. By spending so much time in different parts of India, with so many different kinds of people, I discovered a fundamental change that India was going through. I also changed as a writer—I pushed myself to become a better storyteller to convey the strength, power and emotion behind these stories.

I also learnt that the apple never falls far from the tree. India has a strongly-set culture of family and kinship, and it is impossible to remove it all, in one, two or even three generations. Society is changing, and a lot of our old ideals are being questioned. Though young India has made new India their own through a multiplicity of circumstances, they don't realize how much like their parents they really are. This is what I noticed in the stories of the hundreds of people that I interviewed, the ones that I told in this book, and even in my own. Sometimes when I look in the mirror, I see the face of my mother. Sometimes when I hear myself talking, I hear the words of my father. And I realize that no matter how hard I try, there is only so much that I can change, only so different that I can be.

ACKNOWLEDGEMENTS

This book could not have been written without the voices of those who chose to talk to me. First and foremost I would like to thank all of those people: Kapil, Priya, Shiny, the Love Commandos, Prayag, Tips, Rudy, Gopal Suri, and so many more who bravely shared their stories with me. I also want to thank all those who were my guiding lights along the way—Wendy Doniger, Sudhir Kakar, James McConnachie, Stephanie Coontz, Kong Pat, Kailash Chand, and the many other experts who shared their knowledge with me.

David Davidar lent *India in Love* his unconditional support, editorially and otherwise. Thank you for giving me this chance. There were others too who put their minds, energy and hearts into it—Jean Kim, Simar and Pujitha.

I would never be a writer if it weren't for my family. I thank my parents; Ishani, Anjani and Anant Vijay. I especially want to thank Anjani Trivedi Kotwal, who did a fantastic job with her contribution of The Dark Side. I am so proud of her sparkling journalistic talent. Maybe Whelp had something to do with her scintillating debut, so a shout out to him too.

Then there are all my friends who supported the writing of this book. The lovely Poonam Saxena who supported the idea from the start, the Klein family in Pondicherry—Dimitri, Emilie, Mitya, Tara and Zen, who provided me with the space and love to finish up my draft. My friends and family members who came along with me on the ride—Ritu Pande in Bangalore, Ghazala and Aftab Laiq Ahmed in Bhopal, Seema Gokhale in Shillong, and the many many others around the country.

Thank you to all my Gurus, teachers and friends at the Sivananda Ashram who provided me with peace, calm and blessings when I needed it the most.

At the end I want to thank Vinayak. Thank you for being with me, and holding my hand every step of the way. I could never have done this without you.

NOTES

INTRODUCTION
1. 'The Global Middle Class Revolution', *BBC News,* 25 June 2012.
2. Tripti Lahiri, 'Much of Indian "Middle Class" Is Almost Poor' *Wall Street Journal,* 19 August 2010.
3. 'India in the Super Cycle', Standard Chartered Bank, 25 May 2011.
4. Yogita Limaye, 'Caste or Class?' *BBC,* June 2013.
5. 'India in the Super Cycle', Standard Chartered Bank, 25 May 2011.
6. Anand Giridharadas, 'Rumbling Across India to a New Life in the City', *The New York Times,* 25 November 2007.
7. Office of the Registrar General and Census Commissioner, 2001.
8. Kaushik Basu, 'India's Demographic Dividend', *BBC News,* 25 July 2007.
9. J. P. Singh, 'Problems of India's Changing Family and State Intervention', *The Indian Women: Myth and Reality* (New Delhi: Gyan Publishing House, 1996).
10. Shaifali Sandhya, *Love Will Follow: Why the Indian Marriage is Burning* (Noida: Random House India, 2009).
11. Ibid.

THE GATHERING REVOLUTION
12. Wendy Doniger, *On Hinduism* (New Delhi: Aleph Book Company, 2013).
13. Wendy Doniger, Interview.
14. Wendy Doniger, *On Hinduism* (New Delhi: Aleph Book Company, 2013).
15. Pavan Varma, *The Book of Krishna,* (New Delhi: Penguin, 2001).
16. Sources include various spiritualists that I spoke with including Radhanath Swami of ISKON and Sreevats Acharya.
17. Adapted from Ira Trivedi, 'Chastity Begins at Home, and Ends in the Dorm Room', *Outlook,* 24 December 2012.
18. Heidi R. M. Pauwels, *The Goddess as Role Model: Sita and Radha in Scripture*

and on Screen (Oxford: Oxford University Press, 2008).
19. Wendy Doniger, *On Hinduism* (New Delhi: Aleph Book Company, 2013).
20. Ibid.
21. Ibid.
22. James McConnachie, *The Book of Love: The Story of the Kamasutra* (London: Atlantic, 2007)
23. Mamta Gupta, 'Sexuality in the Indian subcontinent', *Sexual and Marital Therapy* Volume 9, Issue 1 (1994) pp. 57–69
24. Geeta Patel, Interview on 10 August 2013
25. Ketu H Katrak, 'Indian Nationalism, Gandhian "Satyagraha", and Representations of Female Sexuality', *Nationalisms & Sexualities*, ed. by Andrew Parker et. al. (New York: Routledge, 1992) pp. 385–406.
26. Michael Connellan, 'Women Suffer from Gandhi's Legacy', *The Guardian*, 27 January 2010.
27. Wendy Doniger, Interview
28. Sreenivas Janyala, 'To Die For', *Indian Express*, Feb 2013.

THE MAKING OF A PORN STAR
29. IMRD survey, 2011.
30. *India Today* Sex Survey, 2008.
31. Ibid.
32. Ibid.
33. Ibid.
34. Jason Overdorf, 'India: soft-core porn makes a comeback', Global Post, 7 September 2011.
35. Tusha Mittal, 'Bhabhi Anticlimax', *Tehelka*, Jul 2009.
36. Anastasia Guha, 'The Beatitudes of a Bountiful Bhabhi' *Tehelka*, May 2008.
37. Ibid.
38. Sharin Bhatti, 'Back with a Bang' *Tehelka*, May 2013.
39. Jason Overdorf, 'An interview with secret creator of Savita Bhabhi', *Global Post*, 4 May 2009.
40. Ibid.
41. Arindam Mukherjee, 'A Sniff And A Heave'O' *Outlook*, Dec 2012.
42. *Outlook* Sex Survey, 2007
43. Bipin Kumar Singh, '50-yr-old woman caught with sex toys at airport', *Mid-Day*, 19 July 2011
44. 'Sex toys recovered from shop in Rajkot', *The Times of India*, 2 February 2011
45. Ashish Sinha, 'In hard times, pills, condoms sold most', *Indian Express*, 16 Jun 2010.

46. 'Global Condoms Market to Reach 27 Billion Units and $6.0 Billion by 2015, New Report by Global Industry Analysts, Inc.' *PRWeb,* 12 Aug 2010.
47. *India Today* Sex Survey, 2011.
48. Sonali Kokra, 'The Vagina Wears Diamonds', *Open Magazine,* 16 June 2012.
49. *India Today* Sex Survey, 2011.
50. Koncept Analytics, 'Indian Lingerie Industry; Trends and Opportunities' Market Research, Sep 2008.
51. Aastha Atray Banan, 'Sheer Laciness', *Open Magazine,* 29 June 2013.
52. Ibid.
53. Ibid.
54. *India Today* Sex Survey, 2012

KINKY IS QUEER

55. This tale is from a Malayalee folk narrative of the Mahabharata and shows that gender variance happened freely in India's mythological past.
56. Devdutt Pattanaik, 'Did homosexuality exist in ancient India?' *Devdutt,* 30 June 2009.
57. Kimberly N. Chehardy, 'Wickedness Breaks Forth: The Crime Of Sodomy In Colonial New England' undated.
58. Ruth Vanita, ed. *Queering India; Same-Sex Love and Eroticism in Indian Culture and Society* (London: Routledge, 2002).
59. Manil Suri, 'How to be Gay and Indian', *Granta,* 25 June 2013.
60. Parmesh Shahani, *Gay Bombay* (New Delhi: Sage Publications, 2008).
61. UNAIDS, 'HIV programmes for MSM and transgendered people gradually being scaled up in India', *UNAIDS Press Centre,* 17 May 2012.
62. *India Today* sex survey, 2010.
63. Manil Suri, 'How to be Gay and Indian, *Granta,* 25 June 2013.
64. Ibid.

PIMPS AND HOES

65. 'Forced Prostitution.' *Half the Sky,* PBS, 2012.
66. Pat Califia, 'Whoring in Utopia' from *Public Sex: The Culture of Radical Sex* (Cleis Press, 1994), pp. 242–48.
67. S.N. Sinha and Nitish K Basu, *The History of Marriage and Prostitution (Vedas to Vatsyayana),* (India: Sage Publications, 1998).
68. Ibid.
69. Rekha Pande, 'Ritualized Prostitution: Devadasis to Jogins—A Few Case Studies', *Prostitution and Beyond; An Analysis of Sex Work in India* (India: Sage Publications, 1998).

70. Ibid.
71. Veena Oldenburg, 'Lifestyle as Resistance: The Case of the Courtesans of Lucknow' (1990)
72. Ibid.
73. Ibid.
74. Ibid.
75. Ibid.
76. Ibid.
77. Upasana Bhat, 'Prostitution "increases" in India', *BBC NEWS,* 3 July 2006.
78. Rohini Sahni and V. Kalyan Shankar, 'The First Pan-India Survey of Sex Workers; A summary of preliminary findings', *Center for Advocacy on Stigma and Marginalisation,* April, 2011.
79. *Outlook* Sex Survey, 2006.
80. *Outlook* Sex Survey, 2011.
81. Ibid.
82. Nicholas Kristof, 'Raiding a Brothel in India', *New York Times,* 25 May 2011
83. A. Koirala, H. K. Banskota, B. R. Khadka, *Cross border interception – A strategy of prevention of trafficking women from Nepal,* Int Conf AIDS; 15. (11-16 July 2004).
84. K. K. Mukherji and S. Muherjee, *Girls and women in prostitution in India Department of Women and Child Development* (New Delhi, 2007).
85. 'Trafficking in Persons Report 2012', *US Department of State.*
86. Prateek Chauhan, 'Nexus sexus interruptus for Sex Baba, it's anti-climax', *Hard News,* April 2010.
87. Chinki Sinha, 'Lady and a Pimp', *Open Magazine,* 16 June 2012.
88. Ibid.
89. Ibid.
90. Ibid.
91. Cordelia Jenkins and Appu Esthose Suresh, 'Catering to middle-class interests', *Live Mint ,* 1 August 2011.
92. Mehboob Jeelani, 'Supply & Demand', *The Caravan,* 1 April 2012.
93. Ibid.
94. Ibid.
95. Ibid.
96. Ibid.
97. Mihir Srivastava, 'The New White Flesh Trade', *India Today,* 21 January 2010.
98. Mehboob Jeelani, 'Supply & Demand', *The Caravan,* 1 April 2012.
99. Mihir Srivastava, 'The New White Flesh Trade', *India Today,* 21 January 2010.

100. *India Today* Sex Survey, 2006.

THE DARK SIDE
101. 'Youth in India; Situation and Needs 2006–2007', International Institute for Population Sciences (IIPS) and Population Council, 2010.
102. Jonathan Ablett et al., 'The "bird of gold": The rise of India's consumer market', McKinsey Global Institute Report, 2007.
103. Nishita Jha, 'The Age of Innocence', *Tehelka*, 30 March 2013.
104. Shveta Kalyanwala, Shireen J. Jejeebhoy, A.J. Francis Zavier, and Rajesh Kumar, 'Experiences of unmarried young abortion-seekers in Bihar and Jharkhand, India' *Culture, Health & Sexuality*. Vol. 14 (3) (March 2012), pp. 241–255.; 'Because abortion is relatively uncommon and because pregnancy among the unmarried is highly stigmatised in India, community survey–based abortion data greatly underestimate the incidence of abortion among unmarried young women, and even a subnational study of youth in six states failed to obtain reliable information.'
105. K. G. Santhya, Rajib Acharya, Shireen J. Jejeebhoy and Usha Ram, 'Timing of first sex before marriage and its correlates; evidence from India', *Culture, Health & Sexuality* Vol. 13 (3), 10 December 2010, pp. 327–341.; 'In their sample, her team found almost a third of the girls had been coerced or persuaded to engage in intercourse. 14.4% of women were persuaded and 17.5% were forced.'
106. Ibid. (The study found that in most cases of unwanted or accidental pregnancies the partners somehow 'supported' the women—emotionally or financially.)
107. John Levi Martin and Matt George, 'Theories of Sexual Stratification; Toward an Analytics of the Sexual Field and a Theory of Sexual Capital', *Sociological Theory*. Vol. 24 (2), June 2006, pp. 107–132.
108. Christophe Z. Guilmoto, 'Characteristics of Sex-Ratio Imbalance in India and Future Scenarios', *United Nations Population Fund*, 29-31 October 2007.
109. Defined in the national census data as all children between the ages of zero and 6 years.
110. Mary E. John, Ravinder Kaur, Rajni Palriwala, Saraswati Raju, and Alpana Sagar, 'Planning Families, Planning Gender; The Adverse Child Sex Ratio in Selected Districts of Madhya Pradesh, Rajasthan, Himachal Pradesh, Haryana, and Punjab', *Action Aid and International Development Research Centre*, 2008.
111. Census of India (2011); Sex Ratio of Total population and child population in the age group 0-6 and 7+ years, 2001 and 2011.

112. Anjani Trivedi and Heather Timmons, 'India's Man Problem', *The New York Times*, 16 Jan 2013.
113. Valerie M. Hudson, e-mail interview, 20 December 2012.
114. Valerie M. Hudson and Andrea M. den Boer, 'A Surplus of Men, a Deficit of Peace; Security and Sex Ratios in Asia's Largest States', *International Security* Vol 26 (4), Spring 2002, pp. 5–38.
115. Shikha Dalmia, 'India Needs A Sexual Revolution', *The Wallstreet Journal*, 24 May, 2013.
116. Christophe Z. Guilmoto, 'Characteristics of Sex-Ratio Imbalance in India and Future Scenarios', United Nations Population Fund, 29-31 October 2007.
117. Valerie M. Hudson and Andrea M. den Boer, 'A Surplus of Men, a Deficit of Peace; Security and Sex Ratios in Asia's Largest States', *International Security* Vol 26 (4), Spring 2002, pp. 5–38.
118. Ross Macmillan and Rosemary Gartner, 'When She Brings Home the Bacon; Labour-Force Participation and the Risk of Spousal Violence against Women' *Journal of Marriage and Family*. Vol. 61 (4) (National Council on Family Relations, November 1999), pp. 947–958.
119. K. G. Santhya, Rajib Acharya and Shireen J. Jejeebhoy, 'Condom use before marriage and its correlates; evidence from India', *International Perspectives On Sexual and Reproductive Health* Vol. 37 (4), December 2011.
120. Ibid. (Only 40% of the 106 women who discussed the risk of pregnancy reported having worried about becoming pregnant. Similarly, only eight of the 51 men who discussed pregnancy reported they had been worried about their partner becoming pregnant.)
121. Deborah Mesce and Donna Clifton, 'Abortion; Facts and Figures 2011', *Population Reference Bureau* (April 2011). (An incomplete abortion, like Aasimah's, is when tissue is left in the uterus, and the treatment usually involves 'removing the remaining tissue in the uterus with vacuum aspiration or, if that is not available, with dilation and curettage,' according to WHO's definition. Unsafe methods include 'prolonged and hard massage to manipulate the uterus, or repeated blows to the stomach,' per the WHO.)
122. The Medical Termination Of Pregnancy Act, 1971
123. E-mail interview with Shireen Jejeebhoy, 18 April, 2013. The Abortion Assessment Project of 2004, one of the largest such studies undertaken in India found 6.7 million unreported abortions outside registered and government recognized institutions took place in India that year. Ravi Duggal and Vimala Ramachandran, 'The Abortion Assessment Project – India; Key Findings and Recommendations', *Reproductive Health Matters* 2004; *12* (24 Supplement), pp. 122–129

124. Deborah Mesce and Donna Clifton. 'Abortion; Facts and Figures 2011', *Population Reference Bureau,* April 2011.
125. Susheela Singh, Deirdre Wulf, Rubina Hussain, Akinrinola Bankole and Gilda Sedgh, 'Abortion Worldwide; A Decade of Uneven Progress.' *Guttmacher Institute* (New York; Guttmacher Institute 2009).
126. David A. Grimes, Janie Benson, Susheela Singh, Mariana Romero, Bela Ganatra, Friday E. Okonofua and Iqbal H. Shah, 'Unsafe abortion: The Preventable Pandemic', *The Lancet,* Volume 368, Issue 9550, 25 November 2006.
127. Meena Menon, 'Unsafe Abortions Killing a Woman Every Two Hours', *The Hindu,* 6 May 2013.
128. Heather D. Boonstra, 'Advancing Sexuality Education in Developing Countries; Evidence and Implications' *Guttmacher Policy Review* Vol. 14, (3), Summer 2011.
129. 'Sex education leads to more crimes against women, says police chief', *The Indian Express,* 15 Jan 2013
130. Heather D. Boonstra, 'Advancing Sexuality Education in Developing Countries; Evidence and Implications' Guttmacher Policy Review Vol. 14, (3), Summer 2011. (There is evidence, however, that such programming, which either precludes information about condoms and contraception entirely or permits only negative information, may be making it harder for young people to effectively engage in protective behaviours down the road.)
131. Floyd Whaley, 'Philippine Court Delays Law on Free Contraceptives for Poor' *The New York Times,* 19 March 2013.
132. Laurie Goodstein, 'Catholics File Suits on Contraceptive Coverage', *The New York Times,* 21 May 2012.
133. Connor Simpson, 'India's Rape Problem Is Bad Enough to Jump Out a Window', *The Atlantic Wire,* 19 March 2013.
134. Heather D. Boonstra, 'Advancing Sexuality Education in Developing Countries; Evidence and Implications' *Guttmacher Policy Review* Vol. 14, (3), Summer 2011.
135. Ross Douthat, 'The Great Abstinence Debate', *The New York Times,* 2 February 2010.
136. International Institute for Population Sciences (IIPS) and Population Council, 'Youth in India; Situation and Needs 2006–2007', Mumbai: IIPS 2010.
137. Heather D. Boonstra, 'Advancing Sexuality Education in Developing Countries; Evidence and Implications' *Guttmacher Policy Review* Vol. 14, (3), Summer 2011.

138. William Crowne, 'India's Anti Rape Agenda—Déjà Vu', *Fair Observer,* 15 April 2013.
139. Tom Wright, 'A Short History of Indian Rape-Law Reforms', *The Wall Street Journal,* 9 January 2013.

THE LOVE REVOLUTION

140. Shaifali Sandhya, *Love Will Follow; Why the Indian Marriage is Burning* (Noida: Random House India, 2009), p. 26.
141. Duleep C. Deosthale and Charles B. Hennon, 'Family and Tradition in Modern India' *Families in a Global Context,* ed. Charles B. Hennon and Stephan M. Wilson (New York: Routledge Taylor & Francis Group, 2008) p. 297.
142. Ibid.
143. Ibid.
144. Catherine Glynn and Ellen Smart, 'A Mughal Icon Re-Examined', *Artibus Asiae* Volume 57 No. ½, 1997, pp. 5–15.
145. Rachel Sturman, *The Government of Social Life in Colonial India; Liberalism, Religious Law, and Women's Rights* (New York: Cambridge University Press, 2012) p. 197.
146. Karen Leonard and Susan Weller, 'Declining Subcaste Endogamy in India; The Hyderabad Kayasths, 1900–75' *American Ethnologist* Volume 7, No. 3, August 1980.
147. Rachel Sturman, *The Government of Social Life in Colonial India; Liberalism, Religious Law, and Women's Rights* (New York: Cambridge University Press, 2012) pp. 112–125.
148. Stephanie Coontz, *Marriage, A History: From Obedience to Intimacy, or How Love Conquered Marriage.* (New York: Viking Press, 2005).
149. International Institute for Population Sciences (IIPS) and Population Council, 2010. 'Youth in India; Situation and Needs 2006–2007'. (Mumbai: IIPS).
150. Pia Heikkila, 'Indian women scale heights of the workforce' *The National,* 5 April 2012.
151. Ibid.
152. Jason Burke, 'Indian superchef Sanjeev Kapoor plans 24-hour TV cooking channel, *The Guardian,* 5 March 2010.
153. Joseph Mathew, *Marriage and Modernity* (New Delhi: Neha Publishers, 2010).
154. Lise Fortier, 'Women, Sex and Patriarchy', *Family Planning Perspectives* Vol. 7, No. 6, November-December 1975, pp. 278–281.

155. Nandan Nilekani, *Imagining India: Ideas for the New Century* (New Delhi: Penguin, 2009)
156. In India, Birth Control Focus Shifts to Women, *The New York Times*, 7 March 1982.
157. Meena Dhanda, 'Runaway Marriages; A Silent Revolution?' *Economic & Political Weekly* Volume XLVII (43), 27 October 2012, pp. 100–108.
158. Ibid.
159. Ibid.
160. Sameer Arshad, 'Only whores choose their partners' *The Times of India*, 8 September 2009.
161. Press Trust of India, 'Haryana Khap panchayats says marry them young to avoid rape cases' *NDTV*, 7 October 2012.
162. Suruchi Sharma, 'Rapes, chowmein and hormonal imbalance' The Times of India, 18 June 2013.
163. Meena Dhanda, 'Runaway Marriages: A Silent Revolution?' *Economic & Political Weekly* Volume XLVII (43), 27 October 2012, pp. 100–108.
164. Aditi Tandon, 'Govt sits on report wanting khap curbs' The Tribune, 14 May 2011.
165. Phyllis Chesler and Nathan Bloom, 'Hindu vs. Muslim Honour Killings' *Middle East Quarterly*, Summer 2012, pp. 43–52.
166. 'Techies Death:"girlfriend" arrested' *The Hindu* (26 May 2012).
167. Vikram Patel et al, 'Suicide mortality in India: a nationally representative survey', *The Lancet*, Volume 379, Issue 9834, 23 Jun 2012
168. Carol Upadhya and A. R. Vasavi, 'Work, Culture, and Sociality in the Indian IT Industry: A Sociological Study', *National Institute of Advanced Studies and Indo-Dutch Programme for Alternatives in Development*, August 2006.
169. Ibid.

MATCHMAKER, MATCHMAKER

170. Rochona Majumdar, *Marriage and Modernity; Family Values in Colonial Bengal* (Duke University Press, 2009).
171. Ibid.
172. Ibid.
173. Ibid.
174. A. K. Sur, *Sex and Marriage in India: An Ethno-Historical Survey* (Bombay: Allied Publishers, 1973).
175. Ibid., p. 20.
176. Ibid., p. 34.

177. Ibid., p. 45.
178. Ibid., p. 47.
179. Ibid., p. 51.
180. George P. Monger, *Marriage Customs of the World; From Henna to Honeymoons* (Santa Barbara [CA]: ABC CLIO, November 2004) pp. 151–152.
181. A. K. Sur, *Sex and Marriage in India; An Ethno-Historical Survey* (Bombay: Allied Publishers, 1973).
182. Ibid.
183. Ibid.
184. Ibid.
185. Rochona Majumdar, *Marriage and Modernity; Family Values in Colonial Bengal* (Duke University Press, 2009), p. 27.
186. Ibid., p. 218.
187. Ibid., p. 219.
188. Nainika Seth and Ravi Patnayakuni, 'Online Matrimonial Sites and the Transformation of Arranged Marriage in India', *IGI Global*, 2009.
189. Meghana Biwalkar, 'Matchmaker, matchmaker...', *The Business Standard*, 3 October 2006.
190. Samantha Iyer, 'Match Fixing in India; Where Tradition Meets Technology', Master's thesis, The University of Texas at Austin, May 2009.
191. Ibid.
192. Rukmini S., "Caste no bar", in words if not in action', *The Hindu*, 5 Aug 2013.
193. Sudhir Kakar, 'Match fixing', *India Today*, 26 October 2007.
194. Prabhu Razdan, 'Ash to Marry Tree First', *Hindustan Times*, 28 November 2006.
195. Rochona Majumdar, *Marriage and Modernity; Family Values in Colonial Bengal* (Duke University Press, 2009), p. 35.
196. Sudhir Kakar, 'Match fixing', *India Today*, 26 October 2007.

THE BIG FAT INDIAN WEDDING

197. Elliot Hannon, 'India's Government Aims to Curb Excessive Weddings', *Time World*, 21 May 2011.
198. Ibid.
199. Sudha Ramachandran, 'An end to big fat Indian weddings?' *Asia Times*, 11 May 2001.
200. Shaifali Sandhya, *Love Will Follow; Why the Indian Marriage is Burning* (Noida: Random House India, 2009).
201. 'Top Ten Most Outrageous Billionaire Weddings' *Forbes*, 26 May 2012.
202. Anupreeta Das, 'Middle-class India plows new wealth into big weddings'

Christian Science Monitor, 29 September 2005.
203. Ibid.
204. Padma Srinivasan and Gary R. Lee, 'The Dowry System in Northern India; Women's Attitudes and Social Change' *Perspectives on Families and Social Change* Volume 66, No. 55, December 2004, p. 1109.
205. Ibid., p. 113
206. Lucy Ash, 'India's dowry deaths' *BBC NEWS*, 16 July 2003.
207. Veena Oldenburg, 'Dowry Murder; The Imperial Origins of a Cultural Crime', (Oxford: Oxford University Press, 2002), p. xxx.
208. Ibid.
209. Ibid.
210. Ibid.
211. Ibid.
212. Rochona Majumdar, *Marriage and Modernity; Family Values in Colonial Bengal* (Duke University Press, 2009), p. 241.
213. Anupreeta Das, 'Middle-class India plows new wealth into big weddings' *Christian Science Monitor*, 29 September 2005.
214. Ibid.
215. Ibid.
216. Shaifali Sandhya, *Love Will Follow; Why the Indian Marriage is Burning* (Noida: Random House India, 2009).
217. Ibid.
218. Shubhangi Swarup, 'Something Happened to the Indian Wedding' *Open Magazine*, 19 June 2010.
219. According to a survey of 1,000 brides by the Fairchild Bridal Group.
220. Sameer Reddy, 'My Big Fat Indian Wedding' *Newsweek*, 12 April 2008.
221. Satish Jha and Ismail Zabha, 'Wedding bells toll communal harmony in Gujarat' *Daily News & Analysis*, 28 February 2011.
222. Prashant Dayal, 'Govt extends support for mass wedding at Wadia' *Times of India*, 27 February 2012.
223. Maitreyee Handique, 'Making mass weddings an earthly affair' *Live Mint*, 12 June 2011.
224. 'Indian Bridal Virginity Tests Spur Criticism' *Huffington Post*, 25 May 2011.
225. Deepali Gaur Singh, 'Mass Marriages and Virginity Testing in India' *RH Reality Check, Asia*, 28 September 2009.

BREAKUP NATION
226. Anand Giridharadas, 'The uncoupling of India Divorces rises, as notions of love changes' *The International Herald Tribune*, 19 February 2008.

227. Ibid.
228. Pallavi Pasricha, 'What makes Delhi the divorce capital?' *Times of India*, 4 August 2007.
229. Viju B., 'Divorce cases in Mumbai soar 86% in less than 10 years' *Times of India*, 27 July 2011.
230. Anand Giridharadas, 'The uncoupling of India Divorces rises, as notions of love changes' *The International Herald Tribune*, 20 February 2008.
231. Vicky Nanjappa, 'Bangalore; The rising divorce rate in the IT sector' *Rediff*, 2 August 2007.
232. Odeal D'Souza, 'Another tag for Bangalore: Divorce Capital' *DNA India*, 14 August 2011.
233. Anand Giridharadas, 'The uncoupling of India Divorces rises, as notions of love changes' *The International Herald Tribune*, 20 February 2008.
234. Ibid.
235. Gaurav Jain, 'The Rearranged Marriage' *Tehelka* 6 (43), 31 October 2009.
236. Ibid.
237. From an IMRB survey in 2011.
238. Survey done by matrimony portal Bharatmatrimony.com. 1,058 respondents were covered in Chennai, Mumbai, Delhi, Kolkata, Hyderabad, Bangalore, Pune, Madurai, Mysore, Tiruchirappalli, Coimbatore and Jaipur. All women were between 20–30 years of age.
239. Gaurav Jain, 'The Rearranged Marriage' *Tehelka* 6 (43), 31 October 2009.
240. Shaifali Sandhya, *Love Will Follow; Why the Indian Marriage is Burning* (Noida: Random House India, 2009).
241. *India Today* Sex Survey, 2011
242. Vineeta Pandey, '55,000 Couples Waiting for Divorce in India' *DNA*, 24 June 2010.
243. Aastha Atray Banan, 'Waiting forever to break free' *Open Magazine*, 1 April 2013.
244. The study was conducted by two NGOs—Save Indian Family Foundation and My Nation.
245. Jane E. Meyers, Jayamala Madathil and Lyne R. Tingle, 'Marriage Satisfaction and Wellness in India and the United States: A Preliminary Comparison of Arranged Marriages and Marriages of Choice', *Journal of Counseling and Development* Volume 83 (2), Spring 2005, pp. 183–190.
246. A period of waiting a Muslim woman observes after the death of her husband or after a divorce. She cannot marry anyone else during this time.
247. Anthony Giddens, *Runaway World; How Globalization is Reshaping Our Lives* (New York: Routledge Chapman & Hall, 2003).

MODERN LOVE
248. Jaspreet Nijher 'I have tried and tested live-in formula: Kareena' *Delhi Times* Vol. 12, No. 324, 21 November 2012.
249. *India Today* Sex Survey, 2010
250. Gaurav Jain, 'The Rearranged Marriage' *Tehelka* 6 (43), 31 October 2009.
251. Sanjay Srivastava, personal interview, 6 November 2012.
252. 'Over 53% children face sexual abuse; Survey', *Times of India,* 10 April 2007.
253. Abhijit Banerjee, 'It's Time to Get Real' *Hindustan Times,* 30 October 2012.
254. *India Today* Sex Survey, 2011.
255. *Outlook* Sex Survey, 2011.
256. A.K. Sur, *Sex and Marriage in India: An Ethno-Historical Survey* (Bombay: Allied Publishers 1973), p. 139.
257. John Hart, 'The Studio 54 of Sex' *The Daily Beast,* 7 April 2009.
258. Pariyaram Mathew Chacko, ed. *Matriliny in Meghalaya; Tradition and Change* (New Delhi: Regency Publications, 1998).
259. Verrier Elwin, The Muria and *Their Ghotul* (Oxford: Oxford University Press, 1992).
260. Ibid.
261. Ibid.
262. Ibid.
263. Meren Longkumer, H. C. Srivastava, Palaniyandi Murugesan, 'Alcohol Abuse and Risky Sexual Behaviour among the indigenous college students in Shillong, India' (Mumbai: IIPC, 2000)
264. Richard Burger, *Behind the Red Door* (Hong Kong: Earnshaw Books Limited, 2012), p. 200.
265. Ibid.
266. Ibid, p. 220.

BIBLIOGRAPHY

Abraham, Janaki, 2010, 'Wedding Videos in North Kerala: Technologies, Rituals, and Ideas About Love and Conjugality', *Visual Anthropology Review* 26 (2): 116–127.

Abraham, Leena, 'Bhai-behen, true love, time pass: Friendships and sexual partnerships among youth in an Indian metropolis', *Culture, Society, and Sexuality*: A Reader. Second Edition. Edited by Richard Parker & Peter Aggleton. (Abingdon: Routledge, 2007)

Abraham, Leena, 'Redrawing the Lakshman Rekha', Srivastava, Sanjay, ed. *Sexual Sites, Seminal Atititudes: Sexualities, Masculinities, and Culture in South Asia*. (New Delhi: Sage Publications, 2004).

Agnihotri, Indu, 'The Expanding Dimensions of Dowry', *Indian Journal of Gender Studies* 10 (2): 307-319, June 2003.

Agnihotri, Satish Balram, *Sex Ratio Patterns in the Indian Population: A Fresh Exploration*. (New Delhi: Sage, 2000).

Ahmad, Imtiaz, *Family, kinship, and marriage among Muslims in India*. (Columbia: South Asia Books, 1976)

Ahmad, Nehaluddin, 'Female feticide in India', *Law and Medicine* 26 (1): 13. Summer 2010.

American Congress of Obstetricians and Gynecologist, 'Vaginal 'Rejuvenation' and Cosmetic Vaginal Procedures', *ACOG Committee Opinion* 378. September 2007.

Anapol, Deborah, 'What Ever Happened to the Sexual Revolution?' *Psychology Today: Love Without Limits*. 15 August 2012.

Ansari, Ghaus, 'Lucknow: The City of Palace Culture', *Urban Symbolism*, Peter J. M. Nas, ed. (The Netherlands: Leiden University, 1993).

Aravamudan, Gita, *Disappearing Daughters: The Tragedy of Female Foeticide*. (New Delhi: Penguin Books India, 2007).

Aravamudan, Gita, *Unbound: Indian Women @ Work*. (New Delhi: Penguin Books India, 2010).

Balch, Oliver, *India Rising* (London: Faber and Faber, 2012).

Banerjee, Abhijit et al, 'Marry for What: Caste and Mate Selection in Modern India', Cambridge: National Bureau of Economic Research Working Paper, May 2009.

Bose, A. N., 'Evolution of Civil Society and Caste System in India', *International Review of Social History* 3 (1): 97-121. April 1958.

Burger, Richard, *Behind the Red Door: Sex in China*. (Hong Kong: Earnshaw Books Ltd, 2012).

Buss, David M, 'International Preferences in Selecting Mates: A Study of 37 Cultures', *Journal of Cross-Cultural Psychology* 21: 5–47. 1990.

Buss, David M., Todd K. Shackelford, Lee A. Kirkpatrick, and Randy Larsen. 2001. 'A Half Century of Mate Preferences: The Cultural Evolution of Values', *Journal of Marriage and Family* 63 (2): 491–503.

Chacko, Pariyaram Mathew, ed. *Matriliny in Meghalaya: Tradition and Change*. (New Delhi: Regency Publications, 1998).

Choudhury, Abhut, 'Descent of the Seven Huts: Folk Narrative as Structure of the Khasi Pnar Consciousness', *Ethno-Narratives: Identity and Experience in North East India*. Sukalpa Bhattacharya and Rajesh Dev, ed. (Delhi: Anshah Publishing House, 2006).

Coontz, Stephanie, *Marriage, A History: From Obedience to Intimacy, or How Love Conquered Marriage*. (New York: Viking Press, 2005).

Dalmia, Sonia and Pareena G. Lawrence, 'The Institution of Dowry in India: Why It Continues to Prevail' *The Journal of Developing Areas* 38 (2): 71-93. Spring 2005.

Dalrymple, William, *The Age of Kali: Indian Travels and Encounters*: 158–177. (New Delhi: Penguin, 1998).

Dalrymple, William, *Nine Lives*. (London: Bloomsbury, 2009).

Das, Kumudin et al, 'Dynamics of inter-religious and inter-caste marriages in India', Population Association of American 2011 Annual Meeting Paper.

Desosthale, Duleep C., and Hennon, Charles B., 'Family and Tradition in Modern India', *In Families in a Global Context*, ed. Charles B. Hennon and Stephan M. Wilson. (New York: Routledge Taylor & Francis Group, 2008).

Dev, S. Mahendra and M. Venkatanarayana, 'Youth Employment and Unemployment in India', Indira Gandhi Institute of Development Research, April 2011.

Dhar, Pulak Naranyan, 'Bengal Renaissance: A Study in Social Contradictions', *Social Scientist* 15 (1): 26-45. January 1987.

Dommaraju, Premchand, 2009, 'Female Schooling and Marriage Change in India', *Population* 64 (4): 667–683.

Dube, Dipa, Dube, Indrajit and Gawali, Bhagwan R., 'Women in BPO Sector in

India: A Study of Individual Aspirations and Environmental Challenges', *Asian Social Science 8* (7): 157-183. 1 June 2012.

Dugar, Subhasish et al, 'Can't Buy Me Love? A Field Experiment Exploring the Trade-off Between Income and Caste-Status in an Indian Matrimonial Market', *Economic Inquiry 50* (2): 534-550. April 2012.

Dwyer, Rachel, 'Zara Hatke (Somewhat Different): The New Middle Classes and the Changing Forms of Hindi Cinema', Being Middle-class in India. Henrike Donner, ed. (London: Routledge, 2011) Pgs. 184-208.

Dwyer, Rachel, 'Yeh Shaadi Nahin Ho Sakti!: Romance and Marriage in Contemporary Hindi Cinema', *(Un)typing the Knot: Ideal and Reality in Asian Marriage.* (Jones, G. W. and K. Ramdas, eds.) (Singapore: Asia Research Institute, National University of Singapore, 2004) Pgs. 59-90.

Fortier, Lise, 'Women, Sex and Patriarchy', *Family Planning Perspectives* 7 (6): 278-281. November - December 1975.

Foucault, Michel, *History of Sexuality, Vol. 1.* (New York: Penguin, 1978).

Foucault, Michel, *Herculin Barbin.* (New York: Pantheon Books, 1980).

Frankl, George, *Failure of the Sexual Revolution.* (London: Kahn and Averill, 1974).

Galatchi, Simona, 'Eroticism or Pornography at the Indian Tntric Temples From the Tenth to Twelfth Centuries', *Romano-Arabica: Discourses on Love in the Orient.* Nadia Anghelescu, ed. Bucharest: Center for Arab Studies, University of Bucharest: 63-71. 2002.

Garg, Yash, 'Representing Culture: Indian Weddings, Family, and Festivals', *In Cross-Cultural Communication: Concepts, Cases, and Challenges*, ed. Francisca O. Norales. (Youngstown: Cambria Press, 2006).

George, Sabu et al, 'Undoing Our Future: Summary of the Report on the Status of the Young Child in India', New Delhi: FORCES, 2009.

George, Annie, 'Embodying identity through heterosexual sexuality—newly married adolescent women in India, Culture', *Health & Sexuality: An International Journal for Research, Intervention and Care* 4 (2): 207-222. 2002.

Giddens, Anthony, *Runaway World: How Globalisation is Reshaping Our Lives.* (London: Profile Books, 2002).

Glynn, Catherine, and Ellen Smart, 'A Mughal Icon Re-Examined', *Artibus Asiae* 57 (1/2): 5–15. 1997.

Gopal, San, *Conjugations: Marriage and Form in New Bollywood Cinema.* (Chicago: University of Chicago Press, 2011).

Gosh, Deepa and Netaji Subhas Mahavidyalaya, 'Eve Teasing: Role of the Patriarchal System of the Society', *Journal of the Indian Academy of Applied Psychology 37*: 100-107. February 2011.

Gupta, Giri Raj, ed. *Family and Social Change in Modern India.* (Durham: Carolina Academic Press, 1971).

Gupta, Mamta, 'Sexuality in the Indian subcontinent', *Sexual and Marital Therapy* 9 (1): 57-69. 1994.

Gupta, Setu, 'The Concept of Divorce Under Muslim Law', *Legal Service India*. 11 September 2009.

Haldar, Partha and Shashi Kant, 'Reading Down of Section 377 of Indian Penal code is a Welcome Move for HIV Prevention and Control Among Men Having Sex with Men in India', *Indian Journal of Community Medicine* 36(1): 57-58. January-March 2011.

Harlan, Lindsey, ed. *From the Margins of Hindu Marriage: Essays on Gender, Religion, and Culture*. (New York: Oxford University Press, 1995).

Heitzman, James and Worden, Robert L., eds. *India: A Country Study*. (Washington: GPO for the Library of Congress, 1995).

Holden, Livia, *Hindu Divorce: A Legal Anthropology*. (Aldershot: Ashgate, 2008).

Hudson, Valerie M. and Boer, Andrea Den, 'A Surplus of Men, A Deficit of Peace: Security and Sex Ratios in Asia's Largest Countries', International Security 26 (4): 5-38. Spring 2002.

Human Rights Watch, 'India: Target-Driven Sterilization Harming Women', 12 July 2012, New Delhi.

Indian Department of Health & Family Welfare, Annual Report for 2010-2011.

International Institute for Population Sciences (IIPS) and Population Council, 2010. 'Youth in India: Situation and Needs 2006–2007', Mumbai: IIPS.

Jha et al, 'Low male-to-female sex ratio of children born in India: national survey of 1.1 million households', *The Lancet 367* (9506): 211–218. January 2006.

Johnston, Wm. Robert, 'India abortions and live births by state and territory, 1971-2011', *Johnston Archives*. 17 October 2012.

Jolly, Susie, 'Why the development industry should get over its obsession with bad sex and start to think about pleasure', *Development, Sexual Rights, and Global Governance*. Amy Lind, ed. Abingdon: Routledge. Chapter 1: 23–38. 2010.

Kakar, Sudhir and Kakar, Katharina, *The Indians: Portrait of a People*. (New Delhi: Penguin India, 2007).

Kant, Anjani, *Women and the Law*. (New Delhi: APH Publishing, 2003).

Katrak, Ketu H, 'Indian Nationalism, Gandhian 'Satyagraha,' and Representations of Female Sexuality', *Nationalisms & Sexualities*, ed. by Andrew Parker et. al. (New York: Routledge, 1992)

Kaur, Ravinder, 'Marriage and Migration: Citizenship and Marital Experience in Cross-border Marriage between Uttar Pradesh, West Bengal, and Bangladesh' *Economics and Politics Weekly* 48 (43). 27 October 2012.

Kellett, Jenna, 'Accessing The Divine Feminine Shakti Cult Worship At The Mother Goddess Kamakhya And Maa Taratarini Shaktipitha Temples', ISP Collection. Paper 1142. 2011.

Kharas, Homi, 'The Emerging Middle Class in Developing Countries', Brookings Institution. 20 June 2011.

Kolsky, Elizabeth, 'The Body Evidencing the Crime': *Rape on Trial in Colonial India*, 1860–1947', Gender & History 22 (1): 109–130. April 2010.

Kugle, Scott, 'Mah Laqa Bai and Gender: The Language, Poetry, and Performance of a Courtesan in Hyderabad' *Comparative Studies of South Asian, Africa, and the Middle East 30* (3). 2010.

Lal, Ruby, *Domesticity and Power in the Early Mughal World*. (New York: Cambridge University Press, 2005).

Lal, Ruby, 'Rethinking Mughal India: Challenge of a Princess' Memoir', *Economic and Political Weekly 38* (1): 53–65. 2003.

Lambert-Hurley, Siobhan, *Muslim Women, Reform and Princely Patronage: Nawab Sultan Jahan Begam of Bhopal*. (London: Routledge, 2007).

Law Commission of India, 'Laws of Civil Marriages in India—A Proposal to Resolve Certain Conflicts', Report No. 212. October 2008.

Lawyers' Collective and Women's Rights Initiative, 'Staying Alive: 5th Monitoring & Evaluation on the Protection of Women from Domestic Violence Act 2005', The International Center for Research on Women. 2012.

Leonard, Karen, and Weller, Susan, 'Declining Subcaste Endogamy in India: The Hyderabad Kayasths, 1900-75', *American Ethnologist* 7 (3): 504–517, 1980.

Luniya, Bhanwarlal Nathuram, *Evolution of Indian Culture*. (Agra: Lakshmi Narain Agarwal, 1967).

Mahapatra, Bidhubhusan et al, 'HIV Risk Behaviors among Female Sex Workers Using Cell Phone for Client Solicitation in India', AIDS and Clinical Research. 14 July 2012.

Maheshwari, Vidhan, 'Same Sex Marriage: Is it Time for Legal Recognition', Legal Service India.com.

Majumdar, Rochona, *Marriage and Modernity: Family Values in Colonial Bengal*. (Durham: Duke University Press, 2009).

McConnachie, James, *The Book of Love: In Search of the Kamasutra*. (London: Atlantic Books, 2007).

McKinsey Global Institute, 'India's Urban Awakening', April 2010.

Menon, Devaki, 'Lessons from Sahayatrika', *Suedasien*. 23 January 2006.

Meyers, Jane E., Marriage Satisfaction and Wellness in India and the United States: A Preliminary Comparison of Arranged Marriages and Marriages of Choice', *Journal of Counseling and Development 83* (2): 183-190. Spring 2005.

Mines, Diana P., *Everyday in South Asia*. (Bloomington: Indiana University Press, 2010).

Ministry of Health and Family Welfare, Government of India. 'HIV Estimations 2012 Report Released', 30 November 2012.

Mishra, Srikanta, *Ancient Hindu Marriage Law and Practice*. (New Delhi: Deep & Deep Productions, 1994).

Monger, George P., *Marriage Customs of the World: From Henna to Honeymoons*. (Santa Barbara: ABC CLIO, 2004).

Myers, Jane E., Jayamala Madathil, and Lynne R. Tingle. 2005. 'Marriage Satisfaction and Wellness in India and the United States: A Preliminary Comparison of Arranged Marriages and Marriages of Choice', *Journal of Counseling & Development* 83 (2): 183–190.

Nag, Moni, 'Anthropological Perspectives on Prostitution and AIDS in India'. *Economic & Political Weekly*. Vol. 36, No. 42 (Oct. 20-26, 2001), pp. 4025–4030.

National AIDS Control Organization, 'National AIDS Control Programme Phase III (2007–2012)', New Delhi. 2007.

Naz Foundation International, 'Section 377: 150 Years and Still Counting', *Pukaar* 77: 1–3. April 2012.

Naz Foundation International, 'Defining 'men who have sex with men' (MSM) in South Asia for the purpose of population size estimation' *Pukaar* 78: 22–23. July 2012.

Ogas, Ogi and Gaddam, Sai, '5 Things That Internet Porn Reveals About Our Brains' *Discover Magazine*. 20 September 2011.

Ogas, Ogi and Gaddam, Sai, *A Billion Wicked Thoughts: What the Internet Tells Us About Sexual Relationships*. (New York: Penguin, 2011).

Oldenburg, Veena, *Dowry Murder: The Imperial Origins of a Cultural Crime*. (Oxford: Oxford University Press, 2002).

Ollman, Bertell, 'Social and Sexual Revolution: from Marx to Reich and Back', *Dialectical Marxism*.

Orsini, Francesca, *Love in South Asia: A Cultural History*. (New Delhi: Cambridge University Press India, 2007).

Pauwels, Heidi R. M., *The Goddess as Role Model: Sita and Radha in Scripture and on Screen*. (Oxford: Oxford University Press, 2008).

Pinto, Sarah, 'The Limits of Diagnosis: Sex, Law, and Psychiatry in a Case of Contested Marriage', *Ethos: Journal of the Society for Psychological Anthropology* 40 (2): 119–141. Programme Working Paper, No 9. New Delhi: Population Council. 2009.

Ramasubramanian, Srividya and Jain, Parul, 'Gender stereotypes and normative heterosexuality in matrimonial ads from globalizing India', *Asian Journal of Communication* 19 (3): 253-269. 23 September 2009.

Ramdya, Kavita, *Bollywood Weddings: Dating, Engagement, and Marriage in Hindu America*. (Lanham: Rowman & Littlefield Publishers, 2010).

Ramu, G., *Family and Caste in Urban India: A Case Study*. (New Delhi: Vikas Publishing House, 1977).

Rao, V. Nandini and Rao, V. V. Prakasa, 'Desired Qualities in a Future Mate in India', *Social Values Among Young Adults: A Changing Scenario*. Man Singh Das and Vijay Kumar Gupta, eds. (New Delhi: M. D. House).

Reddy, Narayan, *Marriages in India*. (Gurgaon: The Academic Press, 1978).

Roy, Anjali Gera. 'Is Everybody Saying 'Shava Shava' To Bollywood Bhangra?' *Bollywood and Globalization: Indian Popular Cinema, Nation, and Diaspora*. Rini Bhattacharya Mehta and Rajeshwari Pandharipande, eds. (London and NYC: Anthem Press, 2001).

Ryali, Rajagopal, 'Matrimonials: A variation of arranged marriages', *International Journal of Hindu Studies* 2 (1): 107-115. April 1998.

Sahni, Rohini and Shankar, V. Kalyan, 'The First Pan-India Survey of Sex Workers: A summary of preliminary findings', Center for Advocacy on Stigma and Marginalisation (CASAM). April 2011.

Sandhya, Shaifali, *Love Will Follow: Why the Indian Marriage is Burning*. (Noida: Random House India, 2009).

Sapovadia, Vrajlal K., 'Controlling HIV/AIDS—a Judicial Measure, Recommendations by Supreme Court of India', HIV/AIDS e-Conference, 2003.

Sastri, A. Mahadeva, *The Vedic Law of Marriage or The Emancipation of Woman*. (New Delhi: Asian Educational Services, 1918).

Save Family Foundation, 'Family against Women or 21st century Women against family?' 30 November 2007.

Saxena, Rachna, 'The middle class in India: Issues and Opportunities', Deutsche Bank Research. 15 February 2010.

Seth, Nainika and Patnayakuni, Ravi, 'Online Matrimonial Sites and the Transformation of Arranged Marriage in India', IGI Global. 2009.

Shah, Vandana, *360 Degrees Back to Life: A Litigant's Humorous Perspective on Divorce*. (London: IdeaIndia.com, 2008).

Shahani, Parmesh, *Gay Bombay*. (New Delhi: Sage Publications, 2008).

Sharma, Bhumika, 'Live-In Relationships: The Indian Perspective', *India Law Journal*. Accessed 12 December 2012.

Sharma, Maya, *Loving Women: Being Lesbian in Unprivileged India*. (New Delhi: Yoda Press India, 2006).

Sharpe, Jenny, 'Gender, Nation, and Globalization in Monsoon Wedding and Dilwale Dulhania Le Jayenge', *Meridians: Feminism, Race, Transnationalism* 6 (1): 58–81, 2005.

Shaw, Alison, 2001, 'Kinship, Cultural Preference and Immigration: Consanguineous Marriage Among British Pakistanis', *Royal Anthropological Institute* 7: 315–334.

Sheel, Ranjana, 'Institutionalisation and Expansion of Dowry System in Colonial

North India', *Economic and Political Weekly* 32 (28). 12 July 1997.

Sheikh, Danish, 'Privacy & Sexual Minorities', Center for Internet & Society. 24 October 2011.

Singh, J.C. et al., 'Prevalence and risk factors for female sexual dysfunction in women attending a medical clinic in south India', *Journal of Postgraduate Medicine* 55 (2): 113-120. 2009.

Singh, Khushwant, *On Women, Sex, Love, and Lust*. Chopra, Ashok, ed. (New Delhi: Hay House India, 2011).

Singh, Susheela, et al., 'Abortion Worldwide: A Decade of Uneven Progress', New York: Guttmacher Institute. 2009.

Sithanna, V., *Immoral Traffic—Prostitution in India*. (Chennai: Jeywin Publications, 2007).

Srinivasan, Padma and Lee, Gary R., 'The Dowry System in Northern India: Women's Attitudes and Social Change', *Perspectives on Families and Social Change*: 1108-1117. December 2004.

Srivastava, Sanjay, 'Non-Gandhian Sexuality, Commodity Cultures, and a 'Happy Married Life',' *Sexual Sites, Seminal Attitudes: Sexualities, Masculinities, and Culture in South Asia*. (New Delhi: SAGE Publications, 2004).

Srivastava, Sanjay. 'Introduction: Semen, History, Desire, and Theory', *Sexual Sites, Seminal Attitudes: Sexualities, Masculinities, and Culture in South Asia*. (New Delhi: SAGE Publications, 2004).

Srivastava, Sanjay, *Passionate Modernity: Sexuality, Class, and Consumption in India*. (New Delhi: Routledge, 2007).

Sturman, Rachel, *The Government of Social Life in Colonial India: Liberalism, Religious Law, and Women's Rights*. (New York: Cambridge University Press, 2012).

Sundar, Ramamani, 'Abortion Costs and Financing: A Review', Mumbai: Centre for Enquiry into Health and Allied Themes. September 2003.

Sutherland, Sally J., 'Sita and Draupadi: Aggressive Behavior and Female Role-Models in the Sanskrit Epics', *Journal of the American Oriental Society* 109 (1): 63-79. January - March 1989.

Tambe, Ashwini, 'Colluding Patriarchies: The Colonial Reform of Sexual Relations in India', *Feminist Studies* 26 (3): 586-600. Autumn 2000.

Tikekar, Aroon, *Mumbai De-Intellectualised: Rise and Decline of a Culture of Thinking*. (New Delhi: Bibliophile South Asia, 2009).

Uberoi, Patricia, *Freedom and Destiny: Gender, Family, and Popular Culture in India*. (Oxford: Oxford University Press, 2006).

UNAIDS, 'HIV programmes for MSM and transgendered people gradually being scaled up in India', UNAIDS Press Centre. 17 May 2012.

Upadhya, Carol and Vasavi, A. R., 'Work, Culture, and Sociality in the Indian IT

Industry: A Sociological Study', School of Social Sciences, Bangalore. August 2006.

Urban, Hugh B., 'Matrix of Power: Tantra, Kingship, and Sacrifice in the Worship of Mother Goddess Kamakhya', *South Asia: Journal of South Asian Studies 31* (3): 500-534. 2008.

Vanita, Ruth and Kidwai, Saleem, Ed. *Same-Sex Love in India: Readings from Literature and History*. (London: Macmillan Press Ltd, 2000).

Vanita, Ruth, ed. *Queering India: Same-Sex Love and Eroticism in Indian Culture and Society*. (London: Routledge, 2002).

Varadpande, M. L., *Love in Ancient India*. (New Delhi: Wisdom Tree, 2007).

Varma, Pavan K. and Mulchandani, Sandhya, *Love and Lust: An Anthology of Erotic Literature from Ancient and Medieval India*. (New Delhi: HarperCollins India, 2004).

Verma, Kaushal K. et al., 'The Frequency of Sexual Dysfunctions in Patients Attending a Sex Therapy Clinic in North India', *Archives of Sexual Behavior 27* (3): 309-314. 1 June 1998.

Whipps, Heather, 'The 300-year History of Internet Dating', *Live Science*. 9 March 2009.

Wilson, Charles Sayer, *Sex and the Devil's Wager: The Armageddon Sex Revolution*. (Central Milton Keynes: AuthorHouse, 2009).

World Bank Group, 'HIV/AIDS in India', World Bank Press Release. 10 July 2012.

World Health Organization: Regional Office for South-East Asia, 'HIV/AIDS among men who have sex with men and transgender populations in South-East Asia: The Current Situation And National Responses', Report, 2010.

INDEX

abortions, 150-151, 158
  India's abortion policy, 159-160
abstinence-focused sexual education, 162
Adolescent Education Programme (AEP), 161, 164–165
Agarwal, Puneet, 52-53
Ahluwalia, Ashim, 48
AIDS Bhedbhav Virodhi Andolan (ABVA), 147
Ajanta and Ellora, 16
All India Institute of Medical Sciences (AIIMS), 147
Aravamudan, Gita, 179
arranged-cum-love marriage, 349
arranged marriages, 2, 174–175, 177-178, 223. *see also* marriage

Bangalore, sexual revolution at work, 201–207
  social lives of IT professionals, 209-215
Bengal Sati Regulation Act in 1829, 227
Bhatt, Pooja, 82
birth control, 182–183
'bit cinema', 49
Bollywood, 43, 141, 184, 186-187, 264-265
  kiss, 186

Book of Leviticus, 76
The Book of Love: The story of the Kamasutra, 29
Boonstra, Heather, 168
Bose, Rahul, 82
Brahmo Samaj, 32
Brazilian wax, 59-60
bridal shopping, 275-278
brothels
  of Chawri Bazar, 103
  of GB Road, 103-104
Buddhacharita, 108
Buddhism, 28
Bwitch, 61

Cadillac Pimp, 139, 142
caste issues and love, 199-200
celebrity wedding dance choreographer, 264-265
celibacy, 28, 33
Centre for Advocacy on Stigma and Marginalisation (CASAM), 118
chat rooms, 345
Child Marriage Restraint Act of 1929, 227
Chopra, Sherlyn, 54
Christian Unitarianism, 32
Cocktail Matches, 253-256
condoms, 59, 81
consensual encounters, 151

Contagious Diseases Act of 1864, 110
Coontz, Stephanie, 177-178, 203
Criminal Law (Amendment) Act of 2013, 169
cunnilingus, 46, 53, 67, 85, 345

designer dresses, 276-278
Devadasis, 107
dharma, 27
Dharmashastras, 224
divorce, 290-291
   in Bangalore, 293
   concept of duty, or dharma and, 307
   double divorcee, 395-302
   getting, 304-305
   in Hindu marriage, 292
   in Kerala, 293
   laws, 294
   mismatch of expectations, 309-310
   Muslim law, 312-318
   mutual consent, 294
   present times, 291
   rates in Indian cities, 292-293
   Shah Bano case, 311
   stories of, 316-317
Dowry Prohibition Act, 1961, 273

endogamy, 177

'fancy' underwear, 60
fear of pregnancy, 182-186
female yoginis, 15
Foreign Marriage Act, 1969, 228
free love, 187

Gaddam, Dr Sai, 54
Gandhi, Mahatma, 33
Gandhi, Prime Minister Indira, 183
gay night at Pegs and Pints, 98-99
gay parties, 71-72

gay terminology, 71
gender imbalance in Asian countries and violence, 153-154
Gitagovinda, 20
Golden Temple, 308-309
Gopalan, Anjali, 83-84
Grover, Rajiv, 61
Guest Control Order, 268
Guilmoto, Christophe Z., 155

hegemony, 32
Hindu caste system, 176
Hinduism, 16, 27
Hindu Marriage Act of 1955, 228, 294
Hindu Married Women's Right to Separate Residence and Maintenance Act of 1946, 228
Hindu mythology, 17, 78
HIV/AIDS prevention in India, 162
Hindu weddings, 291
homophobia, 73, 76–78
homosexuality, 73, 96
   in ancient India, 75-76
   gay social scene, 77
   in Hindu and Muslim traditions, 76
   issues of HIV/AIDS, 80-82
hookers, 137-144
hymen repair surgery, 42

Immoral Traffic Prevention Act (PITA), 115
Indian blue films, 48
Indian IT-BPO industry, 180
Indian Market Research Bureau (IMRB), 181
Iravan, Prince, 75
Islamic Sufism, 32

Jainism, 28

Jaitly, Celina, 82
Jejeebhoy, Dr Shireen, 150-152

Kakar, Sudhir, 67, 234, 261
Kamakhya Devi temple, 12-15
  Ambubachi festival, 15
  Goddess's yearly menstruation, 15
  main idol, 14
  practice of sacrifice, 13
  sanctum sanctorum of, 14
  sexual symbolism at, 15-16
Kamasutra, 26-27, 33-34, 55, 108
  G-spot and woman's climax, 27
  lovemaking, 26-27
  Manusmriti vs, 27-28
  styles of kissing, 26
  use of sex toys, 55
Kapoor, Sanjeev, 182
Kavi, Ashok Row, 79
Khajuraho, 16
Khan, Arif, 140
Khan, Shahrukh, 186, 265
Khandelwal, Dr Rekha, 156-157
Kharbangar, Tipriti 'Tips,' 371-375
Khasi system, 370-371, 363-366
Kidwai, Saleem, 82
Konark Wheel, 46
Kothari, Dr Prakash, 65–69
Krishna, Lord, 17
  Radha-Krishna love story, 17, 19-21
Kurukshetra, 12

labiaplasty, 41
legal system
  gay rights, 81–83
  High Court judgement on Section 377, 82-83
Leone, Sunny, 54
lesbian, 84-88
lesbian organizations, 88-89

LGBT community, 82, 99-100
LGBT rights in India, 73
live-in relationships, 324-337
Love Commandos, 187-194, 199
love failure suicides, 43
love marriages, 203, 209-214
love revolution in India, 177-185, 377-379
  falling in love at work, 201-209
Lucknow Incidents, 82

Macaulay, Lord, 77
Mahabharata, 224
maithunas, 45-46
male psyche, 80
Manu, 27-28
Manusmriti (The Laws of Manu), 27, 31, 76, 225
marriage. *see also* wedding
  arranged in different communities, 223
  arranged *vs* love, 173-175, 177-178
  in *Arthashastra*, 226-227
  astrology and, 243-246
  broker, 220-223
  child, 225
  criteria for breakdown of traditional marriage, 178
  differentiated between Hindus and Muslims, 275
  Facebook and, 246-247
  free-for-all, 279
  history of, 223-226
  Indian culture and, 175-176
  marital practices of Hindus, 225
  matrimonial advertisements, 222, 228-231
  matrimonial sites (e-matrimony), 232-233
  Mughal, 176

occupation of matchmaking by
  ghataks, 223
social reforms on, 227-228
successful matchmaking, 234-243
trouble in traditional marriages,
  246-253
during the Vedic age, 223-224
wealth and marriage market, 253-
  256
massage parlours and prostitution,
  118-124
mass wedding, 279-288
Masterji, Rajender, 264-265
masturbation, 24, 68
Matsya Purana, 107
McConnachie, James, 29, 31
Medical Termination of Pregnancy Act
  in 1971, 159
megamalls, 149
Miss Lovely (movie), 48
Mittal, Lakshmi, 271
modern Indian woman, 25
modern love, 349
Monger, George, 224
monogamy, 344
Motihar, Renuka, 161, 163
mujras, 103
Mukherjee, K. K., 117
Mukherjee, Sutapa, 117
multiple sex partners, 380
Muralidhar, Justice S., 82
mutual consent divorce, 294

Nadvi, Qazi Syed Mushtaq Ali, 313
Nagaswami, Dr Vijay, 293, 344
Narasimhadeva I, King, 45
Nathwani, Suman, 61
National AIDS Control Organization
  (NACO), 80
National Population Education

Project, 162
Naz Foundation, 73, 82-83, 88
neurotic sexual behaviour, 70
Nilekani, Nandan, 183
Nirodh, 59
non-vaginal sex, 75-76
nymphomania, 70

Ogas, Dr Ogi, 54
Oldenburg, Veena, 109, 273-274
online dating sites, 345
online pornography, 47
online sexual behaviour, 54-55
open marriage, 337-348

Pakeezah, 111
panchatattva, 46
Pat, Kong, 363-368
Patel, Bashir, 164
Pattanaik, Devdutt, 76
personal behaviour, 180-181
Pillai, Dr Meena, 49-50
Playboy magazine, 54
pornography
  in India, 47-50
  influence on sexual relationships,
    52-53
  internet and mobile phones, impact
    of, 54
  nicotine-patch porn, 48-49
  online, 47
  pioneers of porn, 49
  proportion of watching porn, 47-48
  of sex-hungry Indian housewife,
    51-52
  shooting of porn, 50
  Western, 60
  women proportion of watching
    porn, 47
Pre-Conception and Pre-Natal

Diagnostic Techniques Act
 (PCPNDT Act), 153
premarital romantic partnership, 25,
 34-35, 43-44
premarital sex, 35-36, 151
prenatal diagnostic technology, 153
prostitution
 in ancient texts, 108
 British soldiers and, 109
 during colonial period, 109-110
 courtesans and prostitutes of
  Lucknow, 109
 cult of prostitute, ancient times,
  106-107
 Devadasi, or temple prostitute
  culture, 107
 ganika, 108
 hookers, 137-144
 in India, 114
 legislation regarding, 114-115
 massage parlours and, 118-124
 during Maurya dynasty, 108
 during Navratri festivities, 111
 nightclubs, 144-146
 organization of sex workers, 116
 pimp and prostitute, 111-117, 124-126
 racket, 128-132, 139-141
 during the reign of Emperor Akbar,
  109
 sex trade, 132-137
 as a soft crime, 134
 in South India, 108
 tawaifs of Mughal courts, 109-110
 trend, 127-128
 woman as pimp and flesh trade,
  132-134
Pushkin's murder, 71-72

Qaziat, 312-313

Queer Pride Parade, 99
queer revolution in India, 79-80, 91-97

Raanjhanaa, 43
Radha-Krishna love story, 17, 19-21
Raghuvamsa, 28
Ram, Lord, story of, 17-19
rape, 154
 Delhi rape case, 147-148, 166
 gang, 169-170
Ravana, 18
're-virginization' techniques for
 women, 42
Roy, Raja Rammohan, 32-33, 227
runaway couples, 194-199

sacrifice, rules of, 13
Samanwaya, Durbar Mahila, 116
Sandhya, Shaifali, 294-295
semen, 28
Seth, Vikram, 82
sex
 history of, 11-16
 Shiva–Parvati, story of, 11-12
sex clinics, 61-65
sex determination, 153
sex doctor, 65-69
sex education, 161-167, 369
sex ratio in India, 153
 and marriage patterns in India, 155-156
sex-selective fertilization, 153
sex talk, 168
sex toys, 55-58
sex trade, 132-137
sexual and marriage revolutions, 1-2
 commercial aspect of, 59
 of middle class, 2-3
 urban *vs* rural youth, 3
sexual behaviour and violence, 151

sexual creatures, 150
sexual culture
   Mughal period (1526-1857), 30
   in Tantric shastras, 29-30
   Victorian influence on Indian, 30–32
sexual expectations, 66-67
sexual experimentation, 67
sexual harassment in India, 154-155
sexually transmitted diseases, 156
sexual performance, 67
sexual problems, 67-68
sexual risk-taking, 167
sexy lingerie, 61
Shah, Justice Ajit Prakash, 82
Shakti peeths, 12
Shikhandi, Princess, 75
Shillong, 361-363
Shiva lingam, 16-17
Singh, Satyapal, 166
Sita, 18-19
   as role model, 25-26
social lives of IT professionals, 209-215
sodomy, 76
soft-core films, 50
Special Marriage Act (1954), 228
Standard Business Conduct (SBC), 209
Sun Temple of Konark, 45-47
Suppression of Immoral Trafficking Act (SITA), 114-115
Suri, Manil, 78
swingers' clubs, 348-359

Tango, 359-360
Tantras, 12, 29-30
Tantric rituals, 15
Taratarini, 12

Thomas, Kuruppasserry Varkey, 268
transgenders (hijras), 76

Uberoi, Patricia, 52
Umrao Jaan, 111
unsafe sex, 160-161
Upanishads, 16
USHA, 116

vaginal beautification, 59-60
Vanita, Ruth, 76
Vatsyayana, 26, 65
Vedic age, 1
violence, unmarried men and, 155–156
Vishnu Samhita, 107
Vivekananda, Swami, 32

wedding. *see also* marriage
   Brahminic customs, 177, 273
   bridal shopping, 275–278
   budget, 271
   celebrity appearance at, 265
   ceremonies, 263-265
   cost of, 278-279
   designer dresses, 277
   dowry, 271-274
   firecrackers, 269, 286
   fresh flowers, use of, 270
   Hindu, 281-283
   mass, 279-288
   package deal, 283-284
   wedding planners, 276
   wedding set, 267
Widow Remarriage Act in 1856, 227
women, categories of, 23-25, 39, 40
women's sexual conduct, 182

Yogini Kaula, 12

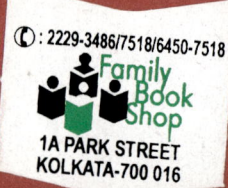